MANUAL of SMALL ANIMAL EMERGENCIES

MANUAL OF SMALL ANIMAL EMERGENCIES

Rhea V. Morgan, D.V.M.
Diplomate
American College of Veterinary Internal Medicine
Clinical Assistant Professor of Internal Medicine
Tufts School of Veterinary Medicine
Staff Clinician in Internal Medicine and Ophthalmology
Angell Memorial Animal Hospital
Boston, Massachusetts

Churchill Livingstone
New York, Edinburgh, London, and Melbourne 1985

Acquisitions editor: *Gene Kearn*
Copy editor: *Kim Loretucci*
Production editor: *Michiko Davis*
Production supervisor: *Joe Sita*
Compositor: *Maryland Composition Company, Inc.*
Printer/Binder: *The Maple-Vail Book Manufacturing Group*

Distributed in the United Kingdom by Churchill Livingstone, Robert Stevenson House, 1–3 Baxter's Place, Leith Walk, Edinburgh EH1 3AF and associated companies, branches and representatives throughout the world.

First published in 1985

Printed in U.S.A.

ISBN 0–443–08322–3

7 6 5 4 3 2 1

Library of Congress Cataloging in Publication Data

Morgan, Rhea Volk.
Manual of small animal emergencies.

Bibliography: p.
Includes index.
1. Veterinary emergencies—Handbooks, manuals, etc.
2. Pets—Diseases—Handbooks, manuals, etc. I. Title.
SF914.3.M67 1985 636.089′6025 84-17499
ISBN 0-443-08322-3

Manufactured in the United States of America

To:

Mom, my role model
Dad, my quiet supporter
Uncle Bud, my inspiration

With love

CONTRIBUTORS

Robert B. Altman, D.V.M.
Staff Clinician, A & A Veterinary Hospital, Franklin Square, New York

Carol S. O'Neill Foil, D.V.M., M.S.
Diplomate, American College of Veterinary Dermatology; Assistant Professor of Small Animal Medicine and Dermatology, Department of Veterinary Clinical Sciences, School of Veterinary Medicine, Louisiana State University, Baton Rouge, Louisiana

Gregory F. Grauer, D.V.M., M.S.
Diplomate, American College of Veterinary Internal Medicine; Assistant Professor of Medical Science, School of Veterinary Medicine, University of Wisconsin, Madison, Wisconsin

Rhea V. Morgan, D.V.M.
Diplomate, American College of Veterinary Internal Medicine; Clinical Assistant Professor of Internal Medicine, Tufts School of Veterinary Medicine; Staff Clinician in Internal Medicine and Ophthalmology, Angell Memorial Animal Hospital, Boston, Massachusetts

Eileen Rowan, V.M.D.
Staff Clinician, A & A Veterinary Hospital, Franklin Square, New York

Don R. Waldron, D.V.M.
Diplomate, American Board of Veterinary Practitioners; Assistant Professor of Surgery, Department of Veterinary Clinical Sciences, School of Veterinary Medicine, Louisiana State University, Baton Rouge, Louisiana

PREFACE

This book was designed and written to be a tool for the practicing veterinarian. It describes the pathogenesis, clinical signs, and diagnosis of the commonly encountered emergencies in veterinary medicine. Step-by-step therapeutic measures are presented in the form of emergency protocols and are accompanied by tables listing commercially available products and their drug dosages. The main goal of this handbook is to provide a systemic and organized approach to the recognition and successful management of the various crises that affect the major body sytems of pet dogs, cats, and birds.

As with most books, this project could not have been accomplished without the help and support of a wide variety of people. I would like to take this opportunity to thank my family and friends who were so understanding when I was not available during the writing of this book. I would also like to thank the Emergency Room staff of Burnham City Hospital, Champaign, Illinois, for introducing me to emergency medicine. From them I learned the necessity of approaching all emergencies in a calm, organized, and precise manner.

The veterinary staff of Angell Memorial Animal Hospital and Tufts School of Veterinary Medicine deserve my deepest gratitude for so generously giving their time to review the chapters of this text. In particular, I want to acknowledge the contribution of Dr. Mary Dulisch, who provided all the illustrations. I am also very appreciative of the diligent efforts put forth by the five veterinarians who contributed the three specialty chapters in this text. Lastly, this book would not be in print without the expertise of my editor, Mr. Gene Kearn, and Churchill Livingstone's belief that this work was a worthwhile endeavor.

The *Manual of Small Animal Emergencies* was not written to be stored away on a library shelf. If in several years you find that your copy is dog-eared and stained, then I will have achieved the goal I set out to accomplish—to provide something useful. This book is for all those veterinarians who find themselves alone, in the middle of the night, trying to bring relief to the sick and injured. I hope it makes your task easier.

Rhea V. Morgan, D.V.M.

CONTENTS

1

Shock

DEFINITION

Shock refers to any condition in which there is inadequate tissue perfusion leading to cellular hypoxia, metabolic acidosis, and cell death.

CLASSIFICATION

I. *Hypovolemic shock* results from loss of circulating blood volume and often follows trauma.

Three major types are seen:

A. Acute blood loss

Major laceration, ruptured abdominal or thoracic organs, surgical procedures

B. Fluid losses

Severe vomiting, diarrhea, plasma depletion accompanying major burns

C. Fluid sequestration

Massive tissue trauma, especially crushing injuries

Note: Losses of 30–40% of circulating blood volume may be compensated for by endogenous vasoconstriction and fluid replacement. Losses of greater than 40% demand intense medical therapy.

II. *Cardiogenic shock* occurs from cardiac insufficiency with lowered cardiac output.

It may result from:

A. Inherent heart diseases such as arrhythmias, myocardial trauma, ruptured chordaetendineae, or terminal CHF

B. Extracardiac diseases such as cardiac tamponade, tension pneumothorax

In contrast with hypovolemic shock, cardiogenic shock usually presents with elevated CVP and venous distention.

III. *Vasculogenic shock* is caused by acute vasodilation.

The effects are mediated through:

A. Autonomic nervous system (*neurogenic shock*)

Shock from CNS depression or trauma is rare in animals. It may follow deep anesthesia with hypotensive agents such as halothane or methoxyflurane via depression of the vasomotor center and loss of vascular tone.

B. Local vasoactive substances (*endotoxic, anaphylactic shock*)

1. Release of endotoxins produces dramatic hypotension and activation of the complement, fibrinolytic, and kinin system.
2. Capillary permeability increases.
3. Large volumes of fluids are sequestered in the hepatoportal system.
4. Endotoxic shock may be caused by peritonitis, pyometra, hemorrhagic gastroenteritis, intestinal strangulation, or volvulus.

In contrast to other forms of shock the mucous membranes are hyperemic, cardiac output initially remains high and the patient may be pyrexic.

PATHOPHYSIOLOGY

I. Although the causes of shock vary, the basic sequence of events is essentially the same:

A. Some precipitating event decreases cardiac output and BP.

B. Stimulation of the adrenal gland and sympathetic nervous system causes peripheral arterial vasoconstriction and contraction of spleen with shunting of blood away from the skin and intestinal viscera.

C. Heart rate and contractility increases, improving cardiac output.

D. The kidney retains sodium and water through an increase in renin-angiotensin, aldosterone, and antidiuretic hormone.

II. On a microvascular level certain compensatory changes become less reversible as shock persists and provide a positive feedback which worsens the circulatory collapse:
   A. Sympathetic constriction of arteriole and precapillary sphincters reduces O_2 delivery to tissues.
   B. Cellular anoxia interrupts oxidative phosphorylation with accumulation of lactic acid.
   C. Cell membrane permeability increases with cell autolysis and release of lysozymes.
   D. Capillary stasis and decreased capillary pH enhances vascular pooling and decreased venous return to the heart.
   E. Hypercoagulability also ensues, which may precipitate DIC.

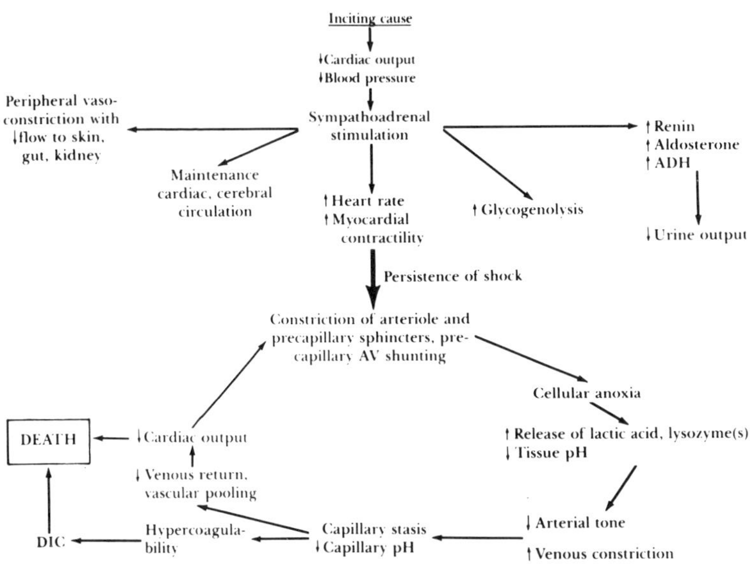

Fig. 1-1. The pathophysiology of shock. (Morgan, RV: Shock, Compend Contin Educ Pract Vet 3(6):533, 1981.)

F. Release of myocardial depressant factor and other chemicals further depress the myocardium.

III. The terminal event in all shock states is cardiac failure (Fig. 1-1).

AFFECTS ON MAJOR BODY ORGANS

Shock is a multisystem disorder which affects the entire body. An understanding of how shock affects the major organs allows the clinician to choose appropriate therapies, anticipate potential complications, and determine an accurate prognosis.

I. Heart

Coronary artery flow is maintained with arterial blood pressures >70 mmHg. (An arterial pulse is palpable at 70 mm Hg.) Direct blood flow to the heart is decreased only if 30–40% of total circulatory volume is lost. Cardiac failure is precipitated by insufficient coronary perfusion, myocardial hypoxia, acidemia, and myocardial depressant factor.

II. Brain

Transient CNS signs occur if mean circulatory blood pressures fall to 45–50 mmHg. Blood pressures of 35 mmHg for 2 or more hours produce chronic brain damage. This reduced functional capacity arises from lowered O_2 tension and depletion of the glucose supply.

III. Kidney

Permanent tubular damage results only if vasoconstriction persists for 12–24 h. Signs of tubular damage include oliguria, onset of glucosuria, and sequential decreases in specific gravity.

IV. Lungs

A. Many of the causes of shock (trauma to thorax and upper abdomen) result in direct physical damage to pulmonary parenchyma. Localized pulmonary contusions and pneumothorax often occur with resuscitative efforts. Released toxins, vasoactive substances, and tissue metabolites all cause dramatic pulmonary pathology. Pulmonary capillaries are also the site where platelet aggregates and microclots in transfused blood are filtered out of the circulation.

B. A syndrome of delayed pulmonary failure has also been recognized in patients that are initially resuscitated successfully and stable for several days. This *shock lung syndrome* was first recognized in human victims of severe crushing injuries, hemorrhage, sepsis, burns, and following major operations. The onset of insufficiency varies from a few hours to several days. It should be suspected in those animals that develop hyperventilation and respiratory alkalosis unresponsive to oxygen therapy. Although the etiology is unknown, overhydration, microembolization, O_2 toxicity, and sepsis are thought to contribute. As yet, no effective therapy has been discovered.

V. Gastrointestinal tract

Vascular stasis, ischemia, and endotoxemia produce mucosal necrosis and hemorrhage. Plasma and tissue fluid are sequestered in the gut lumen. Blood pressures below 45 mmHg for 2 h produce irreversible shock.

VI. Clotting system

Hypotension, capillary stasis and metabolic acidosis, bacterial toxins, and release of thromboplastin from degenerating cells all lead to a state of hypercoagulability during shock. Intravascular activation of the coagulation and fibrinolytic system leads to the phenomenon of DIC. DIC should be suspected if severe protracted bleeding or multiple organ dysfunction occur. The latter develops from microscopic infarction of vital organs secondary to microthrombi. The primary treatment of DIC is to reverse or remove the cause. The use of heparin, fibrinolysin, and ϵ-aminocaproic acid remain controversial in the treatment of DIC. Recent developments suggest that antiplatelet drugs such as aspirin and blood constituent replacement therapy may play a useful role in the treatment of DIC.

CLINICAL SIGNS

I. Tachycardia
II. Hypotension
   A. Prolonged CRT
   B. Weak pulses
III. Rapid respiration
IV. Hypothermia
V. Weakness, restlessness, and depression
VI. Reduced urine output
VII. Coma, dilation of pupils

TREATMENT

I. Objectives:
   A. Support respiration.
   B. Control hemorrhage.
   C. Expand circulatory blood volume.
II. Therapeutic steps
   A. Ensure patent airway. Intubate animal if collapsed or comatose. Deliver O_2 via mask, cannula, cage, or endotracheal tube. (See Table 1-1.)
   B. Stop hemorrhage by direct pressure, bandages, tourniquet, or ligation.
   C. Fluid therapy—three different types of solutions which

TABLE 1-1. TREATMENT PROTOCOL FOR SHOCK

1. Establish patent airway, O_2.
2. Insert IV catheter; check PCV, TS, BUN.
3. Control hemorrhage.
4. Rapid IV infusion of multiple electrolyte solution/Dextrose.
5. Administer corticosteroids, sodium bicarbonate, antibiotics.
6. Maintain body temperature.
7. Note urine output; insert urinary catheter.
8. Monitor color; CRT, pulse, respiration, and CVP.
9. Consider diuretics if there is evidence of overhydration.

are available for volume expansion include crystalloids, whole blood, and colloids such as plasma and dextrans.

1. Multiple electrolyte solutions (crystalloids)
    a) Large volumes are required: 20–50 ml/kg in first 15 min followed by 100–150 ml/kg over next several hours.
    b) Dogs may be given one blood volume (90 ml/kg) in 1 h. Cats given aliquots greater than 150 ml must be monitored closely for development of pulmonary edema.
    c) Maintain PCV between 20 and 50%. Avoid hemodilution and decreased oxygen delivery to tissues which occurs with overhydration. Packed cell volumes greater than 60% result in hyperviscosity of blood and diminished cardiac output.
    d) Add 50 ml of 50% dextrose to each liter of fluids to reduce peripheral resistance, improve ventricular oxygen availability and muscle contraction.
2. Whole blood
    a) Ideal in the anemic patient or to treat shock from blood loss.
    b) Consider transfusion if:
        (1) Rapid loss of 30% total blood volume
        (2) Rapid decline of PCV below 20% in dog and 12–15% in cat
    c) Cross-match or type blood before transfusion. Administer isotonic crystalloids simultaneously to minimize sludging and negative inotropic effects of transfusion.
3. Colloids

    Are hypertonic compounds which expand volume osmotically
    a) *Dextrans* are polysaccharides produced from bacteria.
        (1) Low-molecular-weight dextran (Dextran 40) is osmotically the most active on a weight basis. High-molecular-weight dextran (Dextran 70) is longer-acting.

(2) The use of dextrans in treatment of shock is now unpopular because they may only delay cardiovascular deterioration and have been associated with bleeding disorders which result from platelet dysfunction and an afibrinoplastic effect.

b) *Plasma* is used for protein loss from burns, chronic hemorrhaging, and peritonial and abdominal effusions.

(1) It may be harvested by siphoning from whole blood that has sedimented or collected by centrifugation.

(2) Plasma may be frozen and stored for 6 months.

D. Glucocorticoids

1. Mechanism of action in shock is not well understood. Beneficial effects include:
   a) Increase in cardiac output
   b) Decrease in peripheral resistance
   c) Increase in metabolism of lactic acid
   d) Improved efficiency of glycolytic enzymes
   e) Stabilization of lysosomal enzymes
   f) Interference with endotoxin-induced immune reactions
2. The efficacy varies with the type of shock.
   a) High efficacy
      (1) Septic
      (2) Traumatic—cardiogenic
      (3) Traumatic—hypovolemic
   b) Low efficacy
      (1) Intrinsic cardiac
      (2) Neurogenic
3. The onset of action for various steroids differs.
   a) Hydrocortisone sodium succinate—1–4 min
   b) Prednisolone sodium succinate—1–4 min
   c) Dexamethasone 21-phosphate—$\frac{1}{2}$ to 1 h
   d) Polyethylene glycol suspension of dexamethasone—3–4 h

Note: It is preferable to choose an aqueous corticosteroid in order to ensure a rapid onset of action. The above times are derived from experimental data. Clinical efficacy appears to be good for many forms of corticosteroids.

4. Steroids have minimal effect without adequate fluid therapy.

E. Vasoactive drugs
   1. are used to modify sympathetic and adrenal responses.
   2. may stimulate or block α- and β-receptors.
   3. are difficult to use unless simultaneous measurements of BP can be taken.
   4. *Dopamine* is most popular vasoactive druge used in shock. It selectively causes vasodilatation in the intestines and kidneys and a vasopressor response in peripheral vessels. It may be useful in hypovolemic patients that are not responding to volume expansion, in which a positive inotropic effect is desired.

F. Sodium bicarbonate
   1. Cellular anoxia with accumulation of lactic acid leads to metabolic acidosis.
   2. Determination of bicarbonate need and dosage may be:
      a) Exact, by blood gas measurements:
         Bicarbonate need = 0.3 × kg body weight × base excess
      b) Empirical
         (1) 1–2 mEq/kg IV bolus with
         (2) 1–2 mEq/kg added to each liter IV fluids
            Caution: Cats are sensitive to IV bicarbonate and should be monitored for CNS signs with IV administration. Rapid IV administration of bicarbonate may also aggravate existing hypotension.

G. Other medication
   1. Consider use of antibiotics for infection and diuretics for overhydration or poor urine output.

TABLE 1-2. COMMON DRUG DOSAGES USED IN CASES OF SHOCK

Multiple electrolyte solution
  Dog: 50–150 ml/kg over several hours
  Cat: 100- to 200-ml/aliquot

Dextran 40—20 ml/kg/24 h in 5% D/W IV

Hydrocortisone sodium succinate 8–20 mg/kg IV

Prednisolone sodium succinate 11–25 mg/kg IV

Dexamethasone 1–4 mg/kg IV, SQ

Sodium bicarbonate 2–8 mEq/kg in IV fluids

Dopamine 5 mg in 250 ml 5% D/W IV

Heparin 100–200 IU/kg IV, 600 IU/kg SQ

Aspirin 3–10 mg/kg/day PO

Furosemide 2–4 mg/kg IV, SQ

TABLE 1-3. COMMERCIAL PRODUCTS AVAILABLE FOR USE IN SHOCK

Multiple electrolyte solutions
  Multisol—M, Multisol—R, Abbott Laboratories, N. Chicago, IL 60064
  Lactated Ringers Solution, All Manufacturers
  Plasmalyte, Baxter/Travenol, Deerfield, IL 60615
  Polysol, Cutter Laboratories, Berkeley, CA 94710

Dextran 40—Rheomacrodex, Pharmacia Laboratories, Piscataway, NJ 08854

Hydrocortisone sodium succinate—Solu-Cortef, Upjohn, Kalamazoo, MI 49001

Prednisolone sodium succinate—Solu-Delta-Cortef, Upjohn, Kalamazoo, MI 49001

Dexamethasone—Decadron, Merck, Sharpe & Dohme, West Point, PA 19486
  Azium, Schering, Kenilworth, NJ 07033
  Dexate—SP, Burns Biotec Laboratories, Omaha, NE 68103

Dopamine—Intropin, American Critical Care, McGaw Park, IL 60085

Furosemide—Lasix, American Hoechst, Somerville, NJ 08876

Ultrasonic Doppler sphygmomanometer—Arteriosonde sphygmomanometer, Hoffman LaRoche, Cranbury, NJ 08512

2. Avoid hypotensive tranquilizers. (See Table 1-2 for drug dosages and Table 1-3 for commercial products used in shock.)

PATIENT MONITORING

I. Vital signs
  A. Body temperature
  B. Pulse rate/heart rate
  C. Respiration rate
  D. Color of mucous membranes
  E. Capillary refill time
  F. (See Table 1-4 for normal parameters.)

II. Blood pressure
  A. Methods of measurement:
    1. Digital—pulses are palpable at pressures ≥70 mm Hg
    2. Direct arterial catheterization
    3. Ultrasonic Doppler methods
  B. Blood pressures below 70 mmHg denote shock

III. Central venous pressure

Central venous pressure is the measurement of fluid pressure in the anterior vena cava or right atrium. It is a dynamic function of both cardiac output and venous return to the heart. Any increase in fluid volume or decrease in cardiac output increases the fluid pressure. Any decrease in volume or venous return lowers the fluid pressure.

  A. Technique for measuring central venous pressure
    1. Insert indwelling catheter into external jugular vein.
    2. Bring tip of catheter to rest in right atrium.
    3. Connect catheter to male end of three-way stopcock via extension tubing.
    4. Attach monometer calibrated in centimeters to stopcock, perpendicular to catheter line.
    5. Attach IV infusion solution to third portal of stopcock.

TABLE 1-4. NORMAL PARAMETERS IN PATIENT MONITORING

Body temperature—normal = 101.5°F (37°C)

Heart rate
- Normal in dog = 70–160 beats/min
- Normal in cat = 140–210 beats/min

Respiratory rate
- Normal in dog = 16–20/minute
- Normal in cat = 20–24/minute

CRT = less than 2 sec

Blood pressure—normal = 90–120 mmHg

CVP (cm H_2O)
- Normal = 0–10
- Shock = 0
- Overhydration = 8–12
- Heart failure = 20
- Cardiac tamponade = 22–25

PCV
- Normal in dog = 45–55%
- Normal in cat = 40%

Total solids
- Normal in dog = 7.0
- Normal in cat = 6.0

Urine output—normal = 1–2 ml/kg/h

Arterial blood gases—normal values
- pH = 7.35–7.45
- pco_2 = 40 mmHg
- po_2 = 90 mmHg
- HCO_3 = 25 mEq/L

6. Fill tubing and monometer with heparinized saline or IV solution.
7. Hold manometer so that zero mark is level with the right atrium:
   a) Sternal recumbency—fourth interostal space, 2–3 in. above sternum
   b) Lateral recumbency—parallel to sternum near fourth sternebra
8. Turn stopcock so that infusion set is off and manometer to catheter is free-flowing.
9. Allow liquid in manometer to equilibrate.

10. Note pressure at point where meniscus stops descending.
11. If meniscus falls below zero, refill manometer and lower it so that zero point is now at the 5-cm mark with values between 0 and 5 cm denoting negative measurements.

B. Sources of error in central venous pressure measurement
   1. Incorrect positioning of manometer
   2. Rapid or labored breathing
   3. Kinking of catheter or extension tubing
   4. Clots within the catheter
   5. Malfunctioning of stopcock

C. Central venous pressure is an insensitive test with a margin of error of 2 cm H_2O. Sensitivity can be increased by using minimal lengths of connective tubing and removing all extraneous catheter adapters.

D. Central venous pressure is useful for monitoring adequacy of fluid replacement and the hemodynamic effects of fluid therapy in cardiac patients.

   Note: The trends that develop with sequential CVP recordings are more significant than isolated or individual measurements.

IV. Packed cell volume

Is unreliable early in course due to splenic contraction. The PCV may remain normal even with major blood loss for the first several hours. It becomes a more accurate monitoring tool with time.

A. Continuous decline in PCV—search for sources of persistent blood loss or destruction
B. Persistent elevation of PCV >50%—fluid therapy is inadequate.

V. Total solids

As measured with a refractometer, solid measurements provide an estimation of the total circulating protein level.

A. Serial decrease—overhydration, protein loss
B. Persistent elevation—dehydration (inadequate fluid replacement)—hyperglobulinemia

VI. Urine output

Urine output resumes when successful fluid therapy returns glomular filtration rate to normal.

VII. Electrocardiogram

A. Three types of information determined:

1. Abnormalities in heart rate and rhythm (see Chapter 2)
2. Assessment of myocardial perfusion

   ST segment elevation or depression >2 mV denotes ischemia.
3. Crude evaluation of systemic electrolytes
   a) Hyperkalemia or hypocalcemia
      (1) Spiking of T waves
      (2) Decreased amplitude of P waves
      (3) Prolongation of PR interval and QRS complexes
      (4) Heart block
   b) Hypokalemia
      (1) Small T waves
      (2) Appearance of U waves
      (3) ST segment depression
      (4) Premature ventricular contractions

VIII. Other

A. Blood chemistries—BUN, creatinine, sodium, potassium, chloride

B. Arterial blood gas determination

BIBLIOGRAPHY

Adams HR, Parker TL: Pharmacologic management of circulatory shock: cardiovascular drugs and cortiocosteroids. J Am Vet Med Assoc 175:86, 1979

Brasmer TH: Shock—Basic pathophysiology and treatment. Vet Clin N Am 2(2):219, 1972

Brasmer TH (ed.): Symposium on shock. Vet Clin N Am 6(2):173, 1976

Burch JW, Stanford N, Majerus RP: Inhibition of platelet prostaglandin synthetase by oral aspirin. J Clin Invest 61:314, 1978

Clark DR: Circulatory shock: etiology and pathophysiology. J Am Vet Med Assoc 175(1):77, 1979

Davenport DJ, Carakostas MC: Platelet disorders in the dog and cat—

Part II: Diagnosis and management. Compend Cont Ed Pract Vet 4(10):788, 1982

Dillon R, Hankes GH, Nachreiner RF, Redding RW: Experimental hemorrhage in dogs: effect of prednisolone sodium succinate. JAAHA 14(6):673, 1978

Ettinger SJ, Suter PF: Canine Cardiology. WB Saunders, Philadelphia, 1970

Feldman BF: Disseminated intravenous coagulation. Compend Cont Ed Pract Vet 3(1):46, 1981

Guyton AC: Basic Human Physiology. 6th Ed. WB Saunders, Philadelphia, 1981

Hamlin RL, Kittleson MD, Rice D, et al: Noninvasive measurement of systemic arterial pressure in dogs by automatic sphygmomanometry. Am J Vet Res 43(7):1271, 1982

Hardaway RM III: Cellular and metabolic effects of shock. J Am Vet Med Assoc 175:81, 1979

Johnstone JB: Current concepts of hemostasis. Compend Cont Ed Pract Vet 3(12):1071, 1981

Kolata RJ: The clinical management of circulatory shock based on pathophysiology patterns. Compend Cont Ed Pract Vet 2(4):314, 1980

Kolata RJ, Burrows CF, Sonia LR: Shock pathophysiology and management. p. 32. In Kirk RW (ed.): Current Veterinary Therapy. Vol. 7. WB Saunders, Philadelphia, 1980

Orsher AN, Kolata RJ: Acute respiratory distress syndrome: case report and literature review. JAAHA 18(1):41, 1982

Rawlings CA, Keith JC, Lewis RE, Losonsky TM: Aspirin and prednisone modification of radiographic changes caused by aldulticide treatment in dogs with heartworm infection. J Am Vet Med Assoc 182(2):131, 1983

Ross JN: Comprehensive patient management in shock. J Am Vet Med Assoc 175:92, 1979

Ross JN: Current concepts in the pathophysiology of shock. ACVIM Sci Proc:9, 1980

Ruehl W, Mills C, Feldman BF: Rational therapy in disseminated intravascular coagulation. J Am Vet Med Assoc 181(1):76, 1982

White GL, White GS, Kosanke SD, et al: Therapeutic effects of prednisolone sodium succinate vs. dexamethasone in dogs subjected to E. coli. septic shock. JAAHA 18(4):639, 1982

Wilson JW: Cellular localization of ^{3}H-labelled corticosteroids by electronmicropic autoradiography after hemorrhagic shock. Proc Symp Steroids Shock: 275, 1974

2

Cardiac Emergencies

DEFINITION

A cardiac emergency is any crisis that threatens the integrity of the cardiovascular system. In this chapter four subjects will be discussed: (1) acute CHF, (2) arrhythmias, (3) cardiac arrest, and (4) feline cardiomyopathy.

ACUTE CONGESTIVE HEART FAILURE

Acute congestive heart failure describes a clinical syndrome rather than one specific disease.

I. Etiology

   Acute congestive failure usually develops in a heart that is chronically diseased. Signs occur when the myocardium is unable to maintain adequate cardiac output. Prior compensatory mechanisms such as hypertrophy and dilation are overcome by a precipitative event. Rarely acute failure occurs without previous heart disease.

   Precipitating causes of acute heart failure include:

   A. Systemic infections
   B. Sudden changes in heart rate and rhythm
   C. Environmental heat and humidity
   D. Exertion
   E. Other organ diseases
   F. Mismanagement of drugs
   G. Overzealous fluid therapy

H. Trauma
I. Anesthesia
J. Ruptured chordae tendineae
K. Myocardial infarction
L. Systemic hypertension

All forms of CHF that are not successfully treated end in cardiogenic shock and cardiac arrest.

II. Classification

The heart is a physiologic machine comprised of two pumps in series. Heart failure can be divided into two types depending upon which pump is involved.

A. *Left heart failure* is a more common cause of acute congestive failure than right-sided failure.

Causes of LHF are:

1. Mitral valvular disease
2. Aortic valvular disease
3. Coronary artery disease
4. Arterial hypertension
5. Cardiomyopathy
6. Bacterial or degenerative myocarditis
7. Ruptured chordae tendineae
8. Patent ductus arteriosus
9. Subaortic stenosis
10. Ventricular septal defect

Signs of LHF are summarized in Table 2-1. Left heart failure results in reduced stroke volume and

TABLE 2-1. SIGNS OF CONGESTIVE HEART FAILURE

Left Heart Failure	Right Heart Failure
Exertional dyspnea	Weight gain
Paroxysmal dyspnea	Venous distention
Orthopnea	Subcutaneous edema
Cough	Hydrothorax
Cyanosis	Ascites
Pulmonary edema	Hepatosplenomegaly
Weakness	Cardiac cachexia

pulmonary congestion because the left heart is a high-pressure pump. Murmurs, gallop rhythms, syncope, and arrhythmias may also be noted.

B. *Right heart failure* may arise from long-standing LHF. Other causes include:
   1. Pulmonary valvular disease
   2. Tricuspid valvular disease
   3. Chronic obstructive lung disease
   4. Pulmonary embolization
   5. Dirofilariasis
   6. Tetralogy of Fallot
   7. Right-to-left shunting patent ductus arteriosis
   8. Tumors of the right heart
   9. Pericardial effusion
   10. Cardiac tamponade of any origin

   Right heart failure seldom precipitates acute failure alone. It is usually a component of generalized cardiac decompensation. The right heart is a low-pressure pump which is designed to handle returning blood volumes. Failure results in systemic venous congestion (Table 2-1). Murmurs and arrhythmias are also common. Generalized heart failure will produce clinical signs of both right and left heart failure.

III. Diagnosis

The diagnosis of acute congestive failure is not always easy and relies upon evaluation of:

A. History
B. Physical examination
C. Electrocardiography
   1. Chamber enlargement
   2. Conduction disorders
   3. Arrhythmias
   4. Electrical alternans
D. Radiography of thorax
   1. Enlargement or irregularities of heart chambers
   2. Pulmonary edema, embolization
   3. Pulmonary or aortic vascular abnormalities

4. Pericardial effusion
5. Pleural effusion

E. Echocardiography
1. Valvular diseases
2. Chamber abnormalities
3. Pericardial effusion

F. Measurement of CVP
1. Values of 15–20 cm H_2O = heart failure
2. Values >20 cm H_2O suggestive of pericardial effusion

G. Others:
1. Pleural fluid analysis
2. Arterial blood pressure measurement
3. Cardiac catheterization or nonselective angiography
4. Complete blood count, heartworm test

H. Differential diagnosis:
1. Diffuse pulmonary diseases such as pneumonia, hemorrhage, neoplasia
2. Noncardiac causes of coughing, syncope, pulmonary edema, arrhythmias, weight loss, and generalized fluid retention
3. Other causes of murmurs such as anemia, pyrexia, hyperthyroidism

IV. Treatment

A. Primary objectives are:
1. Increase pumping effectiveness of heart, improve tissue perfusion
2. Relieve respiratory distress, improve oxygenation of blood
3. Reduce fluid accumulation
4. Treat or remove inciting cause

Note: Most animals are extremely susceptible to stress at this time, therefore, separate them from the owner, take them to an emergency treatment area, and handle them with care. Deliver O_2 via mask, cannula, cage, or endotracheal tube. (Table 2-2). Perform physical examination and record standing ECG.

TABLE 2-2. PROTOCOL FOR CONGESTIVE HEART FAILURE

1. Get animal to intensive care immediately and administer oxygen; intubate and establish airway if collapsed
2. Do not stress animal; reduce apprehension and anxiety
    a. Handle carefully
    b. Leave in O_2 cage for a few minutes and call for help
    c. Administer sedatives (morphine, meperidine)
3. Insert IV catheter for administration of IV medications and fluids; keep IV fluids to a minimum; fluid of choice is 5% D/W
4. Start therapy
    a. Diuretics—furosemide IV, IM, SQ
    b. Bronchodilators—aminophylline IV, PO
    c. Correct acidosis—bicarbonate IV
    d. Cardiac glycoside—digitalis IM, IV, PO
    e. Vasodilators—IV, topically, PO
    f. Antibiotics
5. Take ECG tracing, standing if animal is stressed and dyspneic
6. After immediate stabilization, x-ray chest and abdomen
7. If cardiac arrest ensues, treat accordingly
8. If failure to stabilize, consider phlebotomy
    a. In dog—initially remove 8 ml/kg at 2-h intervals; do not remove more than 16 ml/kg total
    b. In cat—remove 6–10 ml/kg

Insert IV catheter for administration of emergency medications. Avoid fluid therapy unless animal is in cardiogenic shock. Avoid infusion solutions containing sodium.

B. Medical therapy should include:

1. Diuretics

   Furosemide—inhibits Na^+ and Cl^- resorption throughout loop of Henle and convoluted tubes; very potent.

2. Bronchodilators

   Xanthine derivatives—also diuretic and positive inotropic effect; potent vasodilators

3. Cardiac glycosides

   Digoxin, digitoxin—increase force of ventricular contraction, increase ventricular diastolic time, improve stroke volume and cardiac output, reduce heart rate by central vagal stimulation and delaying atrioventricular (AV) nodal conduction; may also be arrhythmogenic.

4. Vasodilators
    a) The use of vasodilators in CHF is relatively new in veterinary medicine. Vasodilators lower systemic vascular resistance, thereby reducing ventricular preload and afterload. Cardiac output is usually increased. Because these drugs are potent vasodilators they must be used with caution. Concurrent measurement of arterial blood pressure is advisable.
    b) Examples:
        (1) Nitroprusside—arterial and venous dilator; short half-life, therefore given as continuous IV infusion; monitor blood pressure.
        (2) Nitroglycerin ointment—venodilator; applied topically to skin in inguinal area or ear; wear gloves when applying drug.

TABLE 2-3. DRUG DOSAGES FOR USE IN CONGESTIVE HEART FAILURE

Drug	Dosage
Digoxin	0.007 mg/kg of lean body weight PO, IM q12h
Ouabain	0.01 mg/kg IVq30–120 min
Furosemide	2–4 mg/kg IV, IM, SQ q4–12h
Aminophylline	6–11 mg/kg IV, IM, PO q6–8h
Theophylline	6–11 mg/kg IV, IM, PO q6–8h
Morphine	0.2–0.5 mg/kg SQ
Nitroprusside	5–20 μg/kg/min IV
Nitroglycerin ointment	$\frac{1}{4}$–$\frac{1}{2}$ in. topically q6–8h (small dogs); 2 in. topically q6–8h (giant dogs)
Hydralazine	0.5–1.0 mg/kg PO q8h
Prazosin	1 mg PO q8h

(3) Hydralazine—arterial dilator; causes sustained increase in cardiac output.

(4) Prazosin—arterial and venous dilator; causes profound decrease in systemic vascular resistance and increase in cardiac output. (See Tables 2-3 and 2-4 for drug dosages and commercial products.)

Supportive care with antibiotic, sodium bicarbonate, and manual removal of free thoracic and abdominal fluid should be considered. If the animal fails to stabilize, phlebotomy is indicated (see Table 2-2).

V. Patient monitoring
   A. Electrocardiogram—watch for arrhythmias.
   B. Thoracic radiographs
      1. Watch for progression or resolution of pulmonary edema, pleural effusion.
      2. Note changes in heart size.
   C. Central venous pressure measurement
      Watch for trend toward lower values.
   D. Urine output
   E. Body weight
      Readjust drug dosages as weight declines.

TABLE 2-4. COMMERCIAL PRODUCTS USED IN CONGESTIVE HEART FAILURE

Digoxin—Lanoxin, Burroughs Wellcome, Research Triangle Park, NC 27709
Ouabain—Ouabain, Eli Lilly, Indianapolis, IN 46206
Furosemide—Lasix, National Laboratories, Somerville, NJ 08876
Aminophylline—Aminophyllin, Serle Laboratories, Chicago, IL 60680
Theophylline—Theophyl, Knoll Pharmaceutical, Whippany, NJ 07981
Morphine—Morphine Sulfate Carpuject, Winthrop Laboratories, New York, NY 10016
Nitroprusside—Nipride, Roche Laboratories, Nutley, NJ 07110
2% nitroglycerin ointment—Nitro-Bid ointment, Marion Laboratories, Kansas City, MO 64137
Hydralazine—Apresoline HCl, Ciba Pharmaceutical, Summit, NJ 07901
Prazosin—Minipress, Pfizer Laboratories, New York, NY 10017

F. Biochemical organ profile
   1. Watch for electrolyte abnormalities.
   2. Monitor renal function.

G. Packed cell volume, TS
   Monitor for dehydration.

H. Continue O_2 therapy until pulmonary edema and dyspnea are relieved.

ARRHYTHMIAS

I. Definition
   A. Arrhythmias are disturbances in cardiac rhythm and rate. They may arise from primary heart disease or diseases of other organs. Arrhythmias cause a cardiac emergency when cardiac output is significantly diminished or when myocardial efficiency is severely impaired.
   B. Dogs exhibit a normal sinus arrhythmia. Differences in vagal tone during respiration cause a continuous and cyclic change in the heart rate. The heart rate tends to slow with expiration and quicken during inspiration.

II. Electrocardiography
   A. The ECG is a graphic representation of electrical activity of the heart. The normal ECG must be well understood before arrhythmias can be recognized. Figure 2-1 demonstrates a normal sinus complex as recorded in lead II in the dog.
   B. The following are essential components of the ECG:
      1. P wave
         a) Represents electrical forces occurring during atrial depolarization.
         b) Electrical activity begins in the sinoatrial node and spreads toward the AV node.
      2. P-R segment
         a) Period of isoelectricity which separates atrial and ventricular depolarizations
         b) It denotes conduction through the AV node and bundle of His.

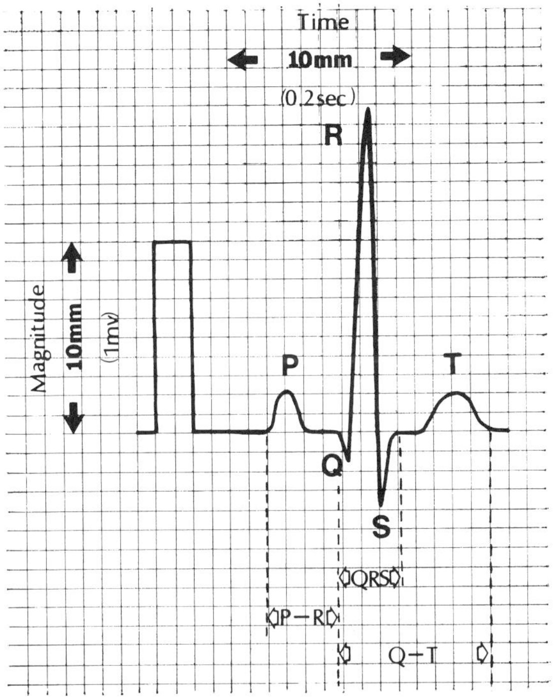

Fig. 2-1. Normal ECG for the dog as recorded in lead II. Time in seconds is plotted on the horizontal axis. Voltage is recorded along the vertical axis. One millivolt is 10 mm. At a paper speed of 50 mm/sec, each horizontal box represents 0.02 sec.

3. P-R interval
   a) Is the time between the beginning of atrial and ventricular depolarizations.
   b) P-R interval = P wave + P-R segment
4. QRS complex
   Represents ventricular depolarization.
5. S-T interval
   a) Portrays part of ventricular repolarization.
   b) Depression or elevation of this segment away from the baseline greater than 0.2 mV is abnormal and signifies ischemia.

6. T wave
   a) Occurs during repolarization of a major part of the ventricles.
   b) It may be negative, positive, or biphasic.
   c) See Table 2-5 for normal electrocardiographic parameters in the dog and cat.

III. Bradyarrhythmias
   A. Normal heart rates:
      1. Dog: 70–160 beats/min
      2. Cat: 140–210 beats/min
      3. Puppies and kittens: 80–200 beats/min
   B. *Sinus bradycardia* is a regular sinus rhythm slower than 70 beats/min in the dog and less than 140 beats/min in the cat.
      1. Causes
         a) Vagal stimulation:
            (1) Athletic animals
            (2) Pharyngeal irritation (especially brachycephalic breeds)
            (3) Cervical, thoracic masses
            (4) Surgical manipulation of vagus nerve
            (5) Gastrointestinal diseases
         b) Central nervous system lesions
         c) Hypothermia
         d) Hyperkalemia, hypokalemia

TABLE 2-5. NORMAL ELECTROCARDIOGRAPHIC PARAMETERS OF THE DOG AND CAT IN LEAD II

ECG Component	Dog	Cat
P wave	0.04 sec × 0.4 mV	0.03 sec × 0.3 mV
P-R interval	0.06–0.12 sec	<0.10 sec
QRS complex	0.04–0.06 sec	0.026–0.036 sec
R-wave height	<3.0 mV	<0.7 mV
S-T interval	<0.24 sec	0.15 sec–0.17 sec
T wave	$\frac{1}{4}$ amplitude of R wave	<0.2 mV
Mean electrical axis	+40–100°	+80°

e) Hypocalcemia
f) Drugs (especially anesthetic agents)

2. Electrocardiogram
   a) Normal sinus rhythm with unusually slow rate (Fig. 2-2)
   b) Electrolyte abnormalities may produce:
      (1) Increased amplitude of T wave
      (2) Prolongation of QRS complex and P-R interval
      (3) ST-segment depression
      (4) Diminution or loss of P wave

C. *Heart block* of the second or third degree produced by conduction abnormalities through the AV node will result in functional bradycardias with slow ventricular rates.
   1. First-degree block
      a) Is a prolongation of P-R interval beyond 0.12 sec.
      b) Is rarely symptomatic.
      c) Commonly occurs with digitalization.
   2. Second-degree block
      a) P wave and QRS complex are normal (Fig. 2-3).

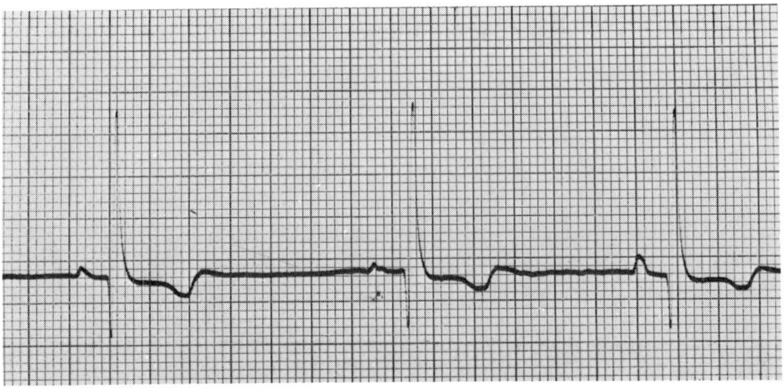

Fig. 2-2. Bradycardia. The PQRST complexes are normal, but are generated at a very slow rate.

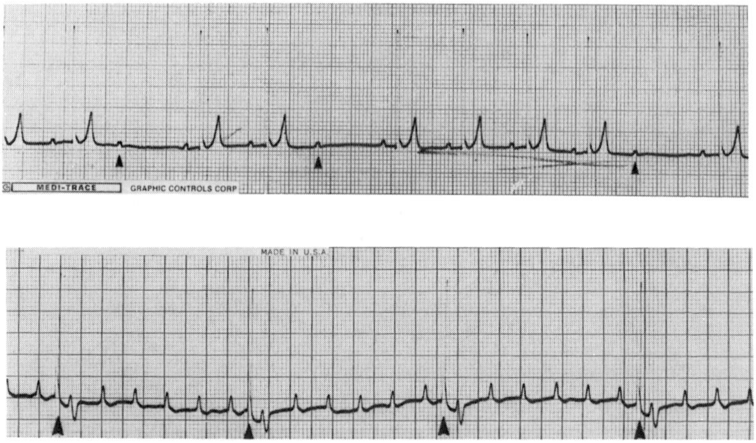

Fig. 2-3. Second-degree heart block. In the top figure the P-R interval becomes progressively longer until the QRS complex fails to follow the P wave (solid arrow). In the bottom figure, conduction through to the ventricle with appearance of a QRS complex (solid arrow) occurs with only one out of every five beats.

b) Two types:
   (1) P-R interval becomes progressively longer until a QRS complex fails to follow the P wave.
   (2) P-R interval is normal, but periodically and with some consistency the QRS complex fails to appear.

3. Third-degree block
   a) P waves occur as expected.
   b) QRS complexes are often wide and irregular due to a change in the pathway of ventricular depolarization.
   c) P wave bears no constant relationship to QRS complexes because there is not apparent conduction from atria to ventricles.
   d) P-P intervals and R-R intervals are often constant (Fig. 2-4).

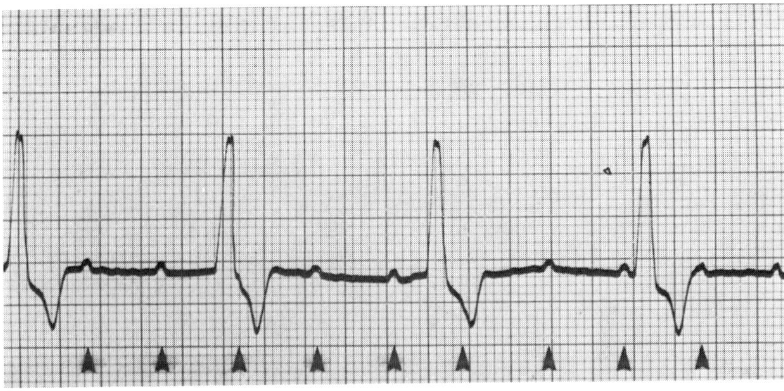

Fig. 2-4. Third-degree heart block. The P waves (solid arrows) bear no constant relationship to the QRS complexes, which in this figure are wider than normal. The P-P intervals and R-R intervals are constant. Some P waves fall within the QRS complexes and are hidden.

4. Sick sinus syndrome
   a) Sinoatrial node is diseased.
   b) Atrioventricular node and junctional myocardium may also be affected.
   c) Electrocardiogram reveals sinus bradycardia, intermittent sinus arrest with or without escape beats, and second-degree heart block.

D. Clinical signs
1. May be absent if bradycardia mild
2. Weakness, syncope
3. Mental dullness, confusion
4. Slow heart rate
5. Slow, ± irregular pulses
6. ± Dyspnea

E. Diagnosis

Bradycardia is usually discovered upon physical examination and can be characterized by electrocardiographic findings. Diagnostic tests that are indicated to determine the cause of the bradycardia include:
1. History
2. Thorough physical examination

3. Biochemical organ profile
4. Radiography of thorax and neck
   a) Rule out cervical, thoracic masses.
   b) Determine heart size and configuration.
5. Atropine response test
   a) 0.044 mg/kg atropine IV, record ECG.
   b) Increase in heart rate by 60–100% = positive response.
   c) Positive response often indicates vagal mechanism as etiology of bradycardia.

F. Treatment

Specific therapy relies on determination of the type and cause of the arrhythmia (Table 2-6).

1. Remove or reverse systemic disease.
   a) Restore K^+ and Na^+ to normal.
      (1) Normal saline or five percent D/W IV.
      (2) Diuretics
      (3) Supplement with mineralocorticoids as needed.
   b) Correct metabolic acidosis.

TABLE 2-6. PROTOCOL FOR BRADYCARDIA

1. Record heart, pulse, and respiratory rates.
2. Record ECG.
3. Consider insertion of IV catheter.
4. Diagnose and treat cause.
   a. Restore K^+ and Na^+ to normal.
      i. IV infusion of normal saline or 5% D/W
      ii. ± Diuretics
      iii. Replacement therapy for hypoadrenocorticism (see Chapter 9)
   b. Correct metabolic acidosis with sodium bicarbonate.
   c. Keep animal warm.
   d. Treat for shock as needed.
5. Decrease vagal tone with atropine.
6. Stimulate heart.
   a. Isoproterenol
   b. Transvenous pacemaker
   c. Permanent pacemaker

c) Correct hypothermia.
2. Decrease vagal tone.
   Atropine
3. Remove depressant drugs.
   a) Stop anesthesia.
   b) Reverse narcotic agents.
4. Stimulate heart.
   a) Isoproterenol
   b) Temporary transvenous pacemaker
   c) Permanent pacemaker

IV. Tachyarrhythmias

Tachyarrhythmias may be supraventricular or ventricular in origin. They are rapid, regular, or irregular heart rhythms.

A. *Sinus tachycardia* is a sinus rhythm with normal conduction to the ventricles at a rate greater than 160 beats/min in the dog and 210 beats/min in the cat.
   1. Causes
      a) Exercise
      b) Excitement
      c) Pyrexia
      d) Anemia
      e) Vagolytic drugs
      f) Shock
      g) Hyperthyroidism
      h) Electrolyte abnormalities
      i) Congestive heart failure
      j) Digitalis intoxication
   2. Electrocardiogram (Fig. 2-5)
      Normal but fast PQRST complexes. P wave may be superimposed on T wave of preceding beat
   3. Clinical signs
      a) If tachycardia is of short duration, animal may be asymptomatic.
      b) Weakness
      c) Anxiety
      d) Weak pulses
      e) Shortness of breath
      f) ± murmurs

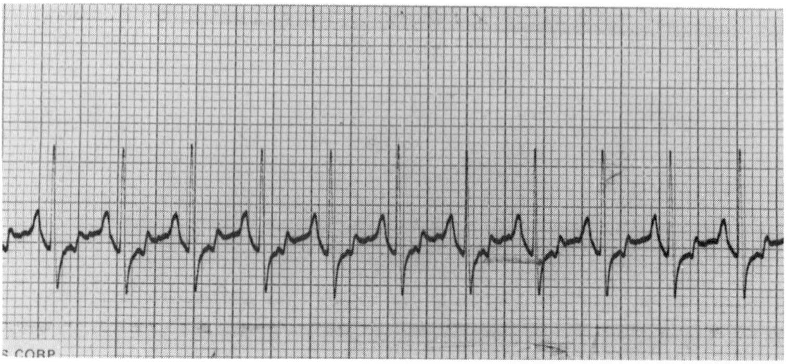

Fig. 2-5. Sinus tachycardia. The PQRST comlexes are normal but occur at short intervals because of the fast heart rate.

4. Treatment

   Remove cause.

B. *Atrial tachycardia* is a fast heart rate that originates in the atria outside the sinoatrial node.

1. Causes
   a) Congestive heart failure
   b) Digitalis intoxication
   c) Pyrexia
   d) Hyperthyroidism
   e) Electrolyte abnormalities
   f) Anemia
2. Electrocardiogram
   a) Configuration of P wave differs from P wave of normal sinus rhythm.
   b) QRS complex normal
   c) P wave may become superimposed on preceding T wave.
   d) Four or more consecutive atrial premature beats may be referred to as *atrial tachycardia*.
3. Clinical signs
   a) If rate is fast enough to compromise ventricular filling, atrial tachycardia will cause:
      (1) Shortness of breath

(2) Cyanosis
(3) Syncope
(4) Weak, thready pulses

b) Murmurs are often found with anemia and hyperthyroidism.

4. Treatment
   a) Vagal maneuver—apply digital pressure to area of carotid sinus or to one of the eyes.
   b) Remove inciting medication—terminate digitalis.
   c) Digitalization—if digoxin is not the cause of atrial tachycardia then it is usually the drug of choice in treatment because it slows conduction through the AV node and improves myocardial efficiency.
   d) Morphine—sedative effect may decrease heart rate.
   e) Propranolol—indicated for tachycardia unresponsive to vagal maneuver or other medical therapy; contraindicated in CHF.
   f) Direct electrical cardioversion—reserved for unresponsive, life-threatening episodes.
   g) See Table 2-7 for treatment protocol for tachyarrhythmias.

C. *Supraventricular premature contractions* arise from ectopic foci within the atria.
   1. Causes
      a) Mitral insufficiency
      b) Left atrial dilatation
      c) Digitalis intoxication
      d) Dirofilariasis
      e) Tricuspid insufficiency
      f) Atrial neoplasia
      g) Endocarditis, myocarditis
      h) Amyloidosis
      i) Arteriosclerosis
   2. Electrocardiogram (Fig. 2-6)
      a) Heart rhythm is irregular.

TABLE 2-7. PROTOCOL FOR TACHYARRHYTHMIAS

1. Record heart, pulse, and respiratory rates; note any pulse deficit.
2. Record ECG; determine type of arrhythmia.
   a. Sinus tachycardia—eliminate cause.
   b. Atrial tachycardia
      i. Vagal maneuver
      ii. Morphine, digoxin
      iii. Propranolol
      iv. Cardioversion
   c. Premature atrial contraction—administer digoxin.
   d. Atrial fibrillation
      i. Digoxin, ± diuretics
      ii. Propranolol
      iii. Cardioversion
   e. Premature ventricular contraction
      i. Withdraw digoxin.
         a) Phenytoin
         b) Propranolol
      ii. Lidocaine
      iii. Procainamide
      iv. Quinidine
      v. Consider new antiarrhythmics.
   f. Ventricular tachycardia
      i. Inset IV catheter.
      ii. Administer O_2.
      iii. Lidocaine—IV bolus, infusion
      iv. Procainamide—IV infusion, IM
      v. See protocol for CHF treatment
3. Start supportive care.
   a. 5% D/W IV
   b. Sodium bicarbonate
   c. Antibiotics
4. Determine and treat underlying cause of arrhythmias.

b) P wave occurs prematurely and is different from normal pacemaker P wave.
c) QRS complexes normal
d) P-R interval is prolonged if P wave reaches AV node during its refractory phase.
e) P-R interval may be shortened if origin of ectopic beat lies close to AV node.

3. Clinical signs
   a) Syncope

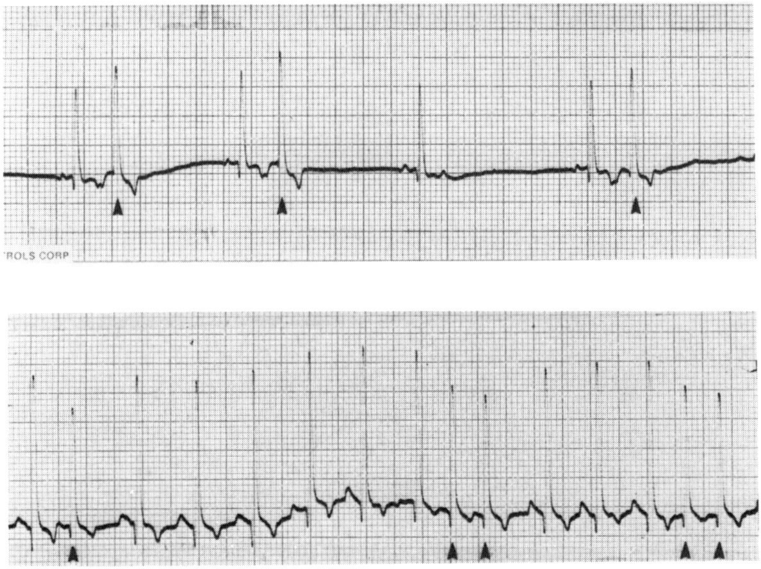

Fig. 2-6. Supraventricular premature beat. Premature beats (solid arrows) can be seen in the top figure. The P wave of the premature beat is superimposed upon the T wave of the normal sinus complex. The heart rate is much faster in the bottom figure, but the supraventricular premature beats (solid arrows) can still be recognized because the P wave is different from the normal P wave and occurs prematurely. The QRS complex remains normal.

b) Paroxysmal weakness

c) Animal may be asymptomatic.

4. Treatment

a) Remove digitalis if it is causing arrhythmia.

b) Digitalization for all other causes

5. Monitoring

Supraventricular premature beats are often evidence of underlying cardiac pathology. These animals are prone to developing other arrhythmias and cardiac decompensation.

D. *Atrial fibrillation* is chaotic electrical activity within the atria arising from ectopic foci. No effective atrial contractions occur. Many of the rapid, irregular impulses fail to be transmitted through the AV node, therefore, the ventricular rate is often irregular.

1. Causes
   a) Cardiomyopathy of large and giant breed dogs.
   b) Chronic mitral insufficiency
   c) Decompensating patent ductus arteriosus
   d) Dirofilariasis
   e) Feline cardiomyopathy (rare)
   f) Advanced heart disease of many origins
2. Electrocardiogram (Fig. 2-7)
   a) Rapid, grossly irregular ventricular rates
   b) Absence of P waves
   c) Presence of baseline oscillations (F waves)
   d) Normal or slightly aberrant QRS complexes
3. Clinical signs
   a) Atrial fibrillation may be insidious and discovered only upon physical examination. More commonly, signs compatible with unilateral or

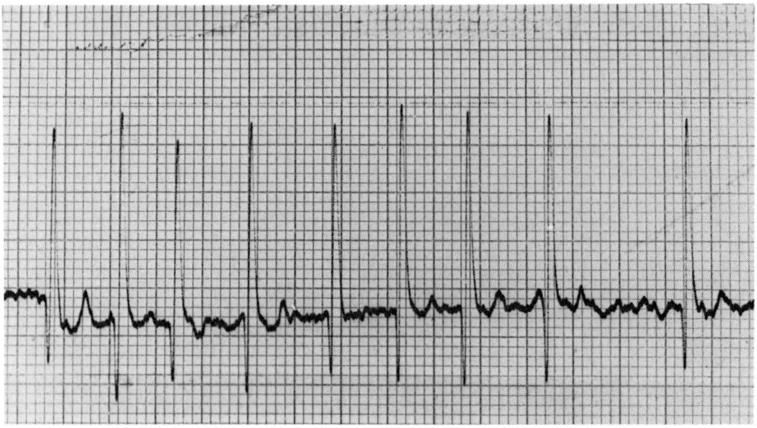

Fig. 2-7. Atrial fibrillation. Note the irregular baseline oscillations (f waves) and the absence of a normal P wave. The QRS complexes are normal but occur at an irregular rate as demonstrated by an irregular R-R interval.

generalized heart failure are present:
(1) Syncope
(2) Coughing
(3) Weight loss
(4) Murmurs
(5) Weakness
(6) Ascites
(7) Limb edema

b) Other classic findings include:
(1) Rapid, irregular heart rates
(2) Heart sounds that vary greatly in intensity
(3) Pulse deficit (disparity between heart rate as felt at apex beat and pulse rate)

4. Treatment
a) For CHF
(1) Digitalization—reduces ventricular rate
(2) ± Diuretics—especially for ascites and pulmonary edema

b) Propranolol—may be added after stabilization of CHF if fast ventricular rate persists despite digoxin therapy; must be used with caution; negative inotropic effect may decompensate the heart failure.

c) Electrical cardioversion—success rate is poor; conversion to normal sinus rhythm may only be transient.

Note: Ventricular arrhythmias are hemodynamically more threatening than atrial arrhythmias. Ineffectual ventricular contractions result in significant changes in cardiac output and blood pressure. It is imperative to quickly diagnose and correct all ventricular arrhythmias.

E. *Premature ventricular contractions* (*PVC*) arise in one or more abnormal foci within the ventricles
1. Cause
a) Traumatic myocarditis
b) Cardiomyopathy

c) Pericarditis
d) Congestive heart failure
e) Cardiac neoplasia
f) Other forms of primary heart disease
g) Digitalis toxicity
h) Any systemic disease that produces toxemia, pyrexia, hypoxia, or release of vasoactive chemicals such as myocardial depressant factor Examples:
   (1) Pyometra
   (2) Postshock state
   (3) Gastric dilatation—volvulus
   (4) Postsurgical procedures
   (5) Uremia
   (6) Pancreatitis

2. Electrocardiogram (Fig. 2-8)
   a) QRS complexes are wide and bizarre in shape.
   b) P wave is absent before QRS complex.
   c) One ectopic focus produces similar QRS complexes.
   d) Multifocal sources result in many types of QRS complexes.
   e) Premature ventricular contractions may be

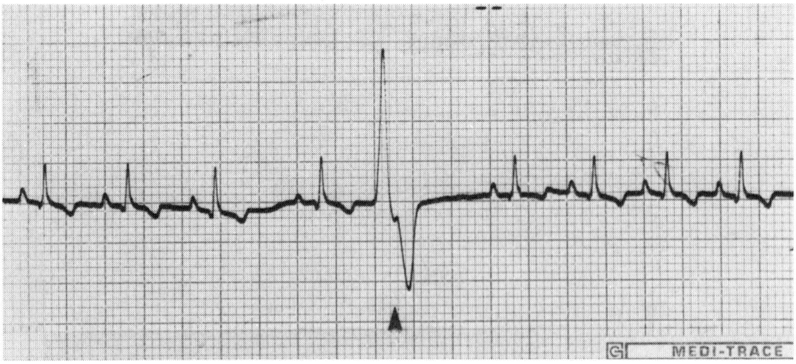

Fig. 2-8. Premature ventricular contraction (solid arrow). The QRS complex is wide and bizarre in shape. There is no P wave prior to the PVC, and it prematurely follows a normal sinus beat.

paired one-to-one with a normal sinus rhythm (bigeminy). This arrhythmias is commonly associated with thiobarbiturate anesthesia (Fig. 2-9).

3. Clinical signs
   a) No clinical abnormalities may occur with single or sporadic, intermittent PVCs.
   b) Frequent or consecutive PVCs produce:
      (1) Pulse deficits
      (2) Varying intensity of heart sounds
      (3) Prolongation of CRT
      (4) ± Cyanosis
      (5) Weakness, collapse, syncope
      (6) Dyspnea
4. Treatment
   a) Single or isolated PVCs do not require medical intervention.
   b) Digoxin toxicity
      (1) Withdraw digoxin
      (2) Phenytoin sodium
      (3) Propranolol
   c) Lidocaine
      Short-term-acting myocardial depressant

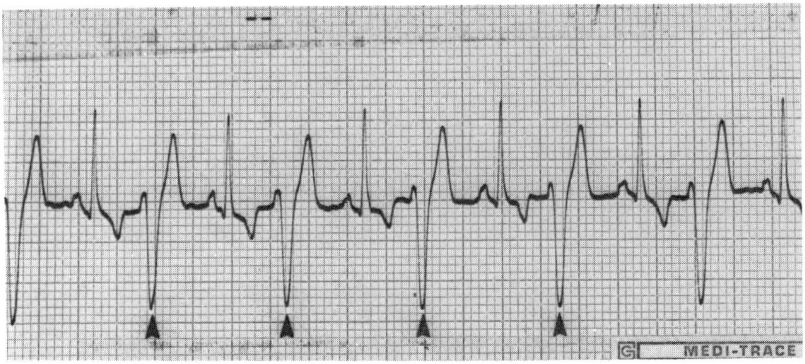

Fig. 2-9. Ventricular bigeminy. There is pairing of a normal sinus rhythmn with a premature ventricular beat (solid arrows).

d) Procainamide

Longer half-life, therefore, effacacious for long-term control of ventricular arrhythmias

e) Quinidine sulfate

Unpredictable, difficult to dose

F. *Ventricular tachycardia* is a series of four or more consecutive premature ventricular contractions with a ventricular rate >100/min.

1. Cause
   a) Any cause of PVCs may lead to ventricular tachycardia.
   b) Some antiarrhythmic drugs will paradoxically cause ventricular tachycardia.
2. Electrocardiogram (Fig. 2-10)
   a) Consecutive ventricular QRS complexes that are wide and bizarre in shape
   b) P wave absent
   c) Unifocal or multifocal
3. Clinical signs
   a) Collapse, weakness
   b) Dyspnea
   c) Weak pulses, pulse deficits

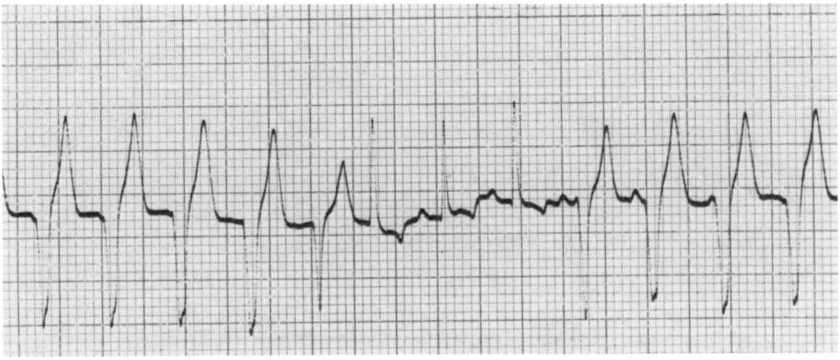

Fig. 2-10. Ventricular tachycardia. This ECG begins and ends in ventricular tachycardia. Three normal sinus beats can be recognized in the middle of the figure. The QRS complexes of ventricular tachycardia are large, wide, and bizarre in conformation and lack P waves.

   d) Jugular cannon—A waves
   e) Signs compatible with CHF
4. Treatment
   a) Lidocaine—rapid IV bolus
   b) Procainamide—continuous IV infusion
   c) Digoxin—for CHF
   d) Propranolol—for digoxin toxicity; also withdraw digoxin
   e) Supportive care—O_2, IV fluids, sodium bicarbonate, antibiotics
5. Prognosis
   a) Is guarded.
   b) Ventricular tachycardia may convert to ventricular fibrillation.
   c) See section on Cardiac Arrest below.
   d) See Tables 2-8 and 2-9 for drug dosages and commercial products useful in treating arrhythmias.

TABLE 2-8. COMMON DRUG DOSAGES USED FOR TREATING ARRHYTHMIAS

Drug	Dosage
Atropine	0.02–0.04 mg/kg IV, SQ, IM
Isoproterenol	1 mg/200 ml 5% D/W IV drip to effect 0.1–0.2 mg SQ, IM q4h
Propranolol	0.25–1.0 mg/200 ml 5% D/W IV 2.5–20 mg PO q6–12h
Phenytoin	50–150 mg IV; do not exceed 50 mg/min
Lidocaine	2 mg/kg IV bolus 1 g in 500 ml D/W drip
Procainamide	500 mg in 500 ml 5% D/W IV drip at 3–25 ml/min 6–20 mg/kg IM q4–6h 6–20 mg/kg PO q8–12h
Quinidine	6–20 mg/kg PO, IM q2h until desired effect, then q6–8h
Sodium bicarbonate	1–2 mEq/kg IV
Digoxin	0.007 mg/kg PO, IM q12h

TABLE 2-9. COMMERCIAL PRODUCTS USED FOR ARRHYTHMIAS AND CARDIAC ARREST

Isoproterenol—Isuprel, Winthrop Laboratories, New York, NY 10016

Propranolol—Inderal, Ayerst Laboratories, New York, NY 10017

Phenytoin—Dilantin, Parke-Davis, Morris Plains, NJ 07950

Lidocaine—Xylocaine, Astra Pharmaceutical Products, Worcester, MA 01606

Procainamide—Pronestyl, E.R. Squibb, Princeton, NJ 08540

Quinidine SO_4—Quinidine, Eli Lilly, Indianapolis, IN 46206

Digoxin—Lanoxin, Burroughs Wellcome, Research Triangle Park, NC 27709

Epinephrine—Adrenalin, Parke-Davis, Morris Plains, NJ 07950

Aminophylline—Aminophyllin, Searle Laboratories, Chicago, IL 60680

Furosemide—Lasix, Hoechst-Roussel Pharmaceuticals, Somerville, NJ 08876

Doxopram—Dopram, A.H. Robbins, Richmond, VA 23220

Mannitol 20%—Mannitol, Abbott Laboratories, N. Chicago, IL 60064

NEW ANTIARRHYTHMIC DRUGS

The reader should be aware that extensive research is underway to develop and test new antiarrhythmic drugs in the dog and cat. Although these drugs are still experimental and the level of safety remains to be proved for some, the reader should be aware of their potential use within the near future. Several examples are listed below:

Drug	Method of Action	Potential Usages
Bretylium tosylate	β-blockers	Ventricular tachycardia
Potassium canrenoate	Diuretic	Digoxin-induced arrhythmia
Verapamil	Slow calcium channel blocker	Atrial tachycardia Supraventricular tachycardia To slow ventricular rate in atrial fibrillation
Nifedipine	Slow calcium channel blocker	Arterial vasodilator

Drug	Method of Action	Potential Usages
Disopyramide PO_4	Myocardial depressant	PVCs Ventricular tachycardia
Aprindine HCl	Myocardial depressant	Resistant ventricular tachycardia Very narrow margin of safety

CARDIAC ARREST

Cardiac arrest is the cessation or absence of any effective ventricular contraction. It is often preceded or accompanied by respiratory arrest.

I. Predisposing causes
    A. Arterial hypoxia
    B. Coronary artery disease
    C. Myocardial disease
    D. Anesthetic agents:
        1. Depress myocardium.
        2. Sensitize myocardium to fibrillating effects of catecholamines.
    E. Toxemia
    F. Head trauma
    G. Electrical shock
    H. Cardiovascular shock
    I. Vagal stimulation by manipulation of head and neck during intubation or surgery
    J. Acid-base disturbances
    K. Electrolyte abnormalities
    L. Primary lung or airway disease
II. Clinical signs
    A. Absence of heart beat and pulse
    B. Signs that precede cardiac arrest:
        1. Shallow respirations
        2. Respiratory rate increased; apneustic gasps
        3. Cessation of respiration
        4. Cyanosis
        5. Prolongation of CRT
        6. Pulse irregularities

- C. Dilatation of pupils
- D. Relaxation of bladder and anus
- E. Absence of bleeding during surgical procedures
- F. Hypothermia
- G. Loss of consciousness

III. Diagnosis

The diagnosis of cardiac arrest must be made qucikly so there is no delay in onset of treatment. Diagnosis is most often recognized by the classic clinical signs. Electrocardiographically four different circumstances may be discovered at the time of arrest:

- A. Asystole
  1. Failure of the pacemaker tissue to propagate an impulse
  2. Absence of P-wave or QRS-T complex
  3. Isoelectricity
- B. Ventricular fibrillation—excitatory impulses arise from many foci and are conducted across random myocardial pathways, resulting in uncoordinated twitching of the ventricles.
  1. No defined QRS complexes
  2. Low-or high-voltage irregular undulations of the baseline (Fig. 2-11)
- C. Ventricular tachycardia

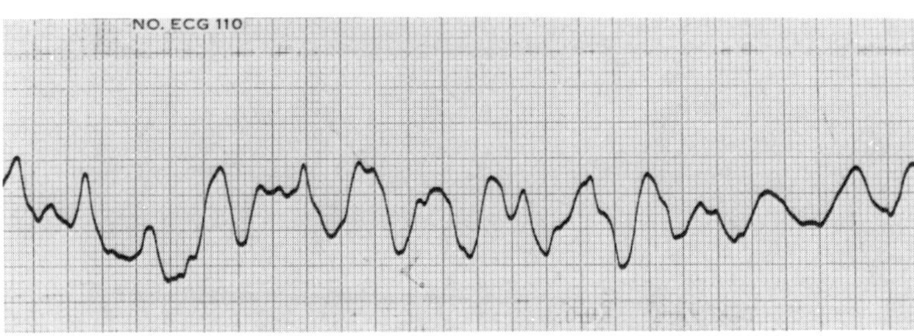

Fig. 2-11. Ventricular fibrillation. There are no well-defined PQRST complexes present. High-voltage, irregular undulations of the baseline are the only electrical activity present.

D. Ineffectual QRS complexes:
Abnormal, sporadic QRS complexes with no cardiac output

IV. Treatment
A. Must be immediate! Irreversible, lethal changes occur in major body organs within 3–4 min.
B. Treatment priorities:
1. Airway
2. Breathing
3. Cardiac compression
C. Therapeutic steps
1. Ensure patent airway
a) Intubate if possible and deliver 100% O_2.
b) Try mouth-to-mouth nostril breathing if circumstances do not allow intubation.
c) Suction any vomitus, blood, mucus, or pulmonary edema fluid from airway (see Table 2-10).
2. External cardiac massage
a) Tap the chest briskly several times in an effort to stimulate deep cardiac centers to begin sinoatrial pacemaker activity.

TABLE 2-10. EQUIPMENT FOR RESUSCITATION

Endotracheal tubes
Laryngoscope
Oxygen
Suction with tubing
ECG monitor and defibrillator
Electrode paste
Hair clippers
Various-sized syringes and needles
IV infusion sets
Emergency drugs (see Table 2-12)

b) Animal is in lateral recumbency.
c) Place one hand on either side of chest caudal to animal's elbow over fourth to sixth intercostal spaces.
d) Apply quick, yet sustained compressions (see Table 2-11).
e) Femoral pulses will become palpable if external compression forces are adequate.
f) Working alone to resuscitate: perform 15 compressions to each breath.

TABLE 2-11. PROTOCOL FOR CARDIAC ARREST

1. Establish patent airway.
   a. Intubate; administer O_2. Positive pressure breathing rate: dog—10–12 breaths/min; cat—12–15 breaths/min
   b. Mouth-to-nostril breathing; see rate under (a).
   c. Suction any mucus or vomitus.
2. Begin external massage; 60–80 compressions/min; test for femoral pulse.
3. Call for help.
4. Insert IV catheter—5% D/W, lactated Ringer's, or multiple electrolyte solution.
5. Record ECG; see Table 2-13.
6. Prepare emergency drugs.
7. Prepare defibrillator.
   a. Shave hair, apply conduction paste
   b. Start with 100–150 watt-sec
   c. Increase to 200–300 watt-sec
8. Continue CPR; if alone—15 compressions to one breath; if working in tandem—7 compressions to one breath.
9. Once stabilized, insert indwelling urinary catheter; x-ray chest; draw blood for electrolytes and blood gases; monitor ECG, CVP, and temperature.
10. Supportive care
    a. Oxygen
    b. Heat
    c. Mannitol
    d. Antibiotics
    e. Diuretics
11. See protocol for CHF.

Abbreviations: CPR, cardiopulmonary resuscitation.

g) Working as a team: perform seven compressions to each breath.

3. Medical therapy
   a) Rapid IV infusion of fluids
   b) Ready emergency drugs (Tables 2-9 and 2-12)
      (1) Intravenous administration
      (2) Intracardiac administration
   c) Terminate all respiratory and cardiac depressant drugs.
   d) Attempt to stimulate respiration with doxopram.
   e) Supportive care
      (1) Diuretics
      (2) Sodium bicarbonate

TABLE 2-12. DRUG DOSAGES USED IN TREATING CARDIAC ARREST

Drug	Dosage
Sodium bicarbonate	1–2 mEq/kg IV, IC
Atropine SO_4	Dog: 0.04 mg/kg IV, IC Cat: 0.02–0.04 mg/kg IV
Epinephrine	Dilute 1 mg in 9 ml saline: Dog: 2–3 ml IV, IC Cat: 1–3 ml IV, IC
Isoproterenol	Dilute 0.2 mg in 9 ml saline: Dog: 1-3 ml IV, IC Cat: 0.5-1.0 ml IV, IC Or, mix 1 to 2 mg in 500 ml 5% D/W slow IV drip to effect
Lidocaine	1–2 mg/kg IV
Procainamide	Dog: 2–4 mg/kg IV slowly; or mix 500 mg 1g in 500 ml 5% D/W—slow IV drip to effect
Calcium	Dog: 0.5–1.0 ml/min IV to total of 5–10 ml; 1–3 ml IC Cat: 0.25–0.5 ml/min IV to total of 3–5 ml; 1.0 ml IC
Aminophylline	Dog: 6–11 mg/kg IV, IM Cat: 3–6 mg/kg IV, IM
Furosemide	2–4 mg/kg IV, IM, SQ
Doxopram	1–4 mg/kg IV

TABLE 2-13. TREATMENT OF CARDIAC ARREST BASED ON ELECTROCARDIOGRAPHIC FINDINGS

Asystole	Normal or Abnormal P-QRS-T Complex; No Cardiac Output	Ventricular Fibrillation	Ventricular Tachycardia; No Cardiac Output
1. Sodium bicarbonate 2 mEq/kg IV	1. Sodium bicarbonate 2 mEq/kg IV	1. Sodium bicarbonate 2 mEq/kg IV	1. Sodium bicarbonate 2 mEq/kg IV
2. Atropine sulfate 0.04 mg/kg IV	2. Treat as for asystole; try isoproterenol first.	2. Hyperventilate with 100% O_2 for 2 min.	2. Cardiac depressant [use (a) or (b)] a. Xylocaine 2% (without epinephrine) 1 mg/kg IV b. Procainamide 2–4 mg/kg IV *cautiously*
3. Give one of the following inotropic drugs (cardiac stimulant). a. Epinephrine—0.2 to 0.3 mg in 2–3 ml saline IV or IC b. Isoproterenol 0.02 mg (0.1 ml) in 1 ml saline IV or IC c. Calcium chloride 10%, 1–3 ml IC	3. Should convert to normal sinus rhythm or one of the other arrhythmias.	3. External defibrillation a. Start at 100–150 w-sec. b. If ineffective, go to 200–300 w-sec.	3. When normal sinus rhythm is established support *cautiously* with isoproterenol 1 mg in 500 ml 5% D/W infusion.
4. Inotropic drugs should convert asystole to normal sinus rhythm or one of the other arrhythmias.	4. If no change, try (a) or (b): a. Epinephrine 0.2–0.3 mg in 2–3 ml saline IV or IC	4. If not effective, repeat above measures; continue cardiac massage.	

	b. Calcium chloride 10%, 1–3 ml IC or 5–10 CC IV at a rate not to exceed 1 ml/min	
5. If asystole persists, repeat inotropic drug given or try a different one.	5. When normal sinus rhythm is established, support with isoproterenol (use as under Asystole—6).	5. If still no effect, give (a) or (b) a. Epinephrine 0.2–0.3 mg in 2–3 ml saline IV or IC b. Calcium chloride 10%, 5 ml IV
6. When normal sinus rhythm is established, support with isoproterenol infusion of 1–2 mg in 500 ml of 5% D/W.		6. If fibrillation reverts to normal sinus rhythm but within a short period reverts back to ventricular fibrillation, or if it reverts initially to ventricular tachycardia, try (a) or (b): a. Xylocaine 2% (without epinephrine) 1 mg/kg IV b. Procainamide 2–4 mg/kg by slow IV injection *cautiously*
		7. When normal sinus rhythm is established, support with isoproterenol (use as under Asystole—6).

(Courtesy of N.K. Harpster, Angell Memorial Animal Hospital, Boston, MA)

    (3) Oxygen
    (4) Heat
4. Record electrocardiogram
  a) Diagnose type of electrical activity present and treat according to Table 2-13
  b) Prepare patient for defibrillation if ventricular fibrillation is found or if medical therapy fails to produce a normal sinus rhythm:
    (1) Shave hair from chest wall over fourth to sixth intercostal spaces.
    (2) Apply electrode conduction paste to shaved area and defibrillation paddles.
    (3) Hold animal in dorsal recumbency between paddles.
    (4) Set defibrillator.
    (5) Turn off, unplug, or disconnect ECG machine.
    (6) If electrical impulse is ineffective in converting fibrillation then increase current and repeat for second and third time.
    (7) With successful conversion to normal sinus rhythm (Fig. 2-12), external cardiac compressions are terminated.

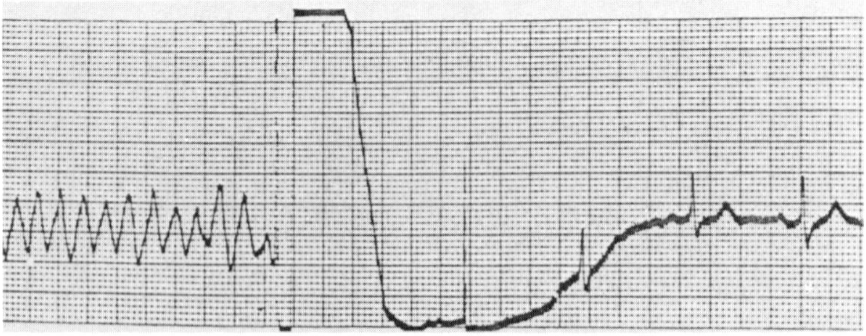

Fig. 2-12. This ECG portrays termination of ventricular fibrillation with direct cardioversion and return to a normal sinus rhythm. (Morgan RV: Cardiac emergencies—part II. Compend Contin Ed Pract Vet 3(9):841, 1981.)

V. Patient monitoring
   A. Maintain heart rate, blood pressure.
      1. Intravenous infusion of fluids
      2. Inotropic drugs as needed
   B. Support respiration.
      1. Assist ventilation until respirations have returned to normal.
      2. Continue O_2 for several hours.
   C. Watch for neurologic deficits from anoxia.
      1. Especially blindness
      2. Consider corticosteroids, mannitol.
   D. Monitor ECG for arrhythmias.
      See protocol for treatment of arrhythmias.
   E. Urine output
      1. Aids in evaluating adequacy of fluid therapy
      2. Aids in detecting renal failure from renal ischemia
   F. Body temperature
   G. Central venous pressure, blood gases, serum electrolytes
   H. Minimize stress and handling.
   I. Radiograph thorax
      Identify residual pulmonary changes from cause of cardiac arrest or resuscitative efforts; that is, contusions, rib fractures, pneumothorax, hemothorax.
   J. Diagnose and eliminate predisposing factors to cardiac arrest.

FELINE CARDIOMYOPATHY

Feline cardiomyopathy is a disorder of heart muscle of unknown etiology. It is often classified into three pathologic types.

I. Classification
   A. Hypertrophic
      1. Young to middle-aged cats
      2. Most often affects males
      3. Consistent pathologic findings are hypertrophy of

the left ventricular wall, papillary muscles, septum, and left atrium.

B. Congestive or dilated
   1. Higher frequency in older cats
   2. Affects males more than females
   3. Pathologic findings include gross dilation of one or both ventricles with flattening of the papillary muscles and trabeculae, and enlargement of both atria.

C. Intermediate
   1. Has pathologic changes seen in both hypertrophic and congestive forms
   2. Left ventricular hypertrophy with dilatation of other areas of the heart is common.
   3. Subendocardial fibrosis may also be seen in the left ventricle.

II. Clinical signs

Three separate clinical syndromes are recognized, but the clinical signs may overlap. Individual cats may show signs from two or more of the syndromes.

A. Acute LHF
   1. Cyanosis, dyspnea
   2. Weakness, collapse
   3. Pulmonary edema with moist crackles
   4. Systolic murmurs
   5. Diastolic gallop rhythm
   6. Hepatomegaly
   7. Weak, peripheral pulses
   8. Subnormal body temperature
   9. Cold distal extremities
   10. Pleural effusion, ascites may occur with generalized heart failure.

B. Arterial embolization
   1. Incidence approaches 50 percent in cats with symptomatic cardiomyopathy.
   2. Signs relate to location and duration of arterial occlusion.
   3. Most common site of embolism is the terminal aorta.

4. Mild signs—pain, weakness, ataxia of limb(s)
5. Severe signs
   a) Total flaccid paralysis with loss of spinal reflexes
   b) Loss of peripheral pulses
   c) Affected leg(s) are cold.
   d) Muscles are painful and hard.
   e) Nail beds may be cyanotic and fail to bleed when cut.
6. General signs
   a) Subnormal temperature
   b) Anxiety, dyspnea
   c) Signs of LHF

C. Syncope
1. Is sudden collapse due to inadequate blood flow to brain.
2. Is the most uncommon form of cardiomyopathy.
3. May occur at regular intervals or be precipitated by physical activity.
4. May or may not show:
   a) Loss of consciousness
   b) Autonomic signs during the episode, for example, urination, defecation, salivation
   c) Vocalization
5. Frequently caused by sinus arrest, sinoatrial block, and AV block

III. Diagnosis

The study of feline cardiomyopathy is relatively new to veterinary medicine and a great deal needs to be learned about this condition. Diagnosis of feline cardiomyopathy relies heavily upon:

A. History
B. Physical examination
C. Electrocardiography
1. Chamber enlargement
2. Conduction disorders
3. Arrhythmias
4. See Figure 2-13 and Table 2-5.

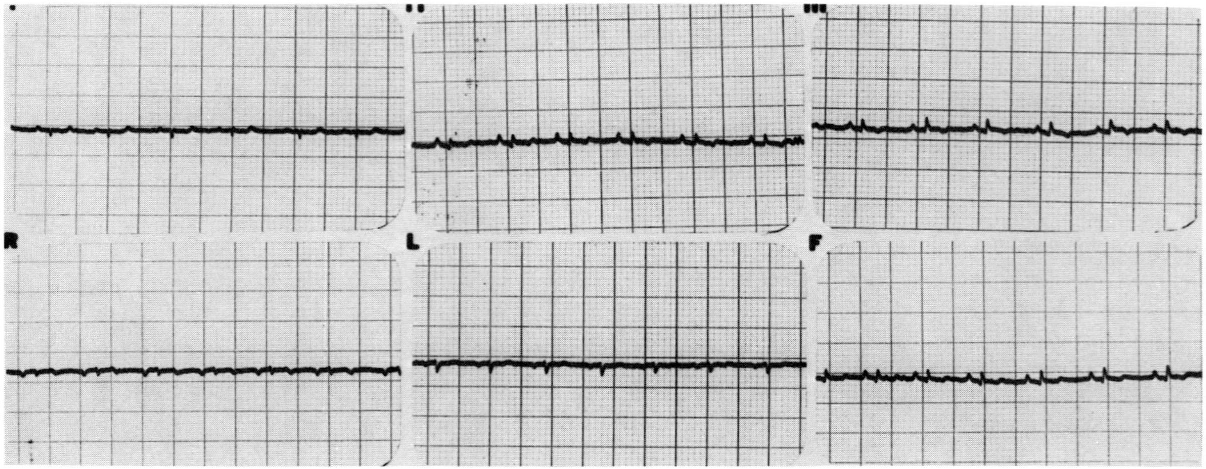

Fig. 2-13. The normal six-lead feline ECG.

D. Plain radiography
   1. Presence of pleural effusion, pulmonary edema
   2. Heart chamber enlargement
      a) Dorsoventral view
         Classic "valentine" shape
      b) Lateral view
         (1) More difficult to interpret
         (2) Heart tends to remain in oblique position with hypertrophic form.
         (3) Heart tends to become upright with less sternal contact in congestive form.
         (4) Loss of caudal waist
   3. Does not allow diagnosis of specific type of cardiomyopathy
E. Angiocardiography
   1. Selective catheterization of left ventricle
   2. Nonselective techniques of injecting radiopaque dye into jugular or cephalic vein
      Rapid-sequence 70-mm film or cassette tunnel exposures are taken.
   3. Allows definition of type of cardiomyopathy.
F. Echocardiography
   1. Chamber abnormalities
   2. Valvular disease
   3. Allows definition of type of cardiomyopathy.
G. Others
   1. Analysis of pleural fluid
   2. Peripheral blood pressure measurement
   3. Positive contrast arteriography

IV. Treatment

Specific therapy depends upon the clinical syndrome and pathologic type of cardiomyopathy present.

A. Immediate considerations
   1. Establish patient airway (Table 2-14).
   2. Administer O_2.
   3. Minimize stress and anxiety.
   4. Sedate as needed for pain, anxiety.
   5. Record ECG.

TABLE 2-14. PROTOCOL FOR FELINE CARDIOMYOPATHY

1. Establish patent airway if necessary (see protocols for cardiac arrest and CHF, administer O_2.
2. Minimize stress; sedate if necessary.
3. Record ECG.
4. Insert IV catheter for administration of IV medications; keep IV fluids to minimum.
5. a. Congestive cardiomyopathy—furosemide; after angiogram—digoxin
   b. Hypertrophic cardiomyopathy—furosemide; after angiogram—propranolol
   c. Aortic embolism—heparin; acepromazine or hydralazine; furosemide
6. After stabilization, begin diagnostic procedures.
   a. Plain radiography
   b. Thoracic, abdominal centesis
   c. Contrast radiography
7. Supportive care
   a. ± Sodium bicarbonate
   b. Antibiotics
   c. Heat
8. Consider embolectomy.

---

6. Consider insertion of IV catheter for administration of emergency medication; fluid therapy is usually contraindicated.

B. Nonspecific therapy
1. Examine closely for body cavity effusions, cardiac gallop rhythms, arterial embolism.
2. Remove thoracic, abdominal fluid by centesis.
3. Institute diuretics.
4. Perform neurologic examination in case of arterial embolization.

C. Surgery
1. Embolectomy should be considered if:
   a) Aorta is occluded above renal arteries.
   b) There is complete neurologic dysfunction of leg(s) with absence of spinal reflexes.
   c) There is failure to improve with medical therapy within 8–12 h.

TABLE 2-15. DRUG DOSAGES USED IN TREATING FELINE CARDIOMYOPATHY

Drug	Dosage
Acepromazine	1.0–2.5 mg SQ q8–12h
Diazepam	2–5 mg IV
Digoxin	0.003–0.005 mg/kg PO, IM q12h
Propranolol	2.5–5.0 mg PO q8h
Heparin	500 U IV, then 100–500 U/kg SQ q4–8h (adjust dosage to prolong clotting time to twice normal)
Hydralazine	2.5 mg PO q12h
Sodium bicarbonate	1–2 mEq/kg IV
Furosemide	2–4 mg/kg IV, IM, SQ, PO

2. Embolectomy may be considered as the primary treatment for arterial occlusion in those patients whose cardiopulmonary status is not compromised.

D. Specific medical therapy

Can be chosen after diagnostic workup has defined type of cardiomyopathy present and presence of embolism (Tables 2-15 and 2-16).

1. Hypertrophic—propranolol
2. Congestive—digoxin

TABLE 2-16. COMMERCIAL PRODUCTS USED FOR FELINE CARDIOMYOPATHY

Acepromazine—Acepromazine, Ayerst Laboratories, New York, NY 10017

Diazepam—Valium, Roche Laboratories, Nutley, NJ 07110

Digoxin—Lanoxin, Wellcome Animal Health Division, Kansas City, MO 64108

Propranolol—Inderal, Ayerst Laboratories, New York, NY 10017

Heparin—Heparin sodium, Med-Tech, Elwood, KS 66024

Hydralazine—Apresoline HCl, Ciba Pharmaceutical, Summit, NJ 07901

Furosemide—Lasix, Hoechst-Roussel Pharmaceuticals, Somerville, NJ 08876

3. Embolism—heparin, acepromazine or hydralazine

E. Supportive care
1. Antibiotics
2. Sodium bicarbonate
3. External sources of heat
4. Padded cages

V. Patient monitoring
A. Respiratory rate
B. Heart rate
C. Status of peripheral pulses
D. Neurologic function of affected legs
E. Urine output

Note: An indwelling urinary catheter may be necessary in cats with atonic bladders following aortic embolization.

F. Packed cell volume, TS, BUN
G. Withhold food until determination of the need for surgery is completed.
H. Repeat survey radiography of thorax.
I. Clotting status
1. Heparin dosages must be adjusted to ensure adequate anticoagulative effects.
2. The following three parameters may be utilized:

Test	Normal	Desired Value
Crude clotting time	1–3 min	2.0 × normal
Activated clotting time	55–80 sec	1.3–1.6 × normal
APTT	12–14 sec	1.5–2.0 × normal

BIBLIOGRAPHY

Bolton GR: Handbook of Canine Electrocardiography. WB Saunders, Philadelphia, 1975

Bolton GR: Bradycardia. p. 376. In Kirk RW (ed.): Current Veterinary

Therapy. Vol. 7. WB Saunders, Philadelphia, 1980

Bonagura JD: Feline cardiovascular emergencies. Vet Clin N Am 7(2):385, 1977

Bonagura JD: Cardiovascular emergencies. Sci Proc AAHA: 49, 1979

Bonagura JD: Acute heart failure. p. 359. In Kirk RW (ed.): Current Veterinary Therapy. Vol. 7. WB Saunders, Philadelphia, 1980

Bonagura JD, Pipers FS, Kittleson ML, Hamlin RS: Introduction to veterinary electrocardiography. Sci Proc ACVIM: 97, 1980

Bond B, Tilley LP: Cardiomyopathy in the dog and cat. p. 307. In Kirk RW (ed.): Current Veterinary Therapy. Vol. 7. WB Saunders, Philadelphia, 1980

Clark DR: Recognition and treatment of cardiac emergencies. J Am Vet Med Assoc 171(1):98, 1977

Davis LE: Pharmacodynamics of digitalis, diuretics, and antiarrhythmic drugs. p. 352. In Kirk RW (ed.): Current Veterinary Therapy. Vol. 7. WB Saunders, Philadelphia, 1980

Detweiler DK, Knight DH: Congestive heart failure in dogs: therapeutic concepts. J Am Vet Med Assoc 171:106, 1977

Ettinger SJ: Cardiac emergencies. Vet Clin N Am 2(2):235, 1972

Ettinger SJ: Cardiac arrhythmias. p. 918. In Ettinger SJ (ed.): Textbook of Veterinary Internal Medicine. Vol. 2. WB Saunders, Philadelphia, 1975

Ettinger SJ, Suter PF: Canine Cardiology. WB Saunders, Philadelphia, 1970

Ettinger SJ, Suter PF: Congential heart disease. p. 865. In Ettinger SJ (ed.): Textbook of Veterinary Internal Medicine. Vol. 2. WB Saunders, Philadelphia, 1975

Green CE, Meriwether E: Activated partial thromboplastin time and activated coagulation time in monitoring heparinized cats. Am J Vet Res 43(8):1473, 1982

Hamlin RL, Kittleson MD: Clinical experience with hydralazine for treatment of otherwise intractable cough with apparent left-side heart failure. J Am Vet Med Assoc 180(11):1327, 1982

Hamlin RL, Smetzer DL, Smith CR: Radiographic anatomy of the normal cat heart. J Am Vet Med Assoc 43(9):957, 1963

Harpster NK: Feline cardiomyopathy. Vet Clin N Am 7(2):355, 1977

Harvey CD, O'Brien JA: Management of respiratory emergencies in small animals. Vet Clin N Am 2(2):243, 1972

Hoffman BF, Sidbens AA, Cranefield PF, Brooks CM: The effects of epinephrine and norepinephrine in ventricular vulnerability. Circ Res 3:140, 1955

Kittleson MD, Hamlin RL: Hydralazine therapy for severe mitral regurgitation in a dog. J Am Vet Med Assoc 179(9):903, 1981

McIntosh JJ: The use of vasodilators in treatment of congestive heart failure: a review. JAAHA 17(2):255, 1981

Mueller HS, Antman EM, Ferst JA, Muller JE: Nifedipine in the treatment of cardiovascular disease. Hospital Pharmacy Forum, New England Medical Center Hospital 11(1):1, 1982

Muir WW, Bonagura JD: Aprindine for treatment of ventricular arrhythmias in the dog. Am J Vet Res 43(10):1815, 1982

Owens JM, Twedt DD: Non-selective angiocardiography in the cat. Vet Clin N Am 7(2):309, 1977

Phibbs B: The Cardiac Arrhythmias. CV Mosby, St. Louis, 1973

Pyle RL: Tachyarrhythmia. p. 381. In Kirk RW (ed.): Current Veterinary Therapy. Vol. 7. WB Saunders, Philadelphia, 1980

Rosen MR, Hoffman BF, Witt AL: Electrophysiology and pharmacology of cardiac arrhythmias. VI. Cardiac effects of verapamil. Am Heart J 89(5):655, 1975

Ross JN: Heart failure and shock. p. 825. In Ettinger SF (ed.): Textbook of Veterinary Internal Medicine. Vol. 2. WB Saunders, Philadelphia, 1975

Suter PF: The radiographic diagnosis of canine and feline heart disease. Compend Contin Ed Pract Vet 3(5):441, 1981

Swan HJC, Parmley WW: Congestive heart failure. p. 273. In Sodeman WA, Jr, Sodeman WA (eds.): Pathologic Physiology—Mechanisms of Disease. 5th Ed. WB Saunders, Philadelphia, 1974

Tilley LP: Feline electrocardiography. Vet Clin N Am 7(2):255, 1977

Tilley LP: Essentials of Canine and Feline Electrocardiography. CV Mosby, St. Louis, 1979

Watter JW: Radiographic signs of cardiovascular disease. Compend Contin Ed Pract Vet 1 (10):766, 1979

Weirich WE: Heart failure. Compend Cont Ed Pract Vet 1:375, 1979

3

Neurologic Emergencies

BRAIN TRAUMA

I Definition

The CNS, comprised of the brain and spinal cord can be injured by intrinsic and extrinsic events. Extrinsic causes of brain trauma include automobile accidents, falling from heights, blunt blows, and bite wounds. Although uncommon, intrinsic brain injury may result from vascular accidents, embolization, and neoplasia.

II. Classification
- A. Direct trauma from compressed skull fractures
- B. Contrecoup contusion—rapid head movement causes the brain to hit the bony skull of the opposite side
- C. Hemorrhage
- D. Hypoxia, anoxia
- E. Edema
- F. Infarction, ischemia
- G. Embolization
- H. Lack of nutrients, primarily glucose

III. Diagnosis
- A. Physical examination findings:
    1. Skull fractures
    2. Scalp lacerations
    3. Epistaxis
    4. Diminished level of consciousness
    5. Pupil abnormalities
    6. Motor dysfunction
    7. Cranial nerve deficits

B. Ancillary tests:
   1. Plain radiography
   2. Electroencephalography
   3. Echoencephalography
   4. Cerebral arteriography
   5. Computerized axial tomography
   6. Isotope scanning

Complex diagnostic procedures are usually unnecessary in assessing most head injuries. Clinical evaluation of neurologic functions is usually accurate and adequate in determining the severity of the head injury.

C. Differential diagnosis in the unconscious animal must include metabolic disorders such as hepatic encephalopathy and intoxication.

IV. Patient evaluation

The severity of brain trauma may be determined by evaluation of five basic neurologic functions. Serial monitoring of these functions will allow assessment of progress toward recovery or signs of deterioration, and will aid in determining the long-term prognosis.

A. *Level of consciousness* is the best indicator of the extent of cerebral hypoxia. Alterations of consciousness in increasing severity:
   1. Alert, oriented; normal or expected behavior and responsiveness
   2. Confused, apathetic; irritable, depressed; little or no vocalization; responsive to normal stimuli
   3. Stuporous, semicomatose; responsive only to noxious stimuli; dementia, unconscious vocalization, erratic behavior, unreponsive to stimuli; waxing/waning signs
   4. Comatose; cannot be aroused; unresponsive to all stimuli

Observe the animal for:
   1. Spontaneous behavior
   2. Responsiveness to normal environmental stimuli, for example, calling its name, petting

3. Responsiveness to noxious stimuli, for example, pain, heat, cold, loud noises
4. Vocalization
5. Aggressiveness
6. Erratic behavior

Note: If the animal was unconscious at the scene of injury but appears normal during the physical examination; it should still be closely monitored for 24–48 h. If an animal remains unconscious and does not improve within 24–48 h following the injury, it has probably sustained an irreversible brainstem injury.

B. *Motor function*—including degree and symmetry of voluntary movements should be noted.

Examine for:
1. Circling
2. Head tilt
3. Loss of righting reflex
4. Ataxia—differentiate paresis from musculoskeletal and spinal cord injuries.
5. Decerebrate rigidity—opisthotonus, extensor rigidity of all four limbs (Fig. 3-1); occurs with herniation of the cerebral hemispheres or severe brainstem lesions; reflects a life-threatening injury—death may follow quickly.

C. *Pupil size*, symmetry, and responsiveness to light are determined.
1. Pupils are normally equal in size and respond quickly to light.
2. Monitor abnormalities in size for several hours.
3. Rule out primary ocular trauma as the cause of pupil changes.

Note: Progressive constriction or dilation, anisocoria, and diminished responsiveness to light are all signs of neurologic deterioration and necessitates careful patient monitoring and reassessment of therapy (Table 3-1).

D. *Cranial nerve* testing aids in localizing the site of brain trauma.

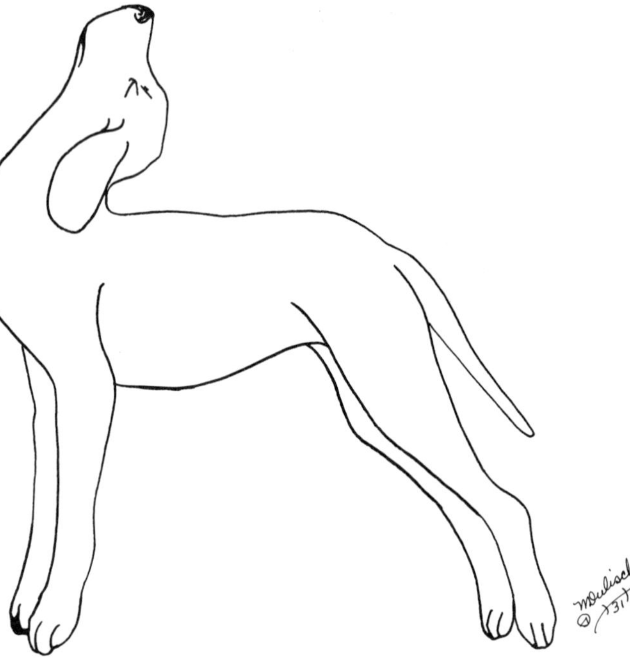

Fig. 3-1. Decerebrate rigidity is portrayed by extensor rigidity of all four limbs and opisthotonus. This posture signifies a life-threatening injury.

Evaluate each of the cranial nerves:

I. Smell

II. Vision

a) Visual deficits with normal pupillary responses suggest a contralateral visual cortex lesion.

b) Diminished vision may also arise from trauma to the eye, optic nerve, and optic tract.

III–V. Ocular movement

Inability to move the globe with rotation of the head from side-to-side and resting strabismus indicate involvement of these nerves.

TABLE 3-1. SIGNIFICANCE OF PUPIL AND OCULAR FINDINGS

Finding	Significance
Pupils equal and responsive	Normal
Unilateral constriction, responsive	Ophthalmic trauma, or concussion; usually resolves with time
Bilateral pinpoint pupils, unresponsive	Contusion to midbrain; prognosis guarded
Bilateral dilated and fixed	Compression, or hemorrhage near oculomotor nerve or nuclei; prognosis grave
Unilateral dilated, unresponsive	Unilateral oculomotor compression, or ipsilateral tentorial herniation with impending irreversible damage; consider surgery
Nystagmus	Cerebellar, vestibular or pontine contusion
Unilateral medial strabismus	Pressure on sixth cranial nerve; high pontine injury
Loss of doll's eye reflex[a]	Brainstem contusion

[a] A normal doll's eye reflex occurs if the eye remains in the center of the palpebral fissure when the head and neck are dorsoflexed.

Loss of corneal reflex and jaw drop denotes dysfunction of the fifth cranial nerve.

VI. Retraction of globe

VII. Movement of eyelid, retraction of lip

Determine presence of ptosis, inability to blink, diminished sensation, and movement of the side of the face.

VIII. Equilibrium, hearing

a) Note any vestibular signs, for example, head tilt nystagmus, ataxia.

b) Deficits of the seventh and eighth nerves may follow fractures of the petrous temporal bone.

IX. Gag and swallow reflex

Abnormalities may develop following bilateral contusion of the medulla.

X. Movement of tongue

Paralysis of the tongue may be uni- or bilateral, and denotes a medullary lesion near the foramen magnum.

Note: When cranial nerve deficits develop slowly from hypoxia and compression at a delayed time after the injury, the prognosis is more guarded than if the deficits arise immediately from the initial insult to the brain.

E. *Vital signs* must be closely monitored.
   1. Respiration
      a) Cheyne-Stokes breathing is rhythmic waxing and waning of the depth of respiration. Short periods of apnea are common. It often results from diencephalic lesions.
      b) Hyperventilation may arise from lesions in the midbrain.
      c) Ataxic or highly irregular respirations can occur with medullary injuries, and often precede respiratory arrest.
      d) Any alteration in respiration necessitates intensive therapy.
      e) Rule out thoracic wall trauma and respiratory tract injuries as the source of labored or irregular breathing.
   2. Pulse, heart beat

      Medullary lesions may produce cardiac depression and arrest (see Chapter 2).
   3. Mucous membrane color is a crude assessment of oxygenation of peripheral tissues.
   4. Capillary refill time reflects peripheral tissue perfusion.

F. *Perform serial testing* of the neurologic functions. Keep a detailed record of findings.

Signs of deterioration that indicate a poor prognosis and require aggressive therapy include:
   1. Decrease in consciousness
   2. Decrease in ambulation; paresis or paralysis
   3. Pupil changes

a) Constriction to dilatation
b) Unilateral to bilateral dilatation
c) Responsive to unresponsive
4. Progressive cranial nerve dysfunction
5. Changes in vital signs—especially respiratory or cardiac abnormalities

V. Treatment
A. Initial therapy
1. Establish patent airway.
2. Correct shock, control hemorrhage.
3. Stabilize systemic injuries.
4. Perform initial neurologic examination.

B. Observation
Observation may be the only treatment necessary if the animal is ambulatory and appears normal.

C. Medical therapy
1. Indicated for neurologic deficits (see Table 3-2)
2. Treatment objectives:
a) Prevent cerebral edema.
b) Relieve intracranial pressure.
3. Type of treatment is proportional to severity of injury:
a) Cortisone (dexamethasone)
(1) Level of consciousness is altered
(2) Patient is ambulatory
b) Cortisone and mannitol
(1) Animal is stuporous, recumbent, or comatose.
(2) Cranial nerve deficits are noted.
c) Diazepam
Used for agitated behavior or seizures

Note: Sedation and tranquilization should be avoided if at all possible because they can mask subtle changes in neurologic functions.

D. Supportive care
1. Oxygen
2. Elevate head with minimal compression of veins of the head.

TABLE 3-2. PROTOCOL FOR BRAIN TRAUMA

1. Establish patent airway.
   a. Oxygen
   b. Assisted ventilation
   c. Elevate head
2. Treat for shock and assess other injuries.
3. Make initial neurologic observations.
   a. Level of consciousness
   b. Movements
   c. Pupil size and response
   d. Vital signs
   e. Obvious skull fractures, trauma
   f. Cranial nerve function
4. Institute treatment.
   a. Dexamethasone 1–4 mg/kg SQ, IV q6–8h
   b. Mannitol 2 g/kg IV slowly over 40–60 min—may be repeated in 3–6 h for a maximum of four doses
   c. Any necessary supportive care:
      i. IV fluids
      ii. Stop hemorrhage
      iii. Control temperature
      iv. Antibiotics
      v. Prevent self-injury; diazepam 5–35 mg/kg IM, IV
5. Monitor changes in neurologic status.
   a. Note any deterioration.
   b. Note vital signs, urine output.
6. Stabilize, x-ray.

3. Maintain low to normal body temperatures to prevent excessive metabolic demands.
4. Hypertonic fluids (mannitol) are contraindicated if active cerebral hemorrhage is suspected.
5. Monitor vital signs, urine output.

E. Reevaluate therapy
1. A favorable response to therapy may occur within 6–8 h.
2. Failure of the unconscious patient to improve within 48 h demands a grave prognosis.
3. Motor and cranial nerve deficits may require days to weeks to return to normal.
4. Intensify medical therapy and consider surgical therapy as the neurologic status deteriorates.

F. Surgery
   1. Craniotomy—accomplishes decompression in the actively bleeding, rapidly deteriorating animal.
   2. Elevation of depressed skull fractures relieves pressure on adjacent brain tissue.
   3. Usually requires referral to a specialty hospital or institution.

SPINAL CORD INJURY

I. Definition

Events that produce neurologic deficits by causing injury to the spinal cord will be included in this discussion. The events are often compression or impaction injuries or insults that result in transection of the cord. Microscopically they result in hemorrhage, edema, cell disruption, leakage of plasma, and catecholamine-induced vascular changes in and around the spinal cord.

II. Etiology
   A. Vertebral fracture, dislocation
   B. Intervertebral disk herniation
   C. Neoplasia
   D. Fibrocartilaginous embolization
   E. Vascular accident

III. Patient evaluation

Because most spinal injuries are not progressive and spinal shock is not clinically significant in animals, initial examination will allow assessment of the injury. Pressure on the spinal cord affects the largest nerve fibers first, sparing the smallest fibers until last. The severity of the lesion is therefore closely correlated to fiber size. Injuries to the spinal cord produce deficits in the following four major nerve functions:

   A. *Conscious proprioception*, also known as "position sense." Conscious proprioception fibers are the largest fibers in the spinal cord and are the first damaged by trauma. Deficits in CP are considered the mildest of the four neurologic dysfunctions.

Test: The foot is forcibly knuckled. All four feet are tested.

1. Normal response: The foot is quickly returned to a weight-bearing position.
2. Abnormality: Delayed response or foot remains knuckled. Knuckling and scuffing of toes occurs with ambulation.

B. *Superficial pain perception* fibers are of medium size and this function is lost after CP. Superficial pain is a very subjective function to evaluate. Testing may be undependable because SPP is also affected by mental awareness, other injuries, and the inherent pain tolerance of the animal.

Test: Prick or pinch skin.

1. Normal response: Visible signs of discomfort
2. Abnormality: No awareness or response to test

C. *Voluntary movement* is the ability to move the limbs at will. Voluntary movement may be difficult to evaluate if muscloskeletal injuries are also present. Loss of VM denotes a severe injury.

Test: The animal is supported and advanced along a flat surface so that purposeful movements can be noted. Strength and ability to support weight are also assessed.

1. Normal response: Completion of normal ambulation
2. Abnormality: Weakness (paresis) to paralysis

D. *Deep pain perception* fibers are the smallest in the spinal cord and absence of DPP signifies a grave prognosis.

Test: Apply noxious stimuli to one of the toes, joints, or deep fascia.

1. Normal response: Conscious demonstration of pain such as crying, turning toward the area stimulated or snapping at the source.
2. Abnormal response: Diminished or lack of awareness of stimulus.

   Note: When the toe is pinched, simple withdrawal of the foot occurs through a local spinal reflex and is *not* indicative of deep pain perception.

IV. Localization
  A. Diagnostic tools:
    1. Physical examination
    2. Testing local spinal reflexes
    3. Plain radiography
    4. Myelography
  B. There are four anatomic divisions of the spinal cord and injuries within these areas produce the following signs or deficits:
    1. C_1–C_5:
      a) Spastic tetraparesis or paralysis
      b) Spinal reflexes are intact and hyperreflexic.
      c) Muscle tone is normal or hypertonic.
      d) Ipsilateral Horner's syndrome occurs with interruption of the lateral tectospinal tract.
      e) Loss of bladder control is uncommon.
      f) Phrenic nerve involvement produces paralysis of diaphragm and severe respiratory distress.
    2. C_6–T_1:
      a) Depression of local spinal reflexes of forelimbs occurs from injury to motor neuron cells.
      b) Ataxia, tetraparesis with forelimbs most affected
      c) Forelimbs: hypo- or arreflexic; hypotonic
      d) Hindlimbs:
        i) Reflexes are normal or hyperactive.
        ii) Muscle tone is normal or slightly hypertonic.
      e) Horner's syndrome may occur with avulsion of roots of T_1.
      f) Paradoxical breathing develops if innervation to intercostal muscles is lost.
    3. T_2–L_3:
      a) Forelimbs: usually normal
      b) Hindlimbs:
        i) Ataxia, paraplegia or paralysis
        ii) Reflexes and tone are normal or hyperactive

c) Schiff-Scherrington posture occurs if the lesion is severe (Fig. 3-2).
d) Analgesia caudal to lesion is common.
e) Severe injuries may cause upper motor neuron paralysis of bladder.

4. L_4–S_3:
a) Depression of local spinal reflexes of the hindlimbs occurs from motor neuron cell injury.
b) Forelimbs: normal
c) Hindlimbs:
    i) Flacid paresis to paralysis
    ii) hypo- or arreflexic; hypotonic or atonic
d) Decreased sensation to tail, perineum is present.

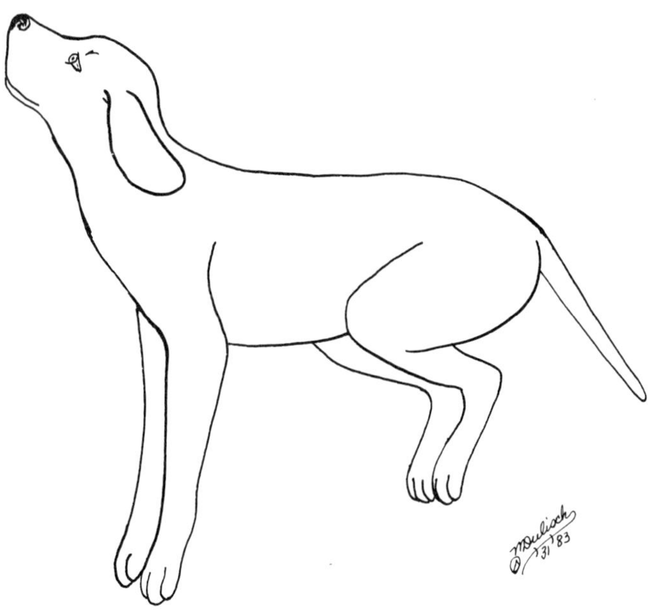

Fig. 3-2. Schiff-Sherrington posture is defined as extensor rigidity of the forelimbs and paralysis of the hindlimbs. It denotes a severe spinal cord lesion caudal to the cervical intumescence.

e) Sacral lesions produce dilation of anus and lower motor neuron paralysis of bladder.

V. Treatment

A. Priorities:

1. Immobilize vertebral column.
2. Prevent edema of spinal cord.
3. Decompress areas under pressure.

B. Therapy is based upon the severity of the lesion as detected by neurologic deficits and instability of the spine. Four types of treatment are available:

1. Cage rest for mild paresis and pain
2. Medical therapy

a) Dexamethasone

For mild neurologic deficits when the vertebral column is stable.

b) Mannitol and dexamethasone (Table 3-3)

i) When CP and SPP are lost.

TABLE 3-3. PROTOCOL FOR SPINAL CORD INJURY

1. Immobilize patient.
   a. Backboard
   b. Strap to cart.
   c. Lift and move animal properly.
2. Treat for shock and assess/treat other injuries.
3. Palpate for obvious fractures.
4. Neurologic examination
   a. CP
   b. SPP
   c. VM
   d. DPP
   e. Schiff-Sherrington posture
   f. Status of bladder, anal tone
   g. Spinal reflexes
5. Stabilize patient, then x-ray; monitor vital signs.
6. Start medical therapy.
   a. Dexamethasone 1–4 mg/kg SQ, IV q6–8h
   b. Mannitol 2 g/kg IV
   c. Supportive care; insert urinary catheter.
7. Prepare for surgery.

ii) When VM is altered but still present.
iii) The vertebral column is stable.

3. Surgical therapy
   a) Decompression
      Is indicated in severe alterations or absence of either VM or deep pain.
      (1) Techniques
         i) Hemilaminectomy
         ii) Total laminectomy
      (2) Perform surgery within 6–24 h following injury or onset of signs.
   b) Vertebral immobilization
      (1) Indicated for vertebral fractures with displacement
      (2) Technique:
         i) Pin and wire
         ii) Bone cement application
         iii) Vertebral body plating
         iv) Dorsal spinus process plating
   c) Visual examination of spinal cord
      (1) Used to confirm suspected total functional cord damage
      (2) May ascertain extent of injury when prognosis is uncertain
4. Euthanasia
   a) Indicated for complete transection of cord as demonstrated by vertebral displacement or at surgery
   b) Loss of voluntary movement and deep pain for greater than 48 h prior to presentation for treatment
   c) Failure of severe neurologic deficits to respond to appropriate therapy within 10–14 days following injury

VI. Patient monitoring
   A. Reevaluate neurologic functions every 6–12 h.
   B. Monitor urine output. If bladder is atonic, utilize an in-

dwelling urinary catheter or manually express the bladder every 6–8 h.

C. Hemorrhagic gastroenteritis and pancreatitis may occur with prolonged cortisone administration. Monitor for tarry stools and vomiting.

D. Provide adequate cage padding and turn the animal frequently to prevent decubitis ulcer formation.

E. Monitor body temperature for evidence of infection.

STATUS EPILEPTICUS

I. Definition

Status epilepticus is a series of rapidly repeating convulsions. Continuous seizures may become life-threatening with side effects such as hyperthermia, lactic acidosis, cerebral edema, laminar necrosis of the cerebral cortex, and terminal hypocalcemia.

II. Causes of seizures

A. Toxins—lead, arsenic, strychnine, organophosphates, ethylene glycol, cyanide, and others

B. Metabolic—hypoglycemia, hypocalcemia, hypernatremia, hepatic encephalopthy

C. Nutritional—thiamine deficiency

D. Structural—neoplasia, vascular malformation, hydrocephalus, ischemia, encephalitis

E. Infectious—canine distemper, tetanus, tick infestation, parasitism

F. Idiopathic—epilepsy

III. Diagnosis

The animal is usually presented during an active major motor seizure. Status epilepticus occurs more often in the dog than in the cat. Frequent seizures in the cat must be differentiated from syncopal episodes. Obtain an accurate history and complete a thorough physical examination. If possible, perform a neurologic exam with careful assessment of cranial nerve function, postural reflexes, and responses to noxious stimuli.

IV. Treatment
  A. Treat seizures intensively when they:
    1. Do not cease within 3–5 min.
    2. Increase in frequency.
    3. Progress to persistent status epilepticus.
    4. Complicate other preexisting diseases.
  B. Ensure patent airway. Prevent self-trauma and injury to animal handlers (see Table 3-4).
  C. Sedation
    1. Diazepam
      a) Drug of choice for short-term sedation
      b) Repeat every 30–60 min as needed.
    2. Barbiturates

TABLE 3-4. PROTOCOL FOR STATUS EPILEPTICUS

1. Prevent self-trauma and injury to animal handlers.
2. Ensure patent airway.
3. Sedate.
   a. Diazepam—dog: 5–40 mg IV to effect; cat: 2.5–5.0 mg IV to effect
   b. Pentobarbital, phenobarbital 3–15 mg/kg IV
   c. Intubation with gas anesthesia
4. Monitor vital signs; assess other injuries or diseases; perform neurologic examination.
5. Immediate diagnostic aids—STAT blood sugar; serum calcium; ECG
6. Draw blood for CBC, blood lead, and biochemical profile.
7. Diagnostic therapy
   a. 50% glucose IV, 2–20 ml to effect
   b. 10% calcium gluconate IV, 2–10 ml slowly
8. Correct hyperthermia.
   a. If temperature is >41°C, lower temperature 1°/h
   b. If temperature is <38°C, apply heat
9. Supportive care
   a. Treat for shock.
   b. O_2
   c. Antibiotics
10. Monitor vital signs, maintain airway.
11. Consider dexamethasone and mannitol for cerebral edema.

TABLE 3-5. COMMERCIAL PRODUCTS USED IN NEUROLOGIC EMERGENCIES

Dexamethasone	Azium, Schering, Kenilworth, NJ 07033 Dexate—SP, Burns Biotec Laboratories, Omaha, NB 68103
Mannitol	Mannitol IV 20%, Abbott Laboratories, N. Chicago, IL 60064
Diazepam	Valium, Roche Laboratories, Nutley, NJ 07110
Pentobarbital	Nembutal sodium solution, Abbott Laboratories, N. Chicago, IL 60064

a) For refractory seizures

b) Pentobarbital is preferred for its rapid onset of action (see Table 3-5)

3. Inhalant anesthetics

Reserved for patients in which other methods fail

D. Collect diagnostic samples

1. Complete blood count
2. Blood sugar, lead, ammonia
3. Serum calcium, electrolytes
4. In the absence of laboratory analysis, the ECG may reveal electrolyte abnormalities. (see Chapter 1.)

E. Diagnostic therapies

Seizures that occur from abnormalities in blood sugar or serum calcium are often poorly responsive to diazepam. If laboratory analysis of blood chemistries is not immediately possible and the seizure fails to respond to diazepam, the following therapies may be tried:

1. Fifty percent dextrose IV

   Cessation of the seizure would allow a tentative diagnosis of hypoglycemia to be made.

2. Ten percent calcium gluconate IV
   a) Administer cautiously.
   b) Terminate therapy with any sign of nausea or elevation of the heart rate.
   c) Positive response to this therapy allows a tentative diagnosis of hypocalcemia.

V. Patient monitoring
  A. Body temperature
    1. Control hyperthermia
    2. Lower temperature 1°C/h until 39°C.
    3. Avoid overzealous cooling; secondary hypothermia is common.
    4. Immerse in cool water momentarily
    5. Cool sponge baths
  B. Vital signs
  C. Maintain airway
  D. Maintain hydration
     Subcutaneous or IV fluid therapy
  E. Consider corticosteroids and mannitol if cerebral edema follows persistent, violent seizures.

Note: Seizures that are refractory or recurrent despite use of the therapeutic protocol warrant a guarded prognosis.

BIBLIOGRAPHY

Averill DR; Intracranial injuries. p. 683. In Kirk RW (ed.): Current Veterinary Therapy. Vol. 5. WB Saunders, Philadelphia, 1974

Bailey CS, Holliday TA: Diseases of the spinal cord. p. 401. In Ettinger SJ (ed.): Textbook of Veterinary Internal Medicine. Vol. 1. WB Saunders, Philadelphia, 1975

Chrisman CL: Problems in Small Animal Neurology. Lea & Febiger, Philadelphia, 1982

Colter SB: Spinal injuries. Vet Clin N Am 11(1):49, 1981

DeLahunta, A. Veterinary Neuroanatomy and Clinical Neurology. WB Saunders, Philadelphia, 1977

Fenner WR: Seizures and head trauma. Vet Clin N Am 11(1):31, 1981

Griffiths IR: Trauma of the spinal cord. Vet Clin N Am 10(1):131, 1980

Hoerlein BF: Canine Neurology. 3rd Ed. WB Saunders, Philadelphia, 1978

Holliday TA: Seizure disorders. Vet Clin N Am 10(1):3, 1980

Moore RW, Withrow SJ: Gastrointestinal hemorrhage and pancreatitis associated with intervertebral disk disease in the dog. J Am Vet Med Assoc 180(12):1443, 1982

Mountcastle VB (ed.): Medical Physiology. 13th Ed., Vol. 1. CV

Mosby, St. Louis, 1974

Oliver JE: Neurologic emergencies in small animals. Vet Clin N Am 2(2):341, 1972

Oliver JE, Knecht CD: Diseases of the brain. p. 357. In Ettinger SJ (ed.): Textbook of Veterinary Internal Medicine. Vol. 1. WB Saunders, Philadelphia, 1975

Parker AJ: Canine spinal disease. p. 2. In Veterinary Scope. Vol. 18. Upjohn, Kalamazoo, MI, 1974

Selcer RR: Trauma to central nervous system. Vet Clin N Am 10(3):619, 1980

Toombs JP, Caywood DD, Lipowitz AJ, Stevens JB: Colonic perforation following neurosurgical procedures and corticosteroid therapy in four dogs. J Am Vet Med Assoc 177(1):68, 1980

4

Ocular Emergencies

INITIAL CONSIDERATIONS

I. Seek immediate veterinary care for any animal exhibiting:
   A. Acute ocular pain
   B. Deformity of the globe
   C. Acute loss of vision
   D. Sudden change in appearance of the eye

II. Obtain thorough and accurate history.

III. Approach the animal gently and carefully; injured eyes are often extremely painful.

IV. Systematically examine the eye:
   A. Start with the extraocular structures.
   B. Observe for visual impairment and ability to maneuver in the examination room.
   C. Discern size and position of globes and palpebral fissures.
   D. Note deformities and laceration of head; photophobia, blepharospasm, ocular discharges.
   E. Check pupil size, responses to light.
   F. Test cranial nerve functions.
   G. Examine lids, membrana nictitans, conjunctiva, cornea, anterior segment, lens and retina for lacerations, hemorrhage, edema, foreign bodies, opacitics, and abnormal anatomic position.

V. Consider use of topical ophthalmic anesthetics, and darkened room to facilitate the examination.
   Diagnostic tools include:
   A. Pinpoint light source

TABLE 4-1. PROTOCOL FOR EYE EMERGENCIES

1. Obtain quick, complete history from owner.
2. Carefully perform systematic examination of structures of eye.
3. Lavage eye vigorously.
4. Correct any obvious problem:
   a. Proptosis—try to replace eye.
   b. Foreign body—remove manually or flush.
   c. Control hemorrhage.
   d. Control swelling of lids with cold compresses.
5. Calm animal and owner.
6. Assess and treat any other injuries.

B. Direct and indirect ophthalmoscope
C. Magnifying loupe
D. Ophthalmic irrigating solutions
E. Fluorescein and Rose Bengal stains
F. Short-acting mydriatic

See Table 4-1 for the protocol for ocular emergencies.

TRAUMATIC PROPTOSIS

I. Definition

Traumatic proptosis is an acute forward displacement of the eye beyond the bony orbit and eyelids.

II. Causes
   A. Blunt blows to the head
   B. Bite wounds
   C. Retrobulbar hemorrhage
   D. Fractures of the orbit
   E. Overzealous manual restraint of the head

III. Clinical signs
   A. Contraction and inward rolling of eyelids behind globe
   B. Protrusion of globe beyond the normal palpebral fissure
   C. Chemosis
   D. Subconjunctival hemorrhage
   E. Drying and ulceration of cornea

F. Deviation of globe with damage to extraocular muscles
G. Proptosis occurs most frequently in the brachycephalic breeds because of their prominent eyes, large palpebral fissures, and shallow orbits.

IV. Diagnosis
  A. Determine cause and duration
  B. Examine for:
    1. Severity of corneal drying
    2. Deviation of globe
    3. Presence of hyphema
    4. Pupil size
  C. It is difficult to accurately determine the prognosis for future vision at initial examination, therefore, all owners should be warned of the potential for blindness.
  D. Prognosis is poor if there is:
    1. Severe facial trauma
    2. Stretching or tearing of optic nerve
    3. Dilation of pupil
    4. Hyphema
    5. Duration of the proptosis greater than 3 h
  E. Prognosis is good if:
    1. Degree of prolapse is mild.
    2. Duration of proptosis is short.
    3. Pupil is miotic.
    4. A mydriatic pupil becomes miotic with replacement of the globe.

V. Treatment
  A. Initial
     Keep eye moist with irrigating solution.
  B. Mild or partial prolapse of globe
    1. Apply gentle retrograde pressure on the globe with moistened cotton.
    2. If mild lagophthalmos is detected after replacement, perform temporary tarsorrhaphy.
  C. Classic proptosis
    1. Attempt surgical replacement with the animal under anesthesia.

2. Techniques for surgical replacement:
   a) Temporary tarsorrhaphy sutures may be preplaced in the eyelids, using an elastic stent to prevent the sutures from pulling through the lids. Three horizontal mattress sutures of 4-0 silk, polyglycolic acid, or polyglactin 910 are passed through the stent and into the eyelid 4–5 mm from the free margin. The sutures exit at the opening of the meibomian glands and care must be used at this point to avoid puncturing the globe with the needle. The sutures then enter the opposite free lid margin at the opening of the meibomian glands. After the three sutures are preplaced, gentle pressure is applied to the globe while the lids are pulled upward and outward by traction on the suture ends. With the globe returned to a normal position, the sutures are tied to maintain closure of the lids (Fig. 4-1).
   b) A strabismus hook is inserted under each folded lid at the medial canthus. Moving laterally, the hooks are used to pull the lids out and away from the globe while gentle pressure is applied to the eye. A temporary tarsorrhaphy is then performed as above.
   c) A lateral canthotomy may be undertaken if the eye cannot be replaced by these two procedures alone.
3. Topical hyperosmotic agents are usually unnecessary and should be avoided.
4. A membrana nictitans flap will cover the eye, but does not provide sufficient support to the globe, therefore, residual exophthalmos and lagophthalmos may follow this procedure.

D. Proptosis with severance of optic nerve
   1. Enucleate the eye.

      Note: Marginal cases should be replaced surgically, as enucleation can be undertaken later if the eye is determined to be unsalvageable.

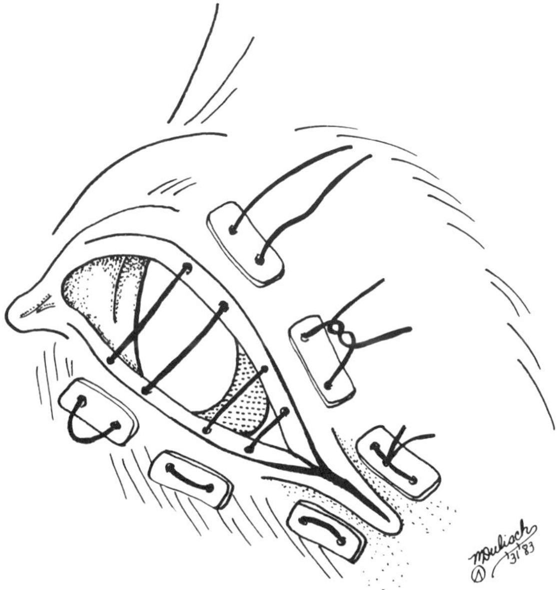

Fig. 4-1. Technique for temporary tarsorrhaphy. Sutures are passed through the lid margins at the opening of the meibomian glands and anchored with elastic stents, effectively closing the eyelids.

E. Postoperative care
   1. Topical atropine (Tables 4-2 and 4-3)
   2. Topical antibiotics for ulceration or drying of cornea
   3. Topical corticosteroids
      Apply *only* if the cornea is intact and has remained moist.
   4. Systemic prednisone
      1 mg/kg BID PO, IM q8–12h for 2–4 doses to reduce inflammation.
   5. Retrobulbar methylprednisone acetate
      a) Two to 4 mg in one injection only
      b) To decrease swelling, inflammation
   6. Warm compresses
   7. Elizabethan collar to prevent self-trauma

TABLE 4-2. EMERGENCY OCULAR MEDICATIONS

Mydriatics
- Atropine 1%—SID to TID
- Epinephrine 1%—QID
- Phenylephrine 10%—TID to QID

Miotics
- Echothiophate iodide 0.03–0.25%—q12–48h
- Philocarpine 1–2%—TID to QID
- Demecarium 0.125–0.25%—q12–48h

Antibiotics
- Topical—chloramphenicol, gentamicin, oxytetracycline, neomycin, polymyxin B, erythromycin
- Subconjunctival—chloramphenicol 15 mg; gentamicin 25 mg, ampicillin 100 mg
- Systemic—chloramphenicol 20–50 mg/kg TID; gentamicin 2 mg/kg BID or TID; ampicillin 20 mg/kg TID

Corticosteroids
- Topical—prednisolone acetate; hydrocortisone; dexamethasone; betamethasone
- Subconjunctival—triamcinolone 8–12 mg; methylprednisolone acetate 2–8 mg
- Systemic—prednisone 1 mg/kg/day divided BID to QID; dexamethasone 1–2 mg/kg/day divided BID to QID

Hyperosmotics
- Mannitol—2 g/kg IV slowly, repeat in 6–12 h; glycerine 50%—2 ml/kg PO

Carbonic anhydrase inhibitors
- Dichlorphenamide
  - Cat: 1 mg/kg BID or TID, PO;
  - Dog: 2–4 mg/kg BID or TID, PO
- Methazolamide—Dog: 2–4 mg/kg TID, PO
- Acetazolamide—Dog: 2–5 mg/kg TID, PO; *caution:* toxicity is common

Antiprostaglandins
- Aspirin
  - Cat: 1¼ g q48h PO
  - Dog: 15 mg/kg BID or TID, PO
- Flunixin meglumine—Dog: 1 mg/kg IV q12–24h for one to two doses; *caution:* not yet licensed for use in dogs

F. Follow-up care
   1. Leave tarsorrhaphy closed for 10–14 days.
   2. Remove tarsorrhaphy earlier if copious mucopurulent discharge occurs, pain persists, systemic malaise is noted, or pyrexia occurs.

VI. Common complications
   A. Blindness
   B. Residual lagophthalmos with exposure keratitis

TABLE 4-3. COMMERCIAL PRODUCTS USED IN OCULAR EMERGENCIES

Fluorescein—Fluori-I-Strip, Ayerst Laboratories, New York, NY 10017

Rose Bengal—1% Rose-Bengal, Maurray Biologic, Los Angeles, CA 90047

Short-acting mydriatics—Mydriacyl 1%, Alcon Laboratories, Fort Worth, TX 76134

4-0 silk suture—4-0 silk, Alcon Laboratories, Fort Worth, TX 76134

Polyglycolic acid suture—Dexon, Haver-Lockart, Shawnee, KS 66201

Polyglactin 910 suture—Vicryl, Pitman-Moore, Washington Crossing, NJ 08560

Collagen suture—plain collagen, Ethicon, Somerville, NJ 08876

Echothiophate iodine—Phospholine iodide, Ayerst Laboratories, New York, NY 10017

Demecarium—Humorsal, Merck Sharpe & Dohme, West Point, PA 19486

Triamcinolone—Kenalog-40, E.R. Squibb, Princeton, NJ 08540

Methylprednisolone acetate—Depo-Medrol, Upjohn, Kalamazoo, MI 49001

Dichlorphenamide—Daranide, Merck, Sharpe & Dohme, West Point, PA 19486

Methazolamide—Neptazane, Lederle Laboratories, Pearl River, NY 10965

Acetazolamide—Diamox, Lederle Laboratories, Pearl River, NY 10965

Flunixin meglumine—Banamine, Schering, Kenilworth, NJ 07033

Acetylcysteine—Mucomyst, Mead Johnson Pharmaceutical Division, Evansville, IN 47721

5% sodium chloride ointment—Muro-128, Muro Pharmaceutical Laboratories, Tewksbury, MA 01876

10% phenylephrine—Phenylephrine HCl 10%, Smith, Miller and Patch, San German, PR 00753

Pilocarpine/epinephrine—E-Pilo-2, Smith, Miller and Patch, San German, PR 00753

Soft contact lens—Softcon, American Optical, Southbridge, MA 01550

Intraocular balanced salt solution—BSS, Alcon Laboratories, Fort Worth, TX 76134

C. Permanent dorsotemporal or dorsolateral deviation of globe from extraocular muscle tearing
D. Phthisis bulbi

EYELID INJURIES

I. Definition
  A. The most common lid injuries are contusions, lacerations, and bite wounds.
  B. Differential diagnosis of swelling and discoloration of the lids should include:
    1. Allergic reactions with angioneurotic edema
    2. Diffuse cellulitis accompanying retrobulbar abscessation
II. Causes
  A. Bite wounds
  B. Blows to the head
  C. Automobile accidents
  D. Any source of trauma to the head
III. Clinical signs
  A. Ocular discharge, lacrimation
  B. Blepharospasm
  C. Swelling, discoloration of lids
  D. Obvious defects of the lids
  E. May be accompanied by:
    1. Subconjunctival hemorrhage, chemosis
    2. Corneal defects
    3. Fractures of the frontal sinus and bony orbit
    4. Cranial nerve deficits
IV. Diagnosis
  A. Accurate history
  B. Ocular examination
    1. Approach cautiously, may be painful
    2. Consider typical anesthetics, sedatives
V. Treatment
  A. Follow two rules:
    1. Attempt repair as soon as possible.
    2. Repair with minimal debridement.
  B. Contusions, ecchymoses

1. Cold compresses
2. Topical antibiotics

C. Lacerations, bite wounds
1. Repair under general anesthesia.
2. Gently clip and clean affected area; avoid soap near the eye.
3. Suture conjunctival lesions separately using 5-0 or 6-0 gut or collagen in a continuous pattern.
4. Suture skin with 4-0 silk, nylon, or polyglactin 910 in a simple interrupted pattern beginning at the lid margin.
5. Allow old or infected wounds to granulate; perform plastic surgery at a later date.

VI. Postoperative care
A. Keep sutured site clean.
B. Consider topical and systemic antibiotics.
C. Prevent self-trauma with Elizabethan collar.
D. Remove sutures in 10 days.

CONJUNCTIVAL INJURIES

I. Classification and etiology
A. Lacerations
Trauma
B. Hemorrhage
1. Trauma
2. Clotting disorders
3. Blood dyscrasias
4. Systemic illness
C. Chemosis (edema)
1. Trauma
2. Upper respiratory infection
3. Exposure to chemicals
4. Systemic illness

II. Clinical signs
A. Many systemic causes of conjunctival deformities will produce minimal clinical signs.
B. Signs that may follow trauma or occur with upper respiratory disorders include:

1. Ocular discharge, lacrimation
2. Blepharospasm, photophobia
3. Swelling and discoloration of eyelids

III. Diagnosis
   A. Accurate history
   B. Physical examination
      1. Complete eye examination
      2. Thorough examination for systemic illness
   C. Laboratory workup
      1. Complete blood count
      2. Clotting survey
      3. Conjunctival culture and sensitivity, cytology

IV. Treatment
   A. Initial
      1. Examine eye closely for accompanying injury to the cornea and intraocular structures.
      2. Remove any foreign material.
      3. Prevent drying with topical antibiotics, lubricants.
   B. Lacerations

      Do not need to be sutured unless extensive or complicated by lacerations of the eyelids or sclera.
   C. Hemorrhage

      Most hemorrhages resolve without treatment within 10–14 days.
   D. Chemosis
      1. Prevent drying
      2. Treat or remove the cause
      3. Prevent self-trauma with Elizabethan collar

V. Complications
   A. Necrosis of conjunctiva
   B. Exophthalmos, lagophthalmos
   C. Self-trauma to eyelids, cornea, skin of face

CORNEAL INJURIES

I. Definitions

   Corneal injuries vary from superficial abrasions to full-thickness lacerations and penetrating wounds. Exposures to chemicals and heat may also result in corneal pathology and are discussed in the following section.

II. Cause
  A. Ectopic cilia, distichiasis
  B. Poor eyelid conformation
  C. Eyelid tumors
  D. Foreign material, projectiles
  E. Infectious diseases
  F. Bite wounds, cat scratches
  G. Unknown

III. Clinical signs
  A. Severe pain, anxiety
  B. Photophobia
  C. Blepharospasm
  D. Lacrimation
  E. May be accompanied by:
    1. Trauma to the eyelids
    2. Subconjunctival hemorrhage, chemosis
    3. Deformity of the globe
    4. Miosis, anterior uveitis

IV. Diagnosis
  A. Accurate history
  B. Ocular examination
    1. Requires topical or regional anesthesia
    2. Fluorescein stain
       Absorbed by stroma
       Note: A descemetocele will not retain stain because stroma is gone.
    3. Note size, location, depth, and regularity of margins of lesion.
    4. Note corneal edema.
       Suggests injury or impairment of normal endothelial function.
    5. Examine lids and membrana nictitans closely.
  C. Perform systemic examination.

V. Classification and treatment
  A. Superficial ulcers
    1. Medical therapy

a) Reserved for superficial abrasions or small corneal ulcers in nonbrachycephalic breeds
b) Topical antibiotics
c) ± Topical atropine
d) Most superficial defects epithelialize within 24–72 h.

2. Surgical therapy
   a) Consider surgery for all ulcers in exophthalmic breeds.
   b) Indicated for recurrent, indolent ulcers.
   c) Protect the eye and promote epithelialization with one of the following procedures:
      (1) Membrana nictitans flap sutured with 4.0 suture to the upper eyelid (Fig. 4-2)—will often provide support for 2 to 4 weeks.
      (2) Membrana nictitans flap sutured to the bulbar conjunctiva (Fig. 4-3)—may be used in exophthalmic dogs with short third eyelids and also restricts movements of the globe; usually stays in place 7–14 days.
      (3) Temporary tarsorrhaphy—for corneal ulcers following traumatic proptosis or exposure keratitis
3. Ancillary therapy
   a) Topical antibiotics, atropine
   b) Topical acetylcysteine—for rapidly "melting" collagenase ulcers caused by collagenase-producing bacteria
   c) Manual debridement of redundant corneal tissue
   d) Topical hyperosmotic saline ointments
   e) Soft contact lenses

   Items c–e above are often indicated in recurrent, indolent epithelial erosions.

Note: Topical steroids are contraindicated in the presence of all corneal ulcers.

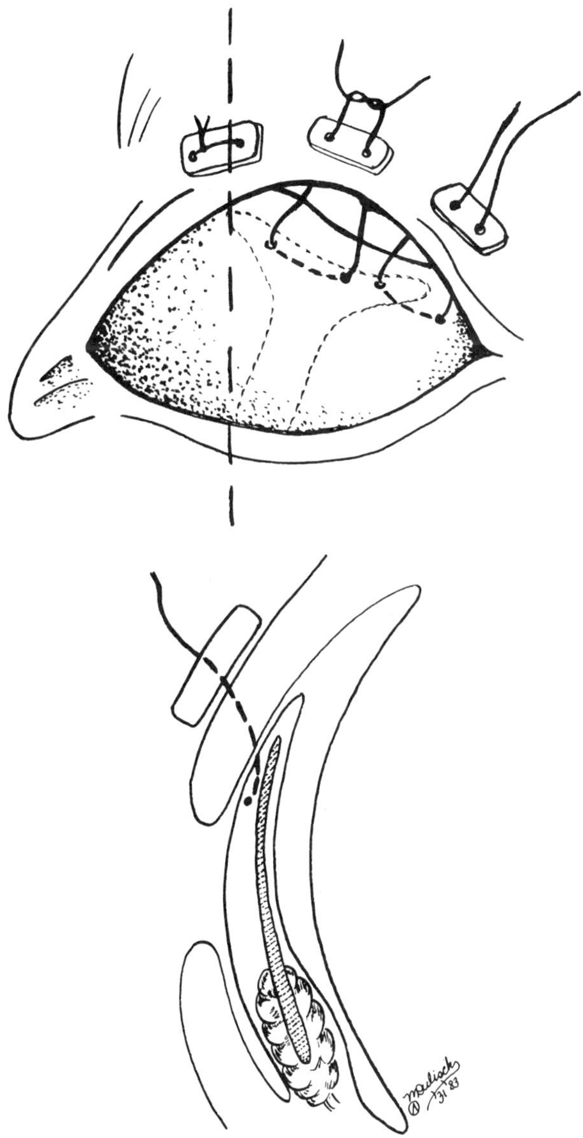

Fig. 4-2. Placement of a membrana nictitans flap by suturing to the upper eyelids.

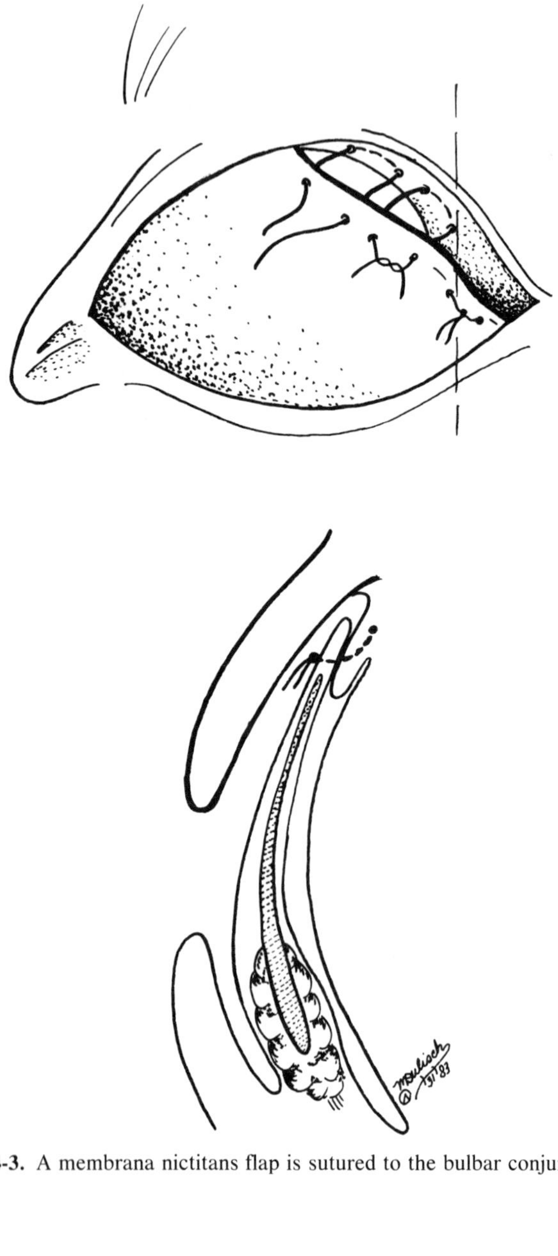

Fig. 4-3. A membrana nictitans flap is sutured to the bulbar conjunctiva.

B. Deep ulcers
  1. Initial therapy
    a) Large or deep stromal injuries potentially threaten the integrity of the globe and must be treated vigorously.
    b) Remove inciting cause.
    c) Obtain conjunctival cultures and cytologic swabs before installation of topical anesthetic.
  2. Medical therapy
    a) Provide specific antibiotics or antiviral therapy as determined by culture.
    b) Increase frequency of application of medications.
    c) Consider subconjunctival and systemic antibiotics.
    d) ± Acetylcysteine
  3. Surgical therapy
    Many large or deep corneal defects require surgical support.
    a) Temporary tarsorrhaphy
    b) Membrana nictitans flap
      Note: Both (a) and (b) above may not provide adequate support for large stromal defects or descemetoceles.
    c) Conjuctival flap
      (1) 360°, 180°, bridge, pedicle types
      (2) Technique: The conjunctiva is incised at the limbus and the incision is extended parallel to the limbus to its desired length. The conjunctiva is bluntly dissected from Tenon's capsule, keeping the conjunctival flap as thin as possible. The conjunctiva is undermined until it can be brought down to cover the corneal defect. The flap is anchored to the cornea with 6-0 suture if it is a pedicle or 180° flap (Fig. 4-4). A 360° flap is anchored by suturing conjunctiva

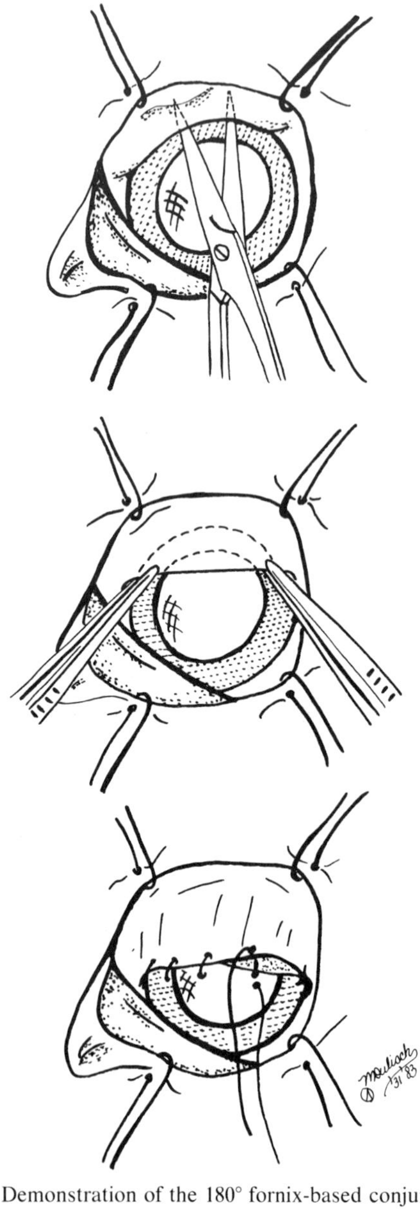

Fig. 4-4. Demonstration of the 180° fornix-based conjunctival flap.

to conjunctiva in a horizontal plane with horizontal mattress sutures of 4-0 or 6-0 suture.

i) A modification of this technique for brachycephalic breeds with excessive tension on the retention sutures is to suture a 180° dorsal fornix-based flap to the free edge of the membrana nictitans.

ii) Remove flap in 14–21 days.

iii) Residual conjunctival tissue which fills corneal defect will recede and remodel with subsequent topical steroid therapy.

d) Lamellar corneal-scleral transposition

(1) This technique is a keratoplasty that does not require a donor and because it is an autograft it is not rejected.

(2) The procedure is more difficult to perform and requires specialized instrumentation.

C. Penetrating wounds

Penetrating wounds are surgical emergencies and should be corrected as soon as possible.

1. Anesthetize animal and prepare for surgery.
2. Avoid topical ointment—if the petroleum base is absorbed into the anterior chamber uveitis may result.

a) Surgical therapy

(1) Reposition viable iris tissue; suture cornea.

i) Excise necrotic iris tissue with electroscalpel.

ii) Lavage anterior chamber with 1:100,000 ocular epinephrine and balanced salt solution.

iii) Suture cornea with 6-0 or 7-0 silk or collagen.

iv) Place sutures 1 mm apart.

v) Transverse two third the thickness of the cornea with sutures.

vi) As the last suture is placed, re-form the anterior chamber with an air bubble.

(2) Conjunctival flap

May be used if the corneal defect is too large or too friable to suture.

b) Adjunct medical therapy

(1) Topical antibiotics

(2) Topical mydriatics

i) Atropine

ii) Phenylephrine

(3) Systemic antiprostaglandin drugs, corticosteroids

(4) Consider topical corticosteroids for postoperative uveitis in uninfected eyes.

CHEMICAL KERATITIS

I. Definition

Active keratitis caused by exposure to chemicals or thermal burns will be discussed in this section.

II. Cause

A. Soaps

B. Aerosol sprays

C. Mace

D. Household cleaners

E. Photolaboratory chemicals

F. Two types:

1. Acids—are precipitated by corneal proteins and are less destructive than alkali.
2. Alkaline chemicals—severely erode corneal epithelium and stroma; polymorphonuclear cells release collagenase which further liquifies the stroma.

III. Diagnosis

A. History of exposure

B. Ocular examination

1. Fluorescein stain outlines defects in the epithelium as it is absorbed by the stroma.
2. Rose Bengal stain will delineate devitalized areas of epithelium even though the epithelium may be intact.

IV. Treatment
  A. Copious lavage
    Use large volume (2L):
    1. Sterile saline
    2. Eye wash solutions
    3. Tap water
  B. Boric acid ointment
    May help to neutralize alkaline compounds.
  C. Topical antibiotics, atropine
    1. Every 4 h
    2. For partial- or full-thickness burns
  D. Anticollagenase drugs (acetylcysteine)
    For evidence of collagenase activity
  E. Soft contact lens
    May help prevent symblepharon when the conjunctiva and lids are also affected.

V. Complications
  A. Perforation of cornea
  B. Persistent corneal edema—if endothelium injured
  C. Permanent scarring of cornea
  D. Symblepharon
  E. Lagophthalmos, exposure keratitis—if lids are involved
  F. Keratoconjunctivitis sicca
    Note: The prognosis for corneal burns depends upon the type and concentration of the insulting chemical, quantity of cornea affected, and time interval between exposure and treatment.

PENETRATING FOREIGN BODIES

I. Cause
  A. Gunshot debris
  B. Wood splinters

- C. Glass
- D. Industrial refuse
- E. Vegetable material

II. Clinical signs
- A. Severe pain—blepharospasm, photophobia
- B. Hemorrhage from area of globe
- C. Miosis
- D. Deformity of globe
- E. May be accompanied by:
  1. Corneal edema
  2. Deviation of globe
  3. Wounds to lids, face
  4. Skeletal deformities of face

III. Diagnosis
- A. History
- B. Physical examination
  1. Locate point of entry and approximate the trajectory taken by the foreign body.
  2. Slit lamp biomicroscopy may be helpful.
- C. Plain radiography to locate radiopaque material
- D. Ancillary tests
  1. Ultrasonography
  2. Computerized axial tomography

IV. Treatment
- A. Initial therapy
  1. Control hemorrhage.
  2. Sedate animal if necessary for thorough ocular examination.
- B. Specific therapy

  Depends upon final location and type of foreign material.
  1. Corneal foreign bodies

     Remove under topical or general anesthesia with irrigation or minimal dissection.
  2. Anterior chamber

     Remove via limbal incision.
  3. Posterior segment
     - a) Removal is difficult and traumatic.

b) Should be attempted for irritating types of material (see Table 4-4).
c) Consider referral to specialty practice or institution.

C. Postoperative therapy
1. Topical antibiotics, mydriatic
2. Systemic antibiotics
3. Systemic antiprostaglandin drugs, corticosteroids
4. Consider topical corticosteroids for active uveitis.
5. Prevent self-trauma with sedation and Elizabethan collars.

V. Complications
A. Uveitis
B. Endophthalmitis
C. Blindness
D. Glaucoma
E. Phthisis bulbi

TABLE 4-4. EFFECTS OF INTRAOCULAR FOREIGN MATERIAL

Material	Effect
Iron and steel (oxidize) Wood Plant debris	Severely irritating—potential loss of eye
Copper Bronze Brass	Local abscessation; endophthalmitis
Mercury Aluminum Nickel Zinc Lead	Moderately irritating
Gold Silver Stone Carbon Glass Plastic Rubber	Inert—usually not irritating

ANTERIOR UVEITIS

I. Definition

Acute uveitis is an inflammatory condition of the anterior vascular tunic of the eye including the iris and ciliary body. It may produce enough pain and ocular abnormalities to prompt an owner to seek immediate veterinary care.

II. Cause
- A. Blunt trauma
- B. Penetrating trauma
- C. Surgical trauma
- D. Allergic reactions
- E. Infectious disease
  1. Leptospirosis
  2. Blastomycosis
  3. Crypotcoccosis
  4. Toxoplasmosis
  5. Feline infectious peritonitis virus
  6. Feline leukemia virus
- F. Immune-mediated diseases
- G. Neoplasia—primary intraocular or metastatic
- H. Leakage of lens material
- I. Other systemic illnesses
- J. Idiopathic

III. Clinical signs
- A. Pain, blepharospasm, photophobia
- B. Redness (episcleral injection)
- C. Miosis
- D. Anterior chamber flare
- E. Ciliary flush, rubeosis iridis
- F. Hypotony

IV. Diagnosis
- A. Classic clinical signs
- B. Ocular examination
  1. Direct ophthalmoscopy
  2. Indirect ophthalmoscopy
  3. Slit lamp biomicroscopy
  4. Gonioscopy
  5. Tonometry

C. Physical examination
D. Laboratory workup
  1. Complete blood count
  2. Biochemical profile
  3. Immune survey
  4. Antibody titers
  5. Specific ELIZA tests

Note: The reader is directed to the bibliography at the end of the chapter for a more detailed discussion of the diagnosis and treatment of uveitis.

V. Treatment
  A. Topical cycloplegics
  B. Topical antibiotics/steroid preparations
  C. Systemic antiprostaglandins
  D. Systemic steroids are indicated in the absence of infection.

VI. Complications
  A. Posterior synechia, iris bombé
  B. Anterior synechia
  C. Endophthalmitis, panophthalmitis
  D. Lens opacities
  E. Glaucoma
  F. Blindness

HYPHEMA

I. Definition

Hyphema is blood (frank hemorrhage) within the anterior chamber. Blood in the anterior chamber may clot and darken or remain unclotted.

II. Cause
  A. Trauma
  B. Glaucoma
  C. Intraocular neoplasia
  D. Congenital ocular lesions
  E. Systemic diseases
  F. Clotting defects
  G. Hypertension

III. Diagnosis
   A. Ocular examination
      1. Direct visualization
      2. Slit lamp biomicroscopy
      3. Tonometry
      4. Direct and indirect ophthalmoscopy whenever possible
   B. Physical examination
   C. Laboratory workup
      1. Complete blood count
      2. Clotting survey
      3. Biochemical organ profile
      4. Immune survey
      5. Arterial blood pressure measurement

IV. Treatment

   The treatment of hyphema is both controversial and enigmatic. The following therapies should be considered:

   A. Topical pilocarpine
      1. Facilitates drainage on intact red blood cells through iridocorneal drainage angle.
      2. Often results in miosis which may predispose to complete posterior synechia.
   B. Topical mydriatics
      1. Indicated for iridocyclitis
      2. May prolong active uveal bleeding
   C. Combination therapy

      The author prefers to use a topical pilocarpine/epinephrine agent for the first 24–72 h followed by atropine.

   D. Topical steroids

      For accompanying uveitis

   E. Sedation, cage rest
   F. Remove cause of bleeding

V. Patient monitoring, complications
   A. Serial measurements of intraocular pressure should be taken.

      Secondary glaucoma is common.

   B. Mild hyphema often resolves within 10–14 days.
   C. Severe, protracted hyphema may result in:

1. Posterior synechiae
2. Cataracts
3. Blindness
4. Glaucoma
5. Phthisis bulbi

LENS LUXATION

I. Definition

Complete displacement of the crystalline lens away from its normal postion in the posterior fossa is termed a *luxation*. Breakage or degeneration of the zonules is necessary to allow movement of the lens. Partial zonule breakage will allow incomplete dislocation of the lens or *subluxation*. The lens may luxate anteriorally or posteriorly. Posterior luxations uncommonly threaten the integrity of the eye. Anterior luxations are alarming because they may cause pupillary block, obstruction of the drainage angle, and secondary glaucoma or may allow prolapse of the vitreous with secondary retinal detachment.

II. Cause

A. Inherited predisposition, especially terrier breeds
B. Secondary to glaucoma
C. Following any dramatic fluctuation in intraocular pressure
D. Trauma
E. Neoplasia
F. Idiopathic

III. Diagnosis

Discovery of the lens in an abnormal position upon examination of the eye allows the diagnosis to be made. Subluxated lenses lie partially in the posterior fossa. An aphakic cresent can usually be visualized through the pupillary aperture in the area where the lens is displaced. Following an anterior luxation the lens will be found resting in the anterior chamber entirely cranial to the iris. Crystalline, cataractous lens are easy to see in the anterior chamber. Transparent lens or cloudiness of the cornea may make the diagnosis more difficult.

IV. Treatment
   A. No treatment necessary
      1. Partial subluxations without pupillary block or intraocular pressure elevation
      2. Posterior luxations with normal ocular tension
      3. Idiopathic, innocuous anterior luxations in cats—often bilateral
      4. Luxations secondary to buphthalmos
   B. Surgical therapy
      1. Indications:
         a) Any luxation followed by elevations in intraocular pressure
         b) Any luxation accompanied by vitreous prolapse
      2. Treatment:
         a) Gentle manual pressure on the cornea may cause an anterior luxation to return to a more normal position. This "couching" technique is performed under topical anesthesia.
         b) Therapy of choice is surgical removal of the lens.
         c) Consider referral of the patient to a specialty practice or institution.

V. Complications
   A. Secondary glaucoma
   B. Vitreous prolapse
   C. Retinal detachment
   D. Intraocular hemorrhage
   E. Corneal edema from disruption of the endothelium
   F. Blindness

ACUTE GLAUCOMA

I. Definition

Glaucoma is an increase in intraocular pressure that is incompatible with normal vision. Normal intraocular tension is 15–27 mmHg. Acute glaucoma is an emergency because the eye does not tolerate elevations in pressure above 50 mmHg for more than 12–24 h without irreversible sequelae such as blindness.

II. Cause
   A. Primary disorders of the drainage angle—often inherited
   B. Secondary to other intraocular disease, for example, hyphema, lens luxation, uveitis, neoplasia

III. Clinical signs
   A. Pain
   B. Cloudy, edematous cornea
   C. Insensitive cornea
   D. Dilated, unresponsive pupil
   E. Palpably hard eye
   F. Episcleral vascular injection
   G. Loss of vision

   Note: Many owners do not immediately notice these changes, especially if the opposite eye is unaffected and visual.

IV. Diagnosis
   A. Classic ocular findings
   B. Suspicious history, breed
   C. Tonometry is necessary to make an accurate diagnosis. Several techniques can be used:
      1. Digital—subjective, often inaccurate
      2. Indention with Schiøtz tonometer—accurate, readily available, inexpensive
      3. Applanation tonometer—most accurate, expensive
   D. Examination of angle with gonioscopy
   E. Tonography—experimental

V. Treatment

   The major priority is to immediately lower the intraocular pressure. Several classes of medicants may be used to accomplish this goal.

   A. Osmotic agents
      1. Reduce the amount of aqueous within the globe.
      2. Mannitol, glycerine (see Tables 4-2, 4-3)
   B. Miotics

1. Enlarge the drainage angle, therefore facilitating removal of aqueous.
2. Pilocarpine, echothiophate iodide, demecarium

C. Carbonic anyhdrase inhibitors
1. Decrease aqueous production
2. Dichlorphenamide, methazolamide, acetazolamide

Note: The long-term medical maintenance of animals with glaucoma is difficult and often unsuccessful. The patient may require referral to a specialty institution for additional surgical therapy.

VI. Patient monitoring
A. Measure serial intraocular pressures
B. Monitor vision
C. Watch for metabolic acidosis which may accompany carbonic anhydrase therapy.
D. Treat or remove the cause of the glaucoma, for example, control uveitis, remove luxated lens.

OPTIC NEURITIS

I. Definition

Optic neuritis is an inflammation of the optic nerve which results in sudden onset of blindness, often in both eyes.

II. Cause
A. Unknown or idiopathic—most common
B. Canine distemper
C. Reticulosis
D. Granulomatous meningoencephalitis
E. Toxoplasmosis
F. Other CNS diseases

III. Clinical signs
A. Acute bilateral blindness
B. Dilated, unresponsive pupils
C. Papillitis
1. May be present if the optic disc is involved.
2. The disc appears swollen with poorly defined margins.

D. The retina may be normal if the inflammation is retrobulbar.
E. The rest of the eye is usually normal.

IV. Diagnosis
  A. Ocular examination
  B. Physical examination
  C. Laboratory workup
    1. Complete blood count
    2. Biochemical organ profile
    3. Cerebrospinal fluid analysis
    4. Serology
  D. Differential diagnosis:
    1. Prechiasmatic neoplasms
    2. Toxic amaurosis

       An ERG and optic nerve thecography or computerized axial tomography may be useful to rule out these disorders.

V. Treatment
  A. Therapy of choice; systemic corticosteroids
  B. Therapy must be instituted immediately in order to maximize the possibility of reversal of blindness.
  C. A favorable response may occur within hours with improvement of pupil response and return of vision.
  D. Untreated optic neuritis will lead to permanent optic nerve atrophy.

VI. Patient monitoring
  A. Central nervous system disease should be suspected if optic neuritis is recurrent.
  B. If the optic neuritis recurs, repeat the cerebrospinal tap.
  C. The prognosis is guarded if the cerebrospinal fluid is abnormal.

BIBLIOGRAPHY

Bistner SJ, Aquirre GD: Management of ocular emergencies. Vet Clin N Am 2(2):359, 1972

Bistner SJ, Aquirre GD, Batik G: Atlas of Veterinary Ophthalmic Surgery. WB Saunders, Philadelphia, 1977

Blogg JR: The Eye in Veterinary Practice. WB Saunders, Philadelphia, 1980

Gelatt KN: Orbit and adnexa: Diagnostic methods in small animal ophthalmology (Part I). Compend Contin Ed Pract Vet 2(5): 413, 1980

Gelatt KN (ed): Textbook of Veterinary Ophthalmology. Lea & Febiger, Philadelphia, 1981

Magrane WG: Canine Ophthalmology. Lea & Febiger, Philadelphia, 1971

Rubin LF: Atlas of Veterinary Ophthalmoscopy. Lea & Febiger, Philadelphia, 1974

Severin GA: Veterinary Ophthalmology Notes. 2nd Ed. College of Veterinary Medicine and Biomedical Sciences, Colorado State University, Fort Collins, 1975

Winston SM: Ocular emergencies. Vet Clin N Am 11(1):59, 1981

Wyman M: Ophthalmic surgery for the practitioner. Vet Clin N Am 9(2):311, 1979

5

Musculoskeletal Emergencies

DEFINITION

True life-threatening emergencies of the MS are confined to skull fractures that result in brain trauma, rib fractures that impair respiratory function, fractures of the mandible and larynx that obstruct the upper airway, and vertebral column injuries that threaten the spinal cord. These respective emergencies are discussed in detail in Chapters 3 and 12. Chapter 5 will discuss the initial evaluation and emergency therapy applied to common orthopedic injuries, such as fractures, dislocations, traumatic amputations, and avulsions.

CAUSES

I. Automobile accidents are the most common
II. Falls from heights or falls during exercise
III. Bite wounds
IV. Gunshot wounds
V. Blows from blunt instruments
VI. Natural disasters
VII. Iatrogenic injury from aggressive manipulation or restraint
VIII. Pathologic fractures from nutritional and neoplastic disorders

CLASSIFICATION OF INJURIES

I. Fractures
  A. Closed
  B. Open

1. Grade I (mild)

   Fracture fragments penetrate the skin from inside to outside.
2. Grade II (moderate)

   Skin penetration occurs as a wound from the outside, with an underlying fracture from violent forces. Accompanying soft tissue injury is common.
3. Grade III (severe)

   Skin penetration occurs from the outside. Fractures are often comminuted. Extensive loss of soft tissue occurs and peripheral nerve injury may be found.

II. Joint luxations, subluxations
   A. Closed
   B. Open

III. Avulsions
   A. Partial amputation of distal extremities
   B. "Degloving" injuries of distal extremities
   C. Amputation of the tail

IV. Traumatic amputation of one or more limbs

CLINICAL SIGNS

I. Lameness, decreased weight bearing
II. Inability to ambulate, paresis
III. Abnormal movement or reduced range of motion
IV. Deformity and angulation
V. Pain
VI. Swelling, crepitance, grating
VII. Soft tissue wounds, contusions, avulsions
VIII. Peripheral nerve deficits
IX. Vascular injury with hemorrhage or impaired peripheral circulation.

DIAGNOSIS

I. Skeletal fractures, even the most obvious and glaring, are rarely life threatening. Although they attract the immediate attention of the owner and veterinarian, other organ systems must take precedence during the initial evaluation of the trauma victim. Detailed examination of appendicular skeletal injuries should be delayed until the clinician is convinced that other organ systems have not sustained serious injury. Tranquilization or sedation to facilitate examination of the MS is contraindicated because it may mask signs of central and peripheral nerve damage and may complicate recovery from shock, cardiovascular, and respiratory emergencies.

II. Once the patient has been stabilized, diagnosis of musculoskeletal injuries involves:
   A. Observation of ambulation
   B. Detection of clinical signs as listed above
   C. Palpation of extremities
   D. Evaluation of peripheral nerve function
   E. Examination of surrounding soft tissue
   F. Assessment of circulation to limb
   G. Plain radiography—multiple views

TREATMENT

See Table 5-1.

I. Priorities:
   A. Ensure a patent airway.
   B. Diagnose and correct life-threatening injuries.
   C. Institute first aid for musculoskeletal injuries.

II. Establish an airway.
   A. Intubate and administer O_2 as needed.
   B. Assess fractures near upper airway and of thoracic rib cage.
   C. Relieve pneumothorax if present.

III. Treat systemic injuries.
   A. Treat for shock.
   B. Control hemorrhage.
      1. Pressure bandage
      2. Direct clamping and ligation of arterial bleeding
      3. Tourniquets may be used for brief periods of time, such as during transportation to the hospital, but

TABLE 5-1. PROTOCOL FOR MUSCULOSKELETAL INJURIES

1. Establish patent airway.
2. Treat for shock and assess other injuries.
   a. Control hemorrhage.
   b. Assist respiration as needed.
      i. See protocol for airway obstruction.
      ii. See protocol for pleural cavity disease.
   c. Assess CNS.
      i. See protocol for brain trauma.
      ii. See protocol for spinal cord and injuries.
   d. Examine soft tissues of abdomen.
3. Apply first aid to injured extremities.
   a. Control hemorrhage.
   b. Perform thorough examination.
      i. Define and classify type of fracture.
      ii. Assess soft tissue damage.
      iii. Evaluate peripheral nerve function.
      iv. Examine circulation to limb.
   c. Open fractures
      i. Clean and cover wound.
      ii. Consider culturing site.
      iii. Immobilize limb.
   d. Closed fractures, dislocations
      i. Confine to cage.
      ii. Consider temporary immobilization of limb.
   e. Avulsions, partial amputations
      i. Clean and debride wound.
      ii. Consider culturing site.
      iii. Cover wound, immobilize limb.
   f. Amputation of limb
      i. Treat for shock, control hemorrhage.
      ii. Clean and dress amputation site.
      iii. Assess all other injuries.
      iv. When stable, prepare for surgery.
4. Start supportive care.
   a. Cage rest
   b. ± Antibiotics
   c. ± Fluid therapy
5. Stabilize other injuries and prepare for surgery.
   a. Radiography
   b. Laboratory workup
   c. Withhold food.

are contraindicated for continuous control of bleeding due to their occlusion of venous return from the limb.

C. Assist respiration.
   1. Examine thorax closely if rib fractures or proximal forelimb fractures are found.
   2. Consider radiography to assess injuries to the diaphragm.

D. Evaluate CNS.
   1. Examine for signs of brain trauma and cranial nerve deficits if fractures of the mandible and skull are present.
   2. Assess spinal cord functions and examine for vertebral injuries if hemiparesis or tetraparesis are present.
   3. Immobilize patient if spinal cord injury is suspected.

E. Examine soft tissues of abdomen.
   1. Ensure that urinary bladder is intact, especially if fractures of the pelvis or proximal hindlegs have occurred.
   2. Ensure patency of urethra if fractures of pelvis are present.
   3. Consider radiography to evaluate diaphragm.

IV. Treat injured extremity.

Note: Use caution when performing examination of MS system. The affected limbs are painful and the animal may attempt to bite.

A. Open fractures
   1. Clip hair away from site of wound.
   2. Lavage wound with sterile saline or multiple electrolyte solution.
   3. Avoid sedation, anesthesia if possible.
   4. Using aseptic techniques, gently remove foreign debris and partially avulzed soft tissue.
   5. Consider culturing wound if grossly contaminated.
   6. Cover exposed area with sterile lubricant (K-Y jelly) and gauze, and apply bandage.
   7. Immobilize limb.

B. Closed fractures, dislocations
   1. Some fractures, particularly limb fractures very close to the trunk may be best treated temporarily with cage confinement because they are difficult to immobilize with splints.
   2. Distal limb fractures may be immobilized with a temporary splint or sling—see Table 5-2.

C. Avulsions, partial amputations
   1. Control hemorrhage.
   2. Treat as open fracture—steps A 1–7.

D. Amputation of one or more limbs
   1. Institute therapy for shock.
   2. Control hemorrhage, consider transfusions.
   3. Treat amputation site as open fracture.
   4. Assess other injuries.
   5. As soon as stable, prepare for surgery.

V. Supportive care
   A. Cage rest with padding, waterbeds, or grates
   B. Antibiotics for grossly contaminated wounds
   C. Intravenous or SQ fluid therapy
   D. Keep temporary splints clean and dry.

TABLE 5-2. TEMPORARY IMMOBILIZATION DEVICES

Location of Fracture, Dislocation	Type of Immobilization
Phalanges, metacarpals, metatarsals, carpus and tarsus	Aluminum spoon splint Wood, plastic, or fiberglass coaptation splint Modified Robert Jones bandage
Radius, ulna, tibia, elbow, and stifle	Modified Robert Jones bandage Schroeder-Thomas splint
Humerus and femur	Over-the-shoulder or over-the-hip spica bandage or coaptation splint Schroeder-Thomas splint for distal femoral fractures
Scapula, shoulder, and coxofemeral joints	Valpeau or shoulder sling Ehmer or figure-of-eight sling
Pelvis	Padded cages with strict confinement

PATIENT MONITORING

I. Stabilize other injuries, pay particular attention to:
    A. Respiration
        1. Monitor chest tubes if inserted.
        2. Serial radiography of thorax
        3. Consider blood gas analysis.
    B. Urinations
        1. Monitor urine output.
        2. Perform contrast radiography if needed to rule out urinary tract trauma.
    C. Fluid therapy and persistent blood loss
        1. Monitor PCV, TS, urine output.
        2. Consider biochemical organ profile, urinalysis, and CBC.

II. Body temperature

III. Drainage or odor from site of open wound

IV. Position and cleanliness of temporary splint or sling

V. Swelling at fracture site, swelling of toes of affected limb

VI. Increasing pain

VII. Onset of neurologic deficits

VIII. Warmth, color, and perfusion of affected limb

IX. Mental alertness and responsiveness, ability to ambulate

X. Withhold food when other injuries are stable in anticipation of surgery.

BIBLIOGRAPHY

Aron DN: Emergency management of the musculoskeletal trauma patient. Compend Contin Ed Proct Vet 4(3):220, 1983

Deuland R: Emergency treatment of limb fractures. Vet Clin N Am 5(2):305, 1975

Engen MH: Initial management of closed fractures and joint injuries. Vet Clin N Am 10(3):691, 1980

Parker RB, Waldron DR: The initial treatment of open fractures. Vet Clin N Am 10(3):707, 1980

Ross GE, Jr: The initial management of skeletal injuries in the dog. Vet Clin N Am 2(2):397, 1972

Withrow SJ, Moore RW: Orthopedic emergencies in small animals. Vet Clin N Am 11(1):171, 1981

6

Dermatologic Emergencies

LACERATIONS

I. Definitions

Lacerations of the skin and subcutis are most commonly treated as emergencies when they are accompanied by active bleeding. Lacerations of arteries may result in dramatic, pulsatile bleeding that does not often terminate spontaneously, and if left untreated can be life threatening. Hypovolemic shock may also occur with persistent bleeding from lacerations of highly vascular, cavernous tissue or from lacerations complicated by systemic clotting disorders.

II. Classification

A. Lacerations with common arterial bleeding
   1. Tongue
   2. Pinnae of ears
   3. Distal extremities
   4. Tail

B. Lacerations with persistent nonpulsatile bleeding
   1. Philtrum and cartilages of nose
   2. Tongue
   3. Footpads
   4. Penis
   5. Mammary glands

C. Clotting disorders which complicate any laceration
   1. Warfarin toxicity
   2. Von Willebrand's disease
   3. Inherited hemophilias
   4. Platelet disorders

III. Diagnosis

The diagnosis of life-threatening skin lacerations is usually obvious to the emergency clinician upon physical examination of the animal. For a review of the diagnosis and clinical signs of shocks, see Chapter 1. For further discussion of clotting disorders, see Chapter 11.

IV. Treatment

A. Therapeutic objectives:
   1. Control hemorrhage.
   2. Control hypovolemic shock.

B. Control hemorrhage
   1. Tourniquets
      a) Most useful during transportation of animal
      b) Easily applied to distal extremities
      c) Can be fashioned from readily available materials
      d) Ischemic necrosis may occur to tissue distal to injury site if applied too tightly or for prolonged time.
      e) Limit use to 30–45 min.
   2. Clamping, ligation
      a) Hemostats are used to clamp exposed bleeding arteries.
      b) May be performed in the awake animal if necessary.
      c) Vessel is then ligated with sterile suture.
   3. Direct pressure
      a) Most common means of controlling hemorrhage
      b) May be applied to any site on body.
      c) Fewer potential complications than with the use of tourniquets
      d) Accomplished by application of manual pressure, tight wrap, or bandages
   4. Application of cold
      a) Promotes local vascular constriction.
      b) Helpful in areas of persistent seepage of blood, especially from highly vascular tissue

        c) Also minimizes soft tissue swelling in surrounding traumatized areas.
        d) May be used in addition to direct pressure.
        e) Ice or chemical cold packs are readily available.
    5. Topical hemostatic agents
        a) Good for bleeding from nail beds
        b) Examples
            (1) Silver nitrate
            (2) Styptic
            (3) Epinephrine
C. Combat hypovolemic shock
    1. Institute fluid therapy—consider use of both crystalloid solutions and whole blood.
    2. Consider glucocorticoids.
    3. Maintain respiration.
    (See Table 6-1.)

V. Patient monitoring
    A. Examine for other systemic injuries.
    B. Monitor vital signs for evidence of shock.
    C. Watch tissue distal to tourniquet sites for warmth and evidence of discoloration.

TABLE 6-1. PROTOCOL FOR BLEEDING LACERATIONS

1. Immediately stop hemorrhage.
    a. Direct pressure
    b. Clamping and ligation
    c. Tourniquet
    d. Application of cold
    e. Topical hemostatic
    f. ± Tranquilization
2. Combat shock if present.
    a. Rapid fluid therapy
    b. Whole blood transfusions
    c. Glucocorticoids
3. Examine closely and treat other systemic injuries.
4. When animal is stable, repair laceration surgically.

D. Delay sedation or anesthesia for repair of laceration until animal is hemodynamically stable.
E. Postoperatively monitor for contamination and evidence of infection at the site.

ALLERGIC REACTIONS

I. Definition

The *allergic reactions* discussed here, angioneurotic edema, and urticaria, are actually immunologic diseases with dermatologic manifestations. Because they develop acutely with rather dramatic physical changes, they often require rapid therapeutic intervention. Both conditions arise following exposure to an allergen with subsequent release of histamine and other vasoactive substances. Histologically they are characterized by a localized increase in vascular permeability.

II. Cause

A. Insect bites and stings
B. Foods:
   1. Berries
   2. Nuts
   3. Chocolate
   4. Green vegetables
   5. Shellfish
   6. Tomatoes
C. Blood transfusion
D. Drugs
E. Antibiotics, especially penicillin, tetracyclines
F. Analgesics, especially salicylates
G. Tranquilizers
H. Adriamycin
I. Vaccinations
J. Contrast media used in radiography
K. Vitamin K

Although rarely documented in animals, nonallergic factors have been known to contribute to the development of urticaria in man.

Such factors include:

A. Friction
B. Cold
C. Heat
D. Emotional stress

III. Clinical signs
   A. Urticaria (hives)
      1. Generalized erythema and wheal formation
      2. Appear as localized, raised, and edematous blotches
      3. May be pruritic
   B. Angioneurotic edema
      1. Dramatic swelling and edema (usually pitting) of lips, face, eyelids, and pinnae of ears
      2. Laryngeal edema and dyspnea are uncommon but potential sequelae.

IV. Diagnosis
   A. Typical history
      1. Acute onset, rapid progression
      2. Other systemic signs are rare.
      3. Known exposure to allergen is uncommon, but owner should be thoroughly questioned.
   B. Clinical signs

      Examine closely for evidence of insect bite or sting.

V. Treatment
   A. Remove or isolate cause.
      1. Withdraw offending medications.
      2. Limit exposure to insects and offensive food.
      3. Stop blood transfusion.
   B. Counteract allergic reaction.

      Regimen of therapy depends upon extent of clinical signs. (See Tables 6-2 and 6-4.)

      1. Dermatologic signs only
         a) Corticosteroids
            (1) Dexamethasone
            (2) Prednisolone
         b) Antihistamines

TABLE 6-2. PROTOCOL FOR ALLERGIC REACTIONS

1. Obtain quick, thorough history from owner.
2. Perform complete physical examination.
   a. Determine extent of clinical signs.
   b. Rule out respiratory involvement.
   c. Watch for evidence of inciting cause.
3. Remove or isolate cause.
4. Counteract allergic reaction.
   a. Dexamethasone 0.1–0.5 mg/kg IV or SQ q 4–8 h
   b. Prednisolone 0.1–0.25 mg/kg IM or PO q 4–8 h
   c. Hydrocortisone sodium succinate 8–20 mg/kg IV
   d. Prednisolone sodium succinate 11–25 mg/kg IV
   e. Diphenhydramine HCl 0.25–0.5 mg/kg IV or IM q 12 h
5. Maintain patent airway.
   a. Administer O_2.
   b. Perform tracheotomy for any upper airway obstruction.
6. Monitor for anaphylactic shock.
   a. Treat for shock as in Chapter 1.
   b. Epinephrine HCl
      i. Infiltrate site of exposure to allergen: 0.2–0.5 ml of 1:10,000 SQ
      ii. 0.5–1.5 ml of 1:1,000 IV
7. Monitor patient.
   a. Watch for progression of signs.
   b. Hospitalize if signs are progressive, facial involvement is dramatic, or respiratory signs are present.
8. Warn owner to avoid future contact with allergen.

---

(1) Diphenhydramine HC1
(2) Most effective within first several hours

2. Dermatologic and respiratory signs

   Immediate-acting corticosteroids should be used in addition to the above medications:

   a) Hydrocortisone sodium succinate
   b) Prednisolone sodium succinate

C. Maintain patent airway.

   If laryngeal edema develops:

   1. Administer O_2.
   2. Consider tracheotomy.

D. Monitor for anaphylaxis.

   Watch for signs of hypotension and circulatory shock,

dyspnea, restlessness, vomiting and diarrhea, seizures or collapse.

1. Administer corticosteroids as above.
2. Administer epinephrine HC1.
    a) Local infiltration
    b) Intravenous bolus
    c) See Table 6-2.
3. Treat for shock.

VI. Patient monitoring

A. Vital signs
B. Progression of clinical signs
C. Hospitalization for observation is recommended.
D. Warn owner to avoid further contact with suspicious allergens in the future.

ACUTE MOIST DERMATITIS

I. Definition

Acute moist dermatitis, often known as acute eczema or "hotspots," is an inflammatory skin disease characterized by denuding of the epithelium, erythema, extreme pruritis, and watery exudation followed by crustiness and matting of the hair. Acute moist dermatitis begins as a local irritation, but the self-trauma induced by licking, scratching, and biting soon overshadows the inciting cause and establishes a vicious cycle of continued irritation and inflammation. The lesions develop rapidly and may progress to involve large areas of the body within several hours.

II. Cause

The causes of acute moist dermatitis are innumerable. Any event producing localized pruritis, particularly in an area of the body that can be reached for licking or scratching, may incite this problem. The areas of the body that are involved may give some clue as to the origin of the problem:

A. Head and neck
    1. Cheilitis
    2. Otitis externa

        3. Ectoparasites
        4. Foreign bodies such as plant awns
    B. Trunk
        1. Ectoparasites
        2. Allergies such as urticaria and Arthus-like reactions
        3. Chemical irritants
        4. Bacterial hypersensitivity reactions
    C. Base of tail and perineum
        1. Ectoparasites
        2. Anal sacculitis
        3. Perivulvar dermatitis
    D. External genitalia
        1. Chemical irritation
        2. Perivulvar dermatitis
        3. Trauma

III. Clinical signs
    A. Classic appearance of lesion: localized, denuded, red exudative lesions which may be crusted and matted with hair.
    B. Extreme pruritis with persistent licking, biting, scratching
    C. Restlessness, anxiety
    D. Malaise, pyrexia may also develop.

IV. Diagnosis
    A. Suspicious history
        1. Sudden onset
        2. Rapid progression
        3. Worsened by self-trauma
        4. ± Seasonal occurrence
    B. Appearance of lesion
    C. Evidence of inciting cause
        1. Examine adjacent areas such as ears, lip folds, anal sacs, and vulva for underlying disease.
        2. Examine for fleas, ticks, lice.
        3. Perform skin scrapings.
        4. Consider biopsy with culture and sensitivity if lesions are generalized.

V. Treatment
   A. Objectives:
      1. Remove cause.
      2. Stop self-trauma.
      3. Provide relief from pruritis.
   B. Determine and remove cause of irritation.
      1. Perform thorough physical examination.
      2. Treat underlying medical problems such as otitis externa, anal sacculitis.
      3. Remove ectoparasites.
      4. Limit exposure to irritating chemicals.
      5. Remove foreign bodies.
   C. Stop cycle of self-trauma.
      1. Sedate if necessary.
      2. Apply Elizabethan collars.
   D. Treat the lesion and accompanying pruritis.
      1. Remove hair from affected area.
      2. Remove crusts with warm, wet compresses.
      3. Wash the site gently with warm water, mild soap.
      4. Begin medical therapy:
         a) Topical antibiotic/steroid ointments or creams
         b) Systemic corticosteroids
            (1) Dexamethasone 0.05–0.1 mg/kg SQ
            (2) Prednisone 0.1–0.4 mg/kg PO or IM BID-TID
            (3) Triamcinolone 0.01–0.04 mg/kg PO or IM BID-TID
         c) Systemic antibiotics (See Table 6-3.)

VI. Potential complications
   A. Systemic bacterial infection
      1. Malaise
      2. Pyrexia
      3. Lymphadenopathy
      4. Leukocytosis
   B. Infiltration of the lesions with fly larvae (maggots)
      1. Increased incidence in:
         a) Hot weather

TABLE 6-3. PROTOCOL FOR ACUTE MOIST DERMATITIS

1. Perform thorough physical examination.
2. Treat acute dermatitis lesion.
   a. Sedate or anesthetize if necessary.
   b. Clip away all hair from area.
   c. Remove crusts with warm, wet compresses.
   d. Wash gently with mild soap.
3. Start medical therapy.
   a. Systemic corticosteroids
   b. Systemic antibiotics
   c. Topical antibiotics, steroids
4. Prevent self-trauma.
   a. Sedation
   b. Elizabethan collars
5. Remove or treat underlying medical problems.

---

   b) Outside animals
   c) Untreated animals
2. May induce toxemia:
   a) Injection of mucous membranes
   b) Pyrexia
   c) Tachycardia
   d) Mental dullness
   e) Weakness, collapse
3. Remove maggots immediately.
   a) General anesthesia
   b) Chemical removal of maggots:
      (1) Hydrogen peroxide
      (2) Ether
   c) Debride necrotic tissue and establish drainage
4. Start supportive care.
   a) Intravenous or SQ fluid therapy
   b) Systemic antibiotics

BURNS

I. Definition

Thermal injuries and chemical burns in animals are not as rare as once suspected. Emergency clinicians may be

TABLE 6-4. COMMERCIAL PRODUCTS USED IN DERMATOLOGIC EMERGENCIES

Dexamethasone
  Azium, Schering, Kenilworth, NJ 07033
  Dexate-SP, Burns Biotec Laboratories, Omaha, NB 68103

Prednisolone—Prednisolone, Purepac Pharmaceutical, Elizabeth, NJ 07207

Hydrocortisone sodium succinate—Solu-Cortef, Upjohn, Kalamazoo, MI 44001

Prednisolone sodium succinate—Solu-Delta-Cortef, Upjohn, Kalamazoo, MI 44001

Diphenhydramine HCl—Benadryl, Parke-Davis, Morris Plains, NJ 07950

Epinephrine HCl—Adrenalin chloride solution, Parke-Davis, Morris Plains, NJ 07950

Triamcinolone—Vetalog, ER Squibb, Princeton, NJ 08540

Heparin—Heparin sodium injection, USP, Eli Lilly, Indianapolis, IN 46206

Tetanus toxoid—Jensal tetanus antitoxin, Jensen-Salsberg Laboratories, Kansas City, MO 64151

Furosemide—Lasix, American Hoechst, Somerville, NJ 08876

Morphine SO_4—Morphine sulfate Carpuject, Winthrop Laboratories, New York, NY 10016

Meperdine HCl—Demerol HCl, Winthrop Laboratories, New York, NY 10016

Pentazocine lactate—Talwin lactate, Winthrop Laboratories, New York, NY 10016

Aloe vera cream—Dermaide Aloe, Dermide Research, Chicago, IL 60611

Aloe vera tablets—Dermaide Aloe tablets, Dermide Research, Chicago, IL 60611

Silver sulfadiazine cream—Silvadene cream, Marion Laboratories, Kansas City, MO 64137

Mafenide—Sulfamylon cream, Winthrop Laboratories, New York, NY 10016

Chlorhexidine—Nolvosan, Fort Dodge Laboratories, Fort Dodge, IA 50501

Gentamicin sulfate—Garamycin cream, Schering, Kenilworth, NJ 07033

called upon to treat a wide variety of these problems from burnt footpads and electrical cord bites to exposure of skin to household chemicals. This section addresses both the pathophysiology and treatment of burns. For a further discussion of smoke inhalation and pulmonary edema following electrical shock, see Chapter 12.

II. Cause
   A. Thermal injuries
      1. Direct heat
         a) Stoves
         b) Radiators
         c) Heating pads
         d) Heat lamps
      2. Flame
         a) House and industrial fires
         b) Campfires
         c) Forest and brush fires
      3. Scalding
   B. Electrical burns
      1. Electrical cord exposure
      2. Lightning
   C. Chemical burns
      1. Acids
      2. Alkalai
      3. Solvents, petroleum distillates
         a) Turpentine
         b) Gasoline
         c) Kerosene
         d) Phenols
      4. Hot tar
      5. Miscellaneous household solutions

III. Classification

A system of categorizing burns as to their severity has been devised. The original system of classifying burns as first, second, or third degree has been changed to the following:

   A. Superficial

      Only the epidermis is affected. Transient erythema and desquamation of the epidermis occurs. The site is hyperesthetic.

   B. Partial thickness

      The depth of the burn extends to the mid-dermis. Loss of the epidermis is complete. Capillaries and venules in the dermis are dilated, congested, and exude plasma. The site is painful, but sensitivity is decreased.

C. Full thickness

The epidermis and dermis are essentially coagulated and nonviable. Severe edema of the subcutis develops from increased permeability of deep vessels. Dry gangrene of the damaged tissues occur, resulting in a dark-brown, leathery eschar. The site is insensitive.

IV. Clinical signs
- A. Thermal burns
  1. Superficial: hyperemia, desquamation, pain
  2. Partial thickness:
     - a) Denuding, exudation, pain, decreased sensitivity
     - b) Normal resistance of hair to pulling
  3. Full thickness:
     - a) Brown, leathery eschar
     - b) Subcutaneous edema
     - c) Little or no pain
     - d) Hair missing or epilates easily
- B. Electrical burns
  1. Well-circumscribed cold, bloodless, pale yellow lesion
  2. No pain
  3. Copper deposit may be present if caused by arcing of current
- C. Chemical burns
  1. Localized to generalized erythema
  2. Pruritis
  3. Pain
  4. Localized alopecia
  5. Denuding of skin secondary to self-trauma
- D. Signs of respiratory distress may arise from:
  1. Laryngeal edema
  2. Smoke inhalation
  3. Carbon monoxide poisoning
- E. With extensive or severe burns, signs of shock often develop.

V. Diagnosis
   A. History
   B. Physical examination
      1. Determine severity of burn.
      2. Determine extent of burn.

$$\frac{\text{Area burned (cm}^2\text{)} \times 100}{\text{Total body surface area (cm}^2\text{)}} = \%\ \text{burned}$$

Note: $1.0\ m^2 = 10{,}000\ cm^2$

$$\text{Surface area (m}^2\text{)} = 0.1 \times \text{body weight (kg)}^{2/3}$$

      3. Perform thorough physical examination. Determine involvement of other organs.
   C. Radiograph thorax for pulmonary injuries.

VI. Pathophysiology
   A. Local pathology
      1. Increased permeability of capillaries with transudation of body water and proteins
      2. Most rapid fluid loss occurs in first 6–8 h and may continue for 48–96 h.
      3. Venous and lymphatic thrombosis occurs.
      4. Interstitial edema develops.
   B. Fluid and electrolyte changes
      1. Fluid losses
         a) Occur rapidly from evaporation and sequestation of body water at site of burn.
         b) More than 50% of surface area involved will usually lead to death.
         c) Hypovolemic shock occurs if >15% of body is involved.
         d) Water loss within first few hours is severe (Davis):

$$\text{Water loss} = 1\ \text{ml/kg body} \times \%\ \text{area burned.}$$

         e) Hemoconcentration is commonly encountered soon after the burn.

2. Electrolyte shifts

   Burned cells lose potassium and gain sodium and water.

C. Hemogram

1. Red blood cells
   a) Widespread hemolysis leads to severe anemia with burns involving 25–45% of body.
   b) Initial hemoconcentration and high PCV is followed by anemia which may persist for 50–60 days.
2. White blood cells
   a) Marked leukocytosis occurs within 12 h and may persist for 10 days.
   b) Eosinophils decrease due to stress.

D. Cardiovascular system

1. Sympathoadrenal system releases epinephrine with subsequent constriction of arteries and rise in arterial BP.
2. Spleen contracts.
3. Heart rate increases and cardiac output may be normal initially.
4. With ensuing water loss and sequestration of body fluid, compensatory mechanisms fail and hypovolemic shock occurs (see Chapter 1).
5. Low-voltage electrical injuries may produce ventricular fibrillation with death from circulatory failure.

E. Respiratory system

1. The source of burn may directly injure the respiratory tract.
2. Pulmonary edema is a common sequela of electrical injuries.
3. High-voltage injuries may also cause respiratory and cardiac arrest.
4. The tendency for pulmonary capillaries to be the site of filtration of circulating debris, combined with massive amounts of fluid therapy, may pre-

dispose to acute respiratory distress syndrome (see Chapter 1).

5. Widespread fibrin embolization of pulmonary capillaries may lead to rapid death in cats with thermal burns.

F. Kidneys
   1. Reflex renal vasoconstriction may result in renal failure when accompanied by shock.
   2. Immediately following the burn, antidiuretic hormone (ADH) and aldosterone activity is high.

G. Liver
   1. Marked congestion, necrosis, and fatty infiltration may occur with severe burns.
   2. Impaired function of the reticuloendothelial cells with altered phagocytosis may promote septicemia.

H. Miscellaneous
   1. Ulceration of the duodenum is common with severe burns (Curling's ulcer).
   2. Widespread intravascular clotting and impaired thrombolytic mechanisms may lead to progressive thrombosis and may predispose to the development of DIC.

VII. Treatment of thermal burns

A. Therapeutic objectives:
   1. Maintain airway.
   2. Treat for shock.
   3. Combat fluid losses.
   4. Treat burn site.
   5. Combat systemic complications.
   6. Relieve pain.

   (See Table 6-5.)

B. Initial therapy
   1. Removal animal from exposure to heat.
      a) Douse any flames.
      b) Remove heat lamps and heating pads.
      c) Note circumstances associated with burn:

TABLE 6-5. PROTOCOL FOR USE IN BURNS

1. Remove animal from source of heat, smoke, or chemicals.
2. Perform initial examination.
3. Establish patent airway.
    a. O_2
    b. Intubate
    c. Tracheotomy
4. Treat hypovolemic shock if present.
    a. Multiple electrolyte solutions
    b. Corticosteroids
    c. ± Sodium bicarbonate
5. Collect samples of blood and urine for analysis.
6. Institute fluid therapy for losses following burn.
    a. Insert IV catheter.
    b. First 24 h
       Multiple electrolyte solutions alternated with 5% D/W
    c. Second 24 h
        i. Continue electrolyte and 5% D/W solutions.
        ii. Consider whole blood transfusion or plasma transfusions.
        iii. Withhold oral water.
7. Begin supportive therapy.
    a. Heparin
    b. Tetanus prophylaxis
    c. Analgesics
    d. ± Antibiotics
    e. Control ambient temperature.
    f. Consider furosemide, sodium sulfate for anuria.
8. Treat site of burn.
    a. Immerse or cover with ice or cold water.
    b. Remove hair and gently clean site.
        i. Sedate or anesthetize if stable.
        ii. Irrigate site with saline.
        iii. Wash with dilute povidone-iodine soap.
    c. Topical antibacterial ointments
        i. Aloe vera cream, tablets
        ii. Silver sulfadiazine cream
        iii. Mafenide cream
        iv. Silver nitrate solution
        v. Chlorhexidine solution
        vi. Gentamicin cream
    d. Subeschar infusion of antibiotics

(1) Quantity of smoke
(2) Exposure occurred in open vs closed space
(3) Type of materials involved in fire and liklihood of production of toxic fumes

2. Perform initial examination.
   a) Determine any exposure of respiratory tract to heat, fumes, or smoke.
   b) Examine extent and severity of burn.
   c) Look for signs of shock.
3. Establish a patent airway.
   a) Administer O_2.
   b) Intubate if animal collapsed or if laryngeal edema is developing.
   c) If intubation is not possible due to extensive airway burns and edema, perform a tracheostomy.
4. Treat for shock.
   a) Hypovolemic shock is likely to occur if more than 15% of body surface is burned.
   b) Fluid of choice is multiple electrolyte solution: 20–100 ml/kg in first 15–60 min.
   c) Consider administering short-acting glucocorticoids.
   d) Consider sodium bicarbonate supplementation if respirations are compromised.
   e) See protocol for shock, Chapter 1.
5. Draw laboratory samples.
   a) Complete blood count
   b) Serum electrolytes
   c) Blood gases
   d) Urinalysis
6. Combat fluid losses
   a) First 24 h

      For the first 24 h, hypovolemia with hemoconcentration and sodium loss is common. Isotonic crystalloid solutions are preferred during this period, especially if serum osmolality is high. Although fluid therapy in burn patients is undergoing considerable review in veterinary medicine, a formula appears below that has been proposed for use in animals:

(1) Alternate electrolyte and dextrose solutions:

i) Electrolyte solutions = body weight (kg) × % burn × 4 ml

ii) 5% D/W = 20–40 ml/kg

(2) Administer one-half total volume in first 8 h. Blood transfusions are contraindicated during this time. Blood given at this time is often extravasated at the burn site and leads to increased deposition of albumin at the burn site.

b) Second 24 h

(1) During this period of time, capillary integrity is often improved and proteins are better retained when administered intravascularly.
(2) Expansion of plasma volume with an attempt to minimize interstitial edema is a major goal.
(3) Decrease the electrolyte dose by one half.
(4) Continue initial dosage of 5% D/W to replace fluid lost from evaporation at burn site. Monitor CVP and urine output carefully.
(5) Consider whole blood transfusions if PCV and TS are decreasing.
(6) Consider plasma transfusions for protein loss only:

0.5 ml × body weight (kg) × % burn

(7) Withhold oral intake of water. Dramatic thirst may occur after the burn once the animal's body begins to detect changes in circulating blood volume. High intake of water during this time may induce vomiting with potential aspiration or cause water intoxication.

7. Other medical therapy
   a) Heparin
      (1) Heparinization may increase the effectiveness of repair mechanisms, decrease thrombosis and the development of gangrene, and protect against development of DIC.
      (2) Heparinization must be elected upon individual considerations.
      (3) The routine use of heparin in *all* patients is of questionable value.
      See Tables 6-4 and 6-6.
   b) Tetanus toxoid
      Tetanus prophylaxis should be considered

TABLE 6-6. COMMON DRUG DOSAGES USED IN BURN PATIENTS

Multiple electrolyte solutions For shock: 20–100 ml/kg IV First 24-h replacement: 4 ml × body weight (kg) × % burn Second 24-h replacement: 2 ml × body weight (kg) × % burn
5% D/W—20–40 ml/kg IV
Plasma transfusion—0.5 ml × body weight (kg) × % burn
Heparin—100–200 IU/kg IV for one to four doses
Tetanus toxin—test dose: 0.2 ml SQ, watch 30 min for signs of anaphylaxis, then give 30,000–100,000 U IV, IM
Furosemide—2–4 mg/kg IV, SQ
Morphine SO_4—0.2–0.5 mg/kg SQ, IM
Meperidine HCl—3–5 mg/kg IM
Pentazocine lactate—0.2–0.5 mg/kg IM

in all animals with burns involving more than 15–20% of the body.

c) Sodium sulfate solutions (Glauber's salts), furosemide:
   (1) Have been recommended to reestablish renal function if anuria occurs.
   (2) See protocol for ARF, Chapter 10.

d) Analgesics

   Consider use of narcotics in low doses.
   (1) Morphine
   (2) Meperdine HC1
   (3) Pentazocine lactate

e) Antibiotics

   Prophylactic antibiotics should be avoided. Studies in both animals and man have shown that use of systemic antibiotics do not often alter mortality rates. Antibiotics usage should be confined to severe burns complicated by septicemia.

f) Environmental temperature

   Improved survival has been noted when ambient temperatures are maintained at 24°C (75°F). Animals should be kept in a cool environment. Overheating within closed O_2 cages must be avoided.

C. Local treatment of burns
   1. Treat site with ice or cold water.
      a) Minimizes coagulation and extent of burn
      b) Decreases depth of burn by dissipating heat
      c) Relieves pain
      d) Helpful within a 2-h period following the burn
      e) Apply cold for 30–45 min, using compresses of water or ice within range of 3–17°C.
   2. Remove hair and gently clean site.
      a) Once the animal is stabilized it may be sedated or anesthetized.
      b) Clip hair from surface.
      c) Remove contaminated debris with saline ir-

rigation and gentle washing with povidone-iodine soap.

   d) Necrotic tissue, especially constrictive eschar lesions, is debrided.
   e) Escharotomy may be performed if circulatory constriction has occurred or excursions of the chest are impaired.

3. Apply topical antibacterial ointments.
   a) Topical antibacterials lower postburn mortality and significantly protect the animal from postburn sepsis.
   b) May be used alone without an overlying dressing (open method) or may be covered by sterile burn pads (closed method).
   c) The author would refer the reader to the Bibliography listed at the end of the chapter for a further discussion of topical long-term burn care, including debridement, types of dressings, and grafting procedures.
4. Several topical commercial products are available:
   a) Aloe vera cream
      (1) The topical application of juice from the Aloe vera plant has been a recognized treatment of burns for thousands of years.
      (2) Extract of Aloe vera juice has bactericidal and antiprostaglandin effects.
      (3) Apply at site to thickness of $\frac{1}{8}$–$\frac{1}{4}$ in. every 6 h for several days, then every 12–24 h.
      (4) Dermaide Aloe tablets are also available and may be administered every 6 h orally.
      (5) No toxicity
      (6) No pain on application
      (7) No staining
   b) Silver sulfadiazine cream
      (1) Water soluble

(2) Low toxicity, high safety margin
(3) Does not cause staining
(4) Is not painful upon application
(5) Apply twice daily for several days, then once daily.
(6) Does delay eschar separation
(7) When applied over large surface areas (>35%), may increase serum osmolality by absorption of propylene glycol

c) Mafenide 10% cream
(1) Apply to thickness of $\frac{1}{4}$–$\frac{1}{2}$ in. twice daily.
(2) Must be washed off completely once daily.
(3) Painful upon application
(4) Is a carbonic anhydrase inhibitor, therefore, may lead to metabolic acidosis if absorbed over large area.
(5) Bacteriostatic
(6) Good penetration of eschar
(7) Does not stain
(8) Sensitivity reactions have been known to occur.

d) Silver nitrate 0.5% solution
(1) Used to saturate wet dressings
(2) Wet dressings are changed every 12–24 h.
(3) Acquired resistance by bacteria to this agent is rare.
(4) Also fungicidal
(5) Low toxicity
(6) Causes black staining of site and nearby objects
(7) May cause electrolyte derangements
(8) Has an adverse effect on potential donor graft sites
(9) Causes delayed exchar separation
(10) Evaporation from bandages may inadvertently concentrate the silver nitrate

at the burn site, resulting in further tissue damage.

- e) Chlorhexidine 0.5% solution
  - (1) Used to saturate wet dressings
  - (2) Dressings are changed every 12–24 h
  - (3) Bacteriostatic
- f) Gentamicin sulfate 0.1% cream
  - (1) Rapid absorption through eschar
  - (2) Application is painless
  - (3) Especially active against Pseudomonas infections
  - (4) Expensive
  - (5) Reported to be ineffective in the presence of exudate
- g) Others
  - (1) Povidine-iodine cream

    When used over a large surface area, will result in very high serum iodine levels from absorption of iodine through the burn
  - (2) Nitrofurazone

    Widespread resistance of Pseudomonas to this medication has limited its use in recent years.

5. Subeschar antibiotic infusions
   - a) Allow concentration of antibiotics directly at site
   - b) Antibiotics should be chosen based on culture and sensitivity results.

D. Maintenance therapy

1. Days 3–14
   - a) Sodium and water reabsorption with diuresis occurs.
   - b) Hemodilution and hypoproteinemia are common.
   - c) Decrease fluid therapy and consider plasma transfusions.
2. Day 5 onward
   - a) Hypermetabolic state occurs due to increased

heat loss through evaporation, increased repair processes, and "resetting" of the hypothalamus.

b) Nutritional adjustments must be made:
   (1) High-caloric, high-nitrogen diet
   (2) Vitamin supplementation
   (3) Hyperalimentation for inappetant animals
   (4) Insert pharyngostomy and force-feed if unable to eat.

c) Consider anabolic steroids and whole blood transfusions for persistent anemia.

d) Hypermetabolic state may persist for several weeks to three months.

VIII. Treatment of electrical burns

A. Initial therapy
   1. Disconnect the patient from the electrical source.
   2. High-voltage injuries may cause respiratory and cardiac arrest. See protocol for cardiac arrest, Chapter 2.

B. Therapy of burn
   Similar to local treatment of thermal burn:
   1. Clip and clean site
   2. Topical antibacterials

C. Hospitalize for respiratory support
   1. Pulmonary edema frequently develops following electrical injuries.
   2. If pulmonary edema is not noted at the initial examination, close monitoring is still warranted because edema may develop up to 24–36 hours after the insult.

   See Table 6-7.

IX. Treatment of chemical burns

A. Initial therapy
   1. Remove animal from source.
   2. Attempt to remove offending chemical from surface of animal.
      a) Acids, alkalies, household solutions
         Wash thoroughly with water.

TABLE 6-7. PROTOCOL FOR USE IN ELECTRICAL AND CHEMICAL BURNS

1. Remove animal from source of burn.
2. Examine for cardiac or respiratory arrest and treat accordingly.
3. Maintain patent airway at all times.
4. Lavage site copiously if contaminated by chemicals.
5. Institute treatment for local burn
   a. Clip and clean site.
   b. Debride if necessary.
   c. Use specific antidotes to remove chemicals.
   d. Start topical antibacterials.
6. Contact National Animal Poison Control Center for specific information.
7. Monitor for pulmonary edema and chemical pneumonia.
8. Treat any systemic signs and prevent self-trauma.

b) Solvents, petroleum products
   (1) Avoid volatilization because fumes may cause pneumonia.
   (2) Wash with strong detergents:
      i) Ivory dishwashing liquid
      ii) Lux industrial detergent
   (3) If evaporation is occurring coat body with light oil, then wash with strong detergents.

c) Hot tar
   (1) Clip matted hair from site.
   (2) Coat the site with any ointment containing the emulsifying agent polyoxyethylene sorbitan.
      For example:
      i) Neosporin ointment
      ii) Other antibiotic ointments
      iii) Polysorbate ointment—Tween 80*
   (3) Wash this mixture away with soap and water.

* Manufactured by Sigma, St. Louis, Missouri.

3. Monitor respirations closely, especially following exposure to volatile chemicals.
4. Contact Animal Poison Control Center for specific information about antidotes and potential complications [(217) 333-3611].

B. Therapy of burn
1. Follow instructions for treatment of thermal burns.
2. Consider use of corticosteroids if pruritis occurs.
3. Prevent self-trauma.
   a) Elizabethan collar
   b) Sedation

X. Patient monitoring
A. First 24 h
1. Vital signs
2. Collect samples of blood and urine prior to fluid therapy for CBC, electrolyte assay and urinalysis.

Note: Hemolysis or hemoglobinuria usually denotes a severe, extensive burn.

3. Packed cell volume and TS
   a) Monitor every 4–6 h
   b) Adjust fluid therapy to maintain PCV $\leq$ 45–50%.
4. Monitor serum osmolality
   a) More accurate tool than PCV
   b) Measure with osmometer or calculate from following formula:

$$2\,(\text{Na} + \text{K mEq/L}) + \frac{\text{glucose mg\%}}{20} + \frac{\text{BUN mg\%}}{3}$$

Normal = 300 mOsm/kg

   c) If osmolality remains > 340 mOsm/kg, increase fluid therapy.
5. Urine output
   a) Is a fair estimate of circulating blood volume and adequacy of fluid therapy.
   b) Note presence of hemoglobinuria.

6. Excessive thirst or restlessness may indicate continued hemoconcentration with need for increased fluid therapy.
7. Serum potassium and sodium
    a) Hyperkalemia is common from hemolysis, tissue necrosis, and metabolic acidosis.
       Treat K^+ levels > 5.5 mEq/L—see protocol for ARF, Chapter 10.
    b) Sodium loss is initially dramatic and should be corrected with balanced electrolyte solutions.
8. Blood gas analysis may be helpful to monitor respiratory involvement.

B. Second 24 h
1. Vital signs
2. Packed-cell volume, TS
    a) Administer whole blood for anemia.
    b) Administer plasma for hypoproteinemia only.
    c) Adjust fluid therapy.
3. Serum osmolality
4. Urine output
5. Serum electrolytes
6. White blood count
    a) White blood cell count commonly increases to > 30,000/mm^3 within 12–24 h.
    b) Neutrophilic leukocytosis usually persists for 5–10 days.
    c) Eosinophils rapidly decline within the first several hours following the burn and usually begin to rise by the third day.
7. Blood urea nitrogen, creatinine
    a) Monitor closely for resolution of prerenal uremia that accompanies hypovolemic state.
    b) Monitor closely for evidence of renal failure.

C. Day 3 onward
1. Vital signs
2. Packed cell volume, TS—monitor daily.

3. Urine output
4. Serum electrolytes—monitor q 48–72 h.
5. White blood cell count
   a) Monitor q 24–72 h.
   b) If eosinophils do not begin to return by third day, prognosis is grave.
6. Blood urea nitrogen, creatinine—monitor q 24–48 h.
7. Body weight
   Causes of decreasing body weight:
   a) Fluid mobilization, improved urine output
   b) Insufficient nutritional intake with increased catabolism

XI. Complications
   A. Two major complications:
      1. Circulatory collapse and renal shutdown
      2. Burn sepsis
   B. Circulatory collapse and renal shutdown
      1. Are most likely to occur within the first 24–48 h following the burn.
      2. It is essential to maintain adequate fluid therapy with correct types of fluids.
      3. Monitor closely for oliguria, anuria, and elevations of BUN and creatinine.
   C. Burn sepsis
      1. Infection is the leading cause of death in those animals who survive the initial injury.
      2. The most common agents cultured from burn sites include Pseudomonas, Staphylococcus, Streptococcus, and Proteus. Candidiasis is also common.
      3. Prevention of burn sepsis is accomplished by:
         a) Early wound cleansing and closure.
         b) Topical antibiotics.
         c) Isolation of the patient in a clean and if possible, sterile environment.
         d) Maintenance of cleanliness at burn site.
         (e) Monitor body temperature and WBC closely.

(f) Note discharges and odors from burn site.
(g) Change dressings frequently using sterile technique.
(h) Institute systemic antibiotics if evidence of infection arises.

D. Other potential complications
1. Liver failure
2. Anemia
3. Pneumonia
4. Seizures
5. Reduction in immunocompetency
6. Wound contracture
7. Excessive scarring

BIBLIOGRAPHY

Alkjaersig N, Fletcher AP, Peden JC, Monafo WW: Fibrinogen catabolism in burned patients. J Trauma 20(2):154, 1980

Bellanti JR: Immunology. WB Saunders, Philadelphia, 1971

Cera LM, Heggers JP, Robson MC, Hagstrom WJ: The therapeutic efficacy of Aloe vera cream (Dermaide Aloe [R]) in thermal injuries: Two case reports. JAAHA 16(5):768, 1980

Davis LE: Thermal burns. p. 214. In Swaim RF (ed): Surgery of Traumatized Skin: Management and Reconstruction in the Dog and Cat. WB Saunders, Philadelphia, 1980

Demling RH, Buerstatte WR, Perea A: Management of hot tar burns. J Trauma 20(3):242, 1980

Farrow CS: Thermal injuries. p. 195. In Kirk RW (ed): Current Veterinary Therapy. Vol. 6. WB Saunders, Philadelphia, 1977

Halbach N: Treatment and management of major burns. Iowa St Univ Vet 41(3):120, 1979

Harris RL, Cottam GL, Johnston JM, Baxter CR: The pathogenesis of abnormal erythrocyte morphology in burns. J Trauma 21(1):13, 1981

Hummel RP (ed): Clinical Burn Therapy—A Management and Prevention Guide. John Wright PSG, Boston, 1982

Hunt JL, Sato R, Heck EL, Baxter CR: A critical evaluation of povidone-iodine absorption in thermally injured patients. J Trauma 20(2):127, 1980

Kulick MI, Lewis NS, Bausal V, Warpeha R: Hyperosmolality in the burn patient: analysis of an osmolal discrepancy. J Trauma 20(3):223, 1980

Leape LL: Kinetics of burn edema formation in primates. Ann Surg 176(2):223, 1972

Loegering DJ: Hemolysis following thermal injury and depression of reticuloendothelial system phagocytic function. J Trauma 21(2):130, 1981

McKeever PJ: Thermal injury. p. 191. In Kirk RW (ed): Current Veterinary Therapy. Vol. 7. WB Saunders, Philadelphia, 1980

McManus WF, Mason AD, Pruitt BA: Subeschar antibiotic infusion in the treatment of burn wound infection. J Trauma 20(12):1021, 1980

Morgan RJ, Jeevendra Martin JA, Philbin DM, et al: Water metabolism and antidiuretic hormone (ADH) response following thermal injury. J Trauma 20(6):468, 1980

Pilarezyk JP: Chemical burn and toxicity in a dog from misuse of flea dip. Canine Pract 6(6):51, 1979

Salisbury RE, Bevin AG, Steinkraus GE, Enterline DS: Burn wound sepsis: effect of delayed treatment with topical chemotherapy on survival. J Trauma 20(2):120, 1980

Swaim SF: Management of contaminated and infected wounds. p. 194. In Swaim SF (ed): Surgery of Traumatized Skin: Management and Reconstruction in the Dog and Cat. WB Saunders, Philadelphia, 1980

Swaim SF: Trauma to the skin and subcutaneous tissues of dogs and cats. Vet Clin N Am 10(3):599, 1980

Willemse A: Acquired cold urticaria in a dog. JAAHA 18(6):961, 1982

7

Gastrointestinal Emergencies

ORAL AND ESOPHAGEAL EMERGENCIES

I. Definition

The most common *oral emergencies* arise following trauma to the face and head or lodgment of foreign bodies within the mouth and pharynx. The most common *esophageal injuries* occur with the swallowing of foreign objects, bite wounds to the neck, or exposure to caustic chemicals. Acute inflammation or abscessation of the mouth, pharynx, or larynx may also cause symptoms severe enough for owners to seek emergency medical attention.

II. Classification

- A. Trauma
    1. Laceration of gingiva, lips, tongue
    2. Fractures of mandible, hard palate, teeth
    3. Bite wounds
- B. Foreign bodies
    1. Bones
    2. Sticks
    3. Fishhooks
    4. Needles
    5. Balls
    6. Porcupine quills
- C. Exposure to agents causing burns
    1. Chemicals
    2. Heat

3. Smoke
4. Electrical current

D. Acute inflammation, infection
1. Bacterial or viral tonsillitis, pharyngitis, laryngitis
2. Sublingual, pharyngeal, cervical abscessation

E. Tumors
1. May occasionally produce severe enough symptoms such as hemorrhage or gagging to warrant immediate attention.
2. Tongue, gingiva, tonsils, skull, and pharynx may be involved.

III. Clinical signs
A. Hemorrhage
B. Salivation
C. Pawing at mouth
D. Rubbing the face
E. Pain upon opening mouth
F. Repeated gagging and retching
G. Dysphagia
H. Regurgitation of solid foods, anorexia
I. Dyspnea
J. Hysteria
K. Lethargy, malaise

IV. Diagnosis
A. History
1. Known trauma to head, fall from height, or fight
2. Exposure to heat, caustic chemicals, or electrical cord
3. Suspected swallowing of objects

B. Physical examination
1. Perform examination of external structures with the animal awake.
2. Sedate or anesthetize for oral examination.
3. It is advisable to wear gloves for oral examination, especially in areas of endemic rabies infections, because this disease can produce similar symptoms.

C. Radiography
1. Of skull, soft tissues of neck, and thorax

2. To locate:
   a) Fractures
   b) Foreign bodies
   c) Soft tissue swelling

   If radiolucent esophageal foreign bodies are suspected, contrast media may be administered and radiographs repeated.

D. Endoscopy
   1. Larynx and upper respiratory tract
   2. Esophagus

E. Other
   1. Biopsy
   2. Culture and sensitivity

V. Treatment

A. Objectives:
   1. Prevent airway obstruction
   2. Control hemorrhage, combat shock
   3. Isolate and remove cause
   4. Relieve pain

B. Ensure a patent airway.
   1. Clean or suction away secretions.
   2. Intubate if animal is collapsed.
   3. Intubate if patency of the upper airway is threatened.

C. Insert IV cathether, treat shock.

   Stabilize animal before diagnostic procedures or anesthesia are performed. (See Table 7-1.)

D. Perform thorough physical examination.

   Note:
   1. Deformities of mouth and skull
   2. Wounds, lacerations to head and neck
   3. Cranial nerve abnormalities or dysfunction
   4. Ocular abnormalities
   5. Respirations
   6. Evidence of pain
   7. Consistency of oral secretions
   8. Presence of other systemic illness

E. Complete diagnostic procedures.

TABLE 7-1. PROTOCOL FOR ORAL AND ESOPHAGEAL EMERGENCIES

1. Ensure patent airway.
2. Treat shock.
3. Perform thorough physical examination.
4. Stabilize patient.
5. Complete diagnostic procedures.
   a. Radiography
   b. Examination of mouth under anesthesia
   c. Endoscopy of esophagus
6. Treat cause.
   a. Stop hemorrhage.
   b. Remove foreign bodies.
      i. Manual extraction
      ii. Retrieval via endoscope
      iii. Surgical removal
   c. Repair lacerations, wounds.
   d. Incise and drain abscesses.
   e. Remove tumors.
7. Start supportive care.
   a. Antibiotics
   b. Withhold food and water.
   c. Provide analgesia.
   d. Consider pharyngostomy.
   e. Decrease salivation.
   f. Administer fluid therapy and hyperalimentation as needed.

---

1. Radiography of head, neck, chest
2. Sedate or anesthetize for oral examination.
3. Examine esophagus with endoscopy.

F. Treat cause
1. Hemorrhage
   a) Apply direct pressure, cold.
   b) Ligate or cauterize arterial bleeding.
2. Foreign bodies
   a) Mouth
      (1) Manual removal
      (2) Surgical removal
   b) Esophagus
      (1) Three common sites of obstruction:
         i) Thoracic inlet

ii) Base of the heart
iii) Hiatus of the diaphragm
(2) If possible, retrieve foreign body via endoscope.
(3) If unable to retrieve object, attempt to push it into the stomach, then perform gastrotomy.
(4) Thoracotomy is reserved for objects that cannot be removed by any other means or when rupture of the thoracic esophagus has occurred.

c) String under tongue
(1) Apply gentle pressure to the string.
(2) If resistance is met or if physical findings suggest entrappment of the string within the intestines, an abdominal exploratory should be performed.

3. Wounds, lacerations
a) Mouth
(1) Clean and leave open small puncture wounds and lacerations.
(2) Suture extensive or through-and-through wounds of lips, gingiva, soft palate, and tongue.

b) Esophagus
(1) Most wounds involve the cervical esophagus because the thoracic portion is protected by the chest wall.
(2) Explore all wounds in the area of the esophagus.
(3) Repair any esophageal tears and establish good drainage.

4. Oral, esophageal burns
See Chapter 6.

5. Acute inflammation, infection
a) Incise and drain any abscesses.
b) Take cultures, biopsies.

6. Tumors

a) Surgical excision
b) Cryosurgical treatment
c) Fulguration via cautery
d) Hyperthermia
e) ± Radiation

G. Supportive care
1. Antibiotics
2. Withhold oral foods and fluids for 24–48 h, then begin soft, soothing foods.
3. Provide analgesia
a) Perforating wounds or foreign bodies of the esophagus with resulting mediastinitis can be extremely painful.
b) Consider use of the following analgesics:
(1) Morphine SO_4 0.2–0.5 mg/kg SQ, IM
(2) Meperidine HC1 3–5 mg/kg IM
(3) Pentazocine lactate 0.2–0.5 mg/kg IM
(4) See Table 7-2.
4. Perform pharyngostomy.

TABLE 7-2. COMMERCIAL PRODUCTS FOR USE IN GASTROINTESTINAL EMERGENCIES

Morphine SO_4—Morphine sulfate Carpuject, Winthrop Laboratories, New York, NY 10016

Meperidine HCl—Demerol HCl, Winthrop Laboratories, New York, NY 10016

Pentazocine lactate—Talwin lactate, Winthrop Laboratories, New York, NY 10016

Atropine—Atropine sulfate injection, Invenex Laboratories, Orlando, FL 32809

Glycopyrrolate—Robinul injection, A.H. Robins, Richmond, VA 23220

Pharyngostomy tube—Foley catheter by Argyle, Sherwood Medical, St. Louis, MO 63103

Gastrografin—E.R. Squibb, Princeton, NJ 08540

Peritoneal dialysis catheter—Stylocath, Abbott Laboratories, N. Chicago, IL 60064

Azostix—Ames Co. of Miles Laboratories, Elkhart, IN 46515

Ictotest—Ames Co. of Miles Laboratories, Elkhart, IN 46515

ACD bottle—Diamond Laboratories, Des Moines, IA 50304

Abbreviations: ACD, acid citrate dextrose.

a) May be needed for feeding animals while ruptures or wounds of the esophagus are healing
b) The tubing used should be soft and should terminate in the mid-thoracic region or just beyond the tear in the thoracic esophagus. This will help minimize irritation from the tube and reflux esophagitis.

5. Decrease salivation
   a) Salivation may be excessive with inflammation or wounds of the esophagus.
   b) Enzymes present in saliva may complicate existing inflammation and irritate the site of wound repair.
   c) Consider use of atropine or glycopyrrolate.
6. Fluid therapy

   If oral intake of food and fluids is prohibited for long periods of time, continuous IV fluid therapy and hyperalimentation may be needed.

VI. Potential complications
   A. Infection
      1. Soft tissue of mouth and neck
      2. Mediastinitis
      3. Occurs following contamination with bacteria and foreign debris
   B. Esophagitis
   C. Dehiscence of esophageal wounds
   D. Strictures of esophagus
      1. Commonly follow wounds or surgery of esophagus.
      2. May not develop for several weeks following the original injury.

BLUNT ABDOMINAL TRAUMA

I. Definition

Trauma to the abdomen is a common emergency in veterinary medicine. The injury may be nonpenetrating (blunt) or penetrating. Nonpenetrating injuries are often caused by automobile accidents, blunt blows, or falls. Penetrating injuries often occur with bites from other animals or wounds from projectiles. All penetrating wounds should be surgically explored. This section is confined to a further discussion of *blunt abdominal trauma*.

II. Types of organ injury
   A. Contusion
   B. Rupture
   C. Hematoma
   D. Avulsion of organ attachments

III. Clinical signs
   A. May range from mild to profound
   B. Wounds or contusions of abdominal wall
   C. Tire track marks on abdomen
   D. Abdominal pain—initial or delayed onset
   E. Abdominal wall deformity
   F. Anorexia, depression
   G. Vomiting, diarrhea
   H. Pyrexia
   I. Hematuria, dysuria, anuria
   J. Dyspnea
   K. Enlargement of abdomen with fluid
   L. Hypovolemic shock
   M. Weakness, collapse

IV. Pathophysiology

The clinical signs and eventual course following abdominal trauma closely correspond to three specific consequences that may arise following the injury:

   A. Hemorrhage
      1. The severity of bleeding is variable:
         a) Mild and clinically inapparent
         b) Severe with hypovolemic shock and abdominal distention
         c) Death prior to arrival at the hospital
      2. Sources of bleeding:
         a) Organs
            (1) Liver

(2) Spleen
(3) Kidney
b) Vessels
(1) Splenic artery and vein
(2) Renal artery and vein
(3) Mesenteric vessels
(4) Vena cava

B. Peritonitis
1. Develops with leakage of bile, intestinal contents, or urine into the abdomen.
2. May also arise with severe inflammation of the pancreas.
3. Common sequela of contaminated penetrating wounds

C. Uremia
1. Occurs with leakage of urine into the abdominal cavity and subsequent absorption of urinary waste products back into the circulation.
2. May also occur with inadequate renal filtration following kidney trauma or prolonged hypovolemia.

V. Diagnosis
A. History
1. Description of accident
2. Time of accident
3. Animal's behavior following injury

B. Physical examination
1. Inspection of external abdomen
2. Evaluation of axial and appendicular skeleton. Note deformities or fractures of spine and pelvis.
3. Assessment of respirations and lung sounds
4. Thorough abdominal palpation
Note:
a) Pain
b) Abdominal masses
c) Inability to palpate organs such as the bladder
d) Ballottement of free fluids
e) Ruptures of abdominal wall

5. Gentle rectal palpation
   Note:
   a) Fractures of pelvis
   b) Rectal tears
   c) Blood in rectum
6. Abdominal auscultation
   Continued absence of normal gut sounds is often indicative of intraabdominal injury.

C. Catheterization of bladder
   1. Perform if urinary signs are present, the bladder is not palpable, or fractures of floor of pelvis are found.
   2. Submit urinalysis.

D. Radiography
   1. Plain radiographs
      a) Abdomen
      b) Thorax—rule out diaphragmatic hernia
      c) Spine
      d) Pelvis
   2. Contrast radiography
      a) Will delineate specific injuries not seen on plain radiography
      b) Urinary tract
         (1) Positive contrast cystogram
         (2) Intravenous pyelogram
      c) Gastrointestinal tract
         Use soluble organic iodine solution—(Gastrografin) because it is less irritating to the abdominal cavity than barium sulfate.

E. Abdominal paracentesis
   1. To obtain evidence of intraabdominal injury and define organ involved
   2. Needle paracentesis
      a) Use 20- or 22-gauge needle and 12-cc syringe.
      b) Perform three to five aspirations.
      c) Begin at umbilicus.
      d) Attempt aspirations in all four quadrants.

e) Negative results may occur if only small amounts of free fluid are present.

3. Abdominal lavage
   a) Should be attempted if needle paracentesis is negative, but other signs are compatible with intraabdominal injury.
   b) Procedure for lavage:
      (1) Empty bladder
      (2) Clip and prepare sterilely the skin around the umbilicus.
      (3) Infiltrate area just caudal to umbilicus with local anesthetic.
      (4) Make small incision in the skin.
      (5) Insert peritoneal dialysis catheter into abdomen in a caudal direction (see Table 7-2).
      (6) Gently aspirate.
      (7) If no fluid is retrieved, infuse 10–20 ml/kg of saline into the abdomen.
      (8) Connect catheter via an extension tube to a vented bottle.
      (9) Place bottle on floor to allow gravity drainage.
      (10) Submit fluid retrieved for analysis.
   c) For good representation of the abdominal fluid, 20–30% of the infusate or at least 10 ml should be retrieved.

F. Analysis of abdominal fluid
   1. Packed cell volume

      Free-flowing, slowly clotting bloody fluid with a PCV approaching that of peripheral blood denotes significant and active organ or vessel bleeding. Lacerations of the spleen and liver are likely.
   2. Red blood cell count

      Repeated retrieval of abdominal fluid with RBC count >20,000/mm^3 in the face of suspicious clinical signs warrants surgical exploration (Hunt).

3. White blood cell count
    a) White blood cells will be increased in the abdominal fluid within 2 h following exposure to the peritonium with blood, urine, bile, feces, and pancreatic secretions.
    b) The WBC count will also rise within several hours following intestinal infarction or strangulation.
4. Blood urea nitrogen, creatinine
    a) If the BUN and creatinine of the abdominal fluid is greater than that of peripheral blood, urinary tract rupture has occurred.
    b) If laboratory analysis of BUN and creatinine is not available, a rough approximation of BUN is possible with the Azostix.
5. Amylase

    High amylase values often indicate pancreatic injury.
6. Bile
    a) Large amounts of bilirubin in the abdominal fluid occur with biliary tract leakage or high intestinal injuries.
    b) If laboratory analysis of bilirubin is not available a rough estimate of the presence of bile can be made with the Ictotest or with any urinary dipstick.
7. Sediment analysis

    Examine for bacteria, vegetable fiber, and other foreign debris.
8. Consider culturing fluid retrieved.

G. Other laboratory tests
1. Packed cell volume

    Is not initially an accurate assessment of blood loss due to splenic contraction (See Chapter 1).
2. Biochemical organ profile

    Note:
    a) Renal function tests
    b) Liver enzymes

c) Amylase, lipase
d) Electrolytes
e) Bilirubin levels
3. Urinalysis
4. Blood gases
5. Central venous pressure

VI. Treatment
A. Objectives:
1. Treat shock
2. Combat internal bleeding
3. Determine extent of intraabdominal injuries
4. Treat other life-threatening injuries
5. Determine need for surgery

B. Ensure a patent airway.

C. Insert IV catheter, treat shock.
1. Start rapid infusion of multiple electrolyte solution with dextrose: 40–90 ml/kg within first hour.
2. Administer corticosteroids for shock.

D. Draw laboratory samples.
1. Packed cell volume, TS
2. Complete blood count
3. Biochemical organ profile
4. Blood gases
5. Urinalysis

E. Perform abdominal paracentesis.
Especially if abdomen obviously distended with fluid.

F. Consider whole blood transfusion
1. See Table 7-3.
2. For active intraabdominal bleeding.
3. For rapid decline of PCV below 20% in dog and 12–15% in cat.
4. For failure to stabilize patient with bleeding despite large amounts of fluid therapy.
5. If time allows, cross-match or type blood before transfusion.
6. Autotransfusion may also be performed by collection of free abdominal blood into a vacuum bottle

TABLE 7-3. PROTOCOL FOR BLUNT ABDOMINAL TRAUMA

1. Ensure patent airway.
2. Insert IV catheter, combat shock.
3. Draw laboratory samples.
4. Perform initial abdominal centesis.
5. Combat intraabdominal hemorrhage.
   a. Continued fluid therapy
   b. Whole blood transfusion
      i. Stored blood: 20–40 ml/kg IV in first hour
      ii. Autotransfusion
6. Catheterize bladder.
   a. Urinalysis
   b. Monitor urine output.
7. Perform other tests.
   a. Plain radiography—abdomen, chest
   b. Contrast radiography
   c. Consider abdominal lavage
   d. Fluid analysis—compare with other laboratory tests
8. Supportive care
   a. Treat other injuries.
   b. Maintain body temperature.
   c. ± Antibiotics
9. Monitor for:
   a. Persistent abdominal pain
   b. Vomiting
   c. Renewed abdominal bleeding
   d. Progressive distention of abdomen
   e. Persistent absence of gut sounds
   f. Enlarging abdominal mass
   g. Decreased urine output
   h. Pyrexia
   i. Leukocytosis
10. Consider exploratory laparotomy.

of acid citrate dextrose (ACD) solution or into heparinized syringes via a peritoneal dialysis catheter and administration back to the animal IV.

G. Catheterize the bladder.

Note: The presence and flow of urine through a urinary catheter does not preclude rupture of the bladder. See Chapter 10.

H. Perform other diagnostic tests.
   1. Radiography of abdomen and chest
   2. Consider contrast radiography.
   3. Consider abdominal paracentesis.
   4. Consider abdominal lavage.
   5. Analyze any fluid retrieved.

I. Start supportive care.
   1. Continue fluid therapy.
   2. Maintain body temperature.
   3. Treat other injuries.
   4. ± Antiobiotics
   5. Supplement fluids with potassium and sodium bicarbonate as needed.

J. Consider exploratory laparatomy.
   Indications for surgery:
   1. Intraabdominal bleeding is not stabilized by fluid therapy and transfusions.
   2. Free gas is seen in the abdomen radiographically.
   3. Contrast radiography delineates a rupture of the intestine or urinary tract.
   4. Fluid containing urine, bile, or fecal material is retrieved from the abdomen.
   5. An enlarging abdominal mass can be palpated.
   6. A stabilized patient begins to deteriorate, that is, renewed intraabdominal bleeding, persistent vomiting, ileus, abdominal tenderness, and/or other signs of peritonitis develop.
   7. See Table 7-4 for types of abdominal injuries encountered and appropriate surgical procedures for their correction.

VII. Patient monitoring

A. Packed cell volume, TS
   1. Maintain PCV between:
      a) Dog—20 and 40%
      b) Cat—15 and 25%
   2. Monitor PCV every 2–4 h for first 8 h then every 6–8 h.
   3. Declining PCV and TS usually reflects active bleeding or overzealous fluid administration.

TABLE 7-4. BLUNT ABDOMINAL TRAUMA AND SURGICAL THERAPY

Organ	Type of Injuries	Corrective Procedures
Diaphragm	Tear, rupture	Suturing of defect
Liver	Fracture, laceration	Suturing of defect, closing of defect with omentum, or resection of isolated lesion or lobe
Gallbladder and bile ducts	Laceration, rupture, avulsion	Ligation of injured ducts, suturing of defects, removal of gallbladder, or anastomosis of gallbladder to intestine
Spleen	Hematoma, laceration, or rupture	Partial or total splenectomy
Pancreas	Crushing injury or hematoma	Partial pancreatectomy
Gastrointestinal tract	Hematoma, laceration, rupture, avulsion of mesenteric attachment, infarction, or incarceration	Suturing of defects, segmental resection, and anastomosis
Urinary tract	Hematoma, contusion, rupture, avulsion of renal blood vessels, obstruction	Repair of blood vessels, suturing of ruptures, nephrectomy, anastomosis of the ureter, catheterization, urethrostomy

B. Central venous pressure
   1. An accurate assessment of adequacy of fluid therapy and correction of shock
   2. Especially helpful in older animals with concurrent heart disease to detect overzealous fluid therapy
C. Peripheral white blood cell count
   1. Becomes elevated within several hours following exposure of the peritoneum to intestinal or urinary tract contents and bile.
   2. Leukocytosis is also common with traumatic pancreatitis.
D. Urine output
   1. Note quantity of output
   2. Note hematuria
E. Biochemical organ profile
   1. Blood urea nitrogen, creatinine—reflect urinary tract trauma, hypovolemia
   2. Liver enzymes, bilirubin—reflect trauma to liver, bile ducts, proximal intestine
   3. Amylase—reflects irritation, inflammation of pancreas, and is secondarily affected by renal function
   4. Electrolytes—watch for abnormalities of potassium, sodium, calcium.
F. Perform repeated examination of abdomen
   Monitor for:
   1. Pain
   2. Distention
   3. Enlarging mass
   4. Gut sounds
G. Monitor closely for vomiting
H. Body temperature

ACUTE ABDOMEN SYNDROME

I. Definition

The term "*acute abdomen*" is used to describe any problem in which severe abdominal pain is a prominent and persistent finding. One of the more difficult diagnostic challenges a veterinarian can face is to determine whether a patient with an acute abdomen has a medical or surgical problem.

II. Differential diagnosis
   A. Surgical causes
      1. Gastrointestinal:
         a) Obstruction
         b) Intussusception
         c) Linear foreign bodies
         d) Ulceration, rupture
         e) Incarceration
         f) Infarction
         g) Volvulus
      2. Splenic torsion
      3. Testicular torsion
      4. Pyometra, usually ruptured
      5. Ruptured bladder
      6. Ureteral calculi
      7. Hepatic abscess
      8. Prostatic abscess
      9. Penetrating abdominal wounds
      10. Ruptured abdominal neoplasia
      11. Generalized peritonitis
   B. Medical causes
      1. Pancreatitis
      2. Gastroenteritis:
         a) Bacterial
         b) Viral
         c) Hemorrhagic
         d) Toxin induced
      3. Acute nephritis
      4. Endometritis
      5. Prostatitis

III. Clinical signs
   A. Abdominal pain
   B. Anorexia
   C. Vomiting
   D. Diarrhea
   E. Dehydration

F. Lethargy, collapse
G. Pyrexia
H. Dysuria
I. Abdominal distention

IV. Diagnosis

The diagnostic workup of specific disorders that cause abdominal pain can be a very complex and difficult process. The emergency clinician should be certain that the animal is exhibiting intraabdominal pain, not pain that arises from lumbar spinal disorders or external abdominal muscle trauma. Utilizing the aids outlined below, information should be gathered and then carefully integrated and interpreted to achieve an accurate and specific diagnosis. Table 7-5 provides an algorithm which may be useful in reaching a diagnosis.

A. History
1. Attempt to localize the problem to a specific system based upon the history and clinical signs.
2. Age of the animal often affects the incidence of specific diseases.
   a) Common in young animals:
      (1) Intussusception
      (2) Ingestion of foreign materials
      (3) Viral gastroenteritis
   b) More common in older animals:
      (1) Testicular torsion
      (2) Abdominal neoplasia
      (3) Nephritis
      (4) Pyometra
3. Sexual status also affects the likelihood of certain disorders.
   a) Intact male: testicular, prostate disease
   b) Intact female:
      (1) Endometritis
      (2) Pyometra
      (3) Ovarian neoplasia
4. Determine exposure to trauma, toxins, and other ill animals.
5. Note suddenness of onset.

TABLE 7-5. DIFFERENTIAL DIAGNOSIS OF ACUTE

Clinical Signs	Physical Findings	Abdominal Radiography
I. Vomiting Diarrhea Abdominal pain	A. No abdominal mass palpable	1. Diffuse fluid or gas within intestines 2. Localized distention of duodenum with gas, angulation of duodenum, decreased contrast in area of pancreas 3. Abnormal localization of gas, persistent ileus, free gas within abdomen, generalized loss of contrast, bunching of intestines
	B. Mass palpable	1. Localized distention of intestines, radiopaque foreign body, bunching of intestines, mass which appears to be transient 2. Unable to visualize mass due to loss of contrast 3. Malpositioning of spleen with or without gastric distention
II. Dysuria Anuria Hematuria Abdominal pain	A. Bladder is not palpable	1. Poor delineation of bladder
	B. Enlarged prostate	1. Enlarged prostate, rest of abdomen appears normal 2. Enlarged prostate, localized decrease in abdominal contrast, loss of abdominal contrast
	C. Urinary tract organs palpable and may be normal	1. No radiographic abnormalities or radiopaque calculi seen 2. Enlargement or asymmetry of kidneys, malpositioning of kidneys
III. Abdominal pain only General malaise	A. Palpable mass	1. Uterine enlargement 2. Unidentified soft tissue mass
	B. Palpable fluid	1. Organs not discernible

ABDOMEN SYNDROME

Tentative Diagnosis	Further Diagnostic Confirmation
1. Acute gastroenteritis	1. Fecal analysis, serology, fecal culture, barium series
2. Acute pancreatitis	2. Serum amylase and lipase, lipemia
3. Intestinal Ulceration Rupture Infarction Linear foreign body	3. Contrast radiography with barium or Gastrografin, examine feces for occult blood
1. Intestinal Obstruction Intussusception Volvulus Linear foreign body	1. Contrast gastrointestinal radiography, exploratory laparotomy
2. Peritonitis Ruptured abdominal neoplasm Hepatic abscess	2. Consider contrast radiography, biochemical assays, exploratory laparotomy
3. Splenic torsion	3. CBC, barium study, exploratory laparotomy
1. Rupture of bladder	1. Positive contrast cystogram
1. Prostatitis	1. UA, urine culture, prostatic fluid analysis, contrast cystography
2. Prostatic abscess Prostatitis complicated by peritonitis	2. UA, urine culture, contrast cystography, exploratory laparatomy
1. Acute nephritis Ureteral calculi	1. UA, urine culture, biochemical profile, IVP
2. Hydronephrosis Renal trauma Renal neoplasia	2. UA, urine culture, biochemical profile, IVP, percutaneous biopsy
1. Pyometra	1. CBC, vaginal examination, exploratory laparotomy
2. Testicular torsion Ovarian neoplasia, granuloma Splenic neoplasia Lymphoid neoplasia	2. IVP, contrast cystogram, exploratory laparotomy
1. Ruptured bladder Peritonitis Ruptured ureter Ruptured abdominal neoplasm	1. Abdominal fluid analysis, CBC, UA, biochemical profile, exploratory laparotomy

B. Physical examination
   1. Perform thorough examination. Pay particular attention to:
      a) Signs of trauma
      b) Type of vomitus, diarrhea
      c) Presence of retained abdominal testis
      d) Presence of vaginal discharge
      e) Body temperature
      f) Note any hernias of body wall
      g) Presence of foreign body under tongue
      h) Size of prostate on rectal examination
   2. Attempt abdominal palpation.
      a) If possible, localize the pain to one area of the abdomen.
      b) Note presence, size, and consistency of hollow organs.
      c) Note position and contours of solid organs.
      d) Localize any masses.

C. Radiography of abdomen
   1. Plain radiography
      a) Detect, localize masses.
      b) Detect enlargement, abnormal position of organ (s).
      c) Note any loss of abdominal contrast.
         (1) Localized or isolated
         (2) Generalized
      d) Note abnormal gas patterns, free gas in abdomen, or emphysematous masses.
      e) Discern presence of radiopaque foreign bodies or calculi.
   2. Contrast radiography
      a) Aids in localizing and defining the specific abnormality.
      b) Intravenous pyelogram:
         (1) Renal trauma, rupture, hematoma, tumors
         (2) Pyelonephritis

    - (3) Hydronephrosis, ureteral obstruction
    - (4) Ureteral rupture
  - c) Double-contrast cystogram:
    - (1) Ruptured bladder
    - (2) Prostate disease
  - d) Barium sulfate or Gastrografin examination of gastrointestinal tract:
    - (1) Obstruction
    - (2) Masses, foreign bodies
    - (3) Volvulus
    - (4) Intussusception
    - (5) Rupture
    - (6) Displacement of spleen
    - (7) May not rule out severe irritation secondary to ingested toxins or acute gastroenteritis

D. Laboratory analysis

1. Complete blood count
   - a) Elevated WBC with a left shift is common in many of these disorders.
   - b) Low WBC frequently occurs with parvo and other viral diseases.
   - c) Nucleated red blood cells (nRBC) may occur with severe anemias, splenic disorders, and lead poisoning.
2. Biochemical organ profile
   May delineate evidence of:
   - a) Pancreatitis
   - b) Renal disease, azotemia
   - c) Liver disease
   - d) Electrolyte abnormalities accompanying gastrointestinal disease
3. Urinalysis, culture, and sensitivity
   Rule out:
   - a) Renal disease
   - b) Lower urinary tract disease
4. Fecal analysis

Determine presence of blood, foreign material, parasites, and WBC.

E. Others
   1. Abdominal paracentesis or lavage and fluid analysis
      a) See section on blunt abdominal trauma, above.
      b) Retrieval of fluid sample with WBC >1,000/mm^3 with toxic degeneration of neutrophils, is a serious finding and often warrants exploration of the abdomen (Crowe).
   2. Abdominal ultrasonography
   3. Serology
      a) For specific viral, bacterial, and parasitic diseases
      b) Results are often delayed, therefore, it has limited application to emergency situations.
   4. Laparoscopy

V. Treatment
   A. Objectives:
      1. Combat shock
      2. Start supportive care
      3. Determine cause
      4. Stabilize animal
      5. Prepare for surgery if necessary
   B. Insert large-gauge IV catheter.
      1. Treat for shock as necessary with large volumes of IV fluids.
      2. Consider use of corticosteroids.
      3. See Table 7-6.
   C. Draw laboratory samples.
      1. Complete blood count
      2. Biochemical organ profile
      3. Urine for analysis and culture
      4. Fecal analysis
      5. Blood gases
   D. Begin supportive care.

TABLE 7-6. PROTOCOL FOR ACUTE ABDOMEN SYNDROME

1. Insert IV catheter.
   a. Begin shock therapy:
      i. Multiple electrolyte solution ± dextrose
      ii. Normal saline
   b. ± Corticosteroids
2. Draw laboratory samples.
   a. CBC
   b. Biochemical profile
   c. UA, culture
   d. Examine feces
   e. Blood gases
3. Begin supportive care.
   a. Antibiotics
   b. Antiemetics
   c. Electrolyte supplementation
   d. Withhold oral liquids.
4. Determine cause.
   a. Plain radiography
   b. Contrast radiography
   c. Abdominal fluid analysis
5. Stabilize the animal.
   a. Correct shock.
   b. Continue fluid therapy.
   c. Correct electrolyte abnormalities.
   d. Return renal function to normal.
6. Prepare for surgery.

1. Antibiotics
2. Antiemetics
3. Electrolyte supplementation
   a) Sodium bicarbonate
   b) Potassium
   c) Calcium
4. Withhold all food and oral liquids.

E. Continue diagnostic workup.
1. Plain radiography
2. Contrast radiography
3. Abdominal fluid analysis

F. Stabilize patient.
   Continue fluid therapy:
   1. Correct shock.
   2. Provide for losses.
   3. Begin maintenance requirements.
   4. Correct electrolyte abnormalities.
   5. Correct hypoglycemia if present.
   6. Correct uremia, return renal function to normal.

G. Prepare for surgery.
   Indications for surgery include:
   1. Correct/relieve surgical problem.
   2. Determine etiology of generalized peritonitis.
   3. Diagnostic tests do not allow an accurate diagnosis to be made and the animal fails to respond to supportive therapy.
   4. Deterioration of a medical problem to a surgical one.

H. Continue medical therapy of nonsurgical causes of acute abdomen.

VI. Patient monitoring

A. Monitor shock therapy with measurements of:
   1. Packed cell volume, TS
   2. Central venous pressure
   3. Blood pressure
   4. Heart and pulse rate

B. Common electrolyte abnormalities include:
   1. Gastrointestinal disease
      a) Hypokalemia
      b) Total body depletion of sodium, chloride
      c) Metabolic acidosis
   2. Urogenital disease
      a) Hyperkalemia
      b) Metabolic acidosis
      c) Hyperphosphatemia
   3. Pancreatitis
      a) Hypokalemia
      b) Hypocalcemia
      c) Hyper- or hypoglycemia may occur

C. Blood urea nitrogen, creatinine
D. Urine output
E. Body temperature
F. Abdominal pain, distention
G. Persistence of vomiting, diarrhea

HERNIAS

I. Definition

A *hernia* is the protrusion of an organ or part of an organ through an abnormal opening. Traumatic diaphragmatic and body wall hernias are the most common hernias presented for emergency therapy in animals. Acute incarceration of abdominal organs within long-standing umbilical, perineal, or inguinal hernias may also require emergency surgical correction.

II. Cause

A. Diaphragmatic hernia

1. Trauma

A forceful blow (automobile accident, fall, blunt blow) causes increased pressure against a tense abdomen. If the glottis is open, there is no equalizing pressure on the thoracic side of the diaphragm and a rupture occurs. Penetrating wounds rarely result in diaphragmatic tears. Most tears occur within the muscular portion of the diaphragm and are ventral to the esophageal hiatus.

2. Congenital malformation

Developmental abnormalities may result in incomplete closure of the diaphragm and persistent connection of the abdomen with the thorax and/or pericardial sac. Rarely do these types of hernias require emergency attention.

B. Body wall hernias

1. Dog fights
2. Penetrating wounds from impalement on sharp objects
3. Automobile accidents

C. Incarceration within a hernia
    1. Increase in intraabdominal contents, such as during pregnancy, with progressive enlargement of the gravid uterus
    2. Increased intraabdominal pressure secondary to stranguria or tenesmus
    3. Idiopathic, in which an exact causal factor cannot be determined.

III. Clinical signs
  A. Diaphragmatic hernia
    1. Traumatic
      a) Signs vary depending upon the size of the tear and the amount of abdominal organs displaced into the chest.
      b) Polypnea
      c) Orthopnea, dyspnea
      d) ± Cyanosis
      e) ± Cough
      f) Exercise intolerance
      g) Muffled heart and lung sounds with dull percussion on the affected side of the chest
      h) Audible gut sounds within the chest
      i) Conspicuous absence of abdominal organs with abdominal palpation
      j) Collapse, shock
    2. Congenital
      Many are clinically silent and are incidentally discovered.
  B. Body wall hernias
    1. Contusion, wound to abdominal wall
    2. Palpable fluctuant, sometimes reducible SQ swelling
    3. Palpable hole in abdominal wall (skin may be open or closed)
    4. ± Abdominal organs palpable beneath skin
    5. Other systemic signs may occur depending upon organ involved in hernia:
      a) Intestines, pancreas:

(1) Vomiting, diarrhea
(2) Anorexia
b) Bladder, kidney:
(1) Hematuria
(2) Dysuria
(3) Anuria
6. Collapse, shock
C. Incarceration within hernia
1. Localized signs at site of hernia:
a) Pain
b) Swelling
c) Redness, discoloration of skin
2. Lethargy, malaise
3. Anorexia
4. ± Pyrexia
5. Other systemic signs may occur depending upon organ incarcerated, as discussed in section Body wall hernias, above.
6. Weakness, collapse, shock are rare, but may occur.

IV. Diagnosis
A. History
1. Evidence of trauma:
a) Dog fight
b) Automobile accident
c) High-rise fall
d) Blunt blow to abdomen
2. Knowledge of pregnancy or impending parturition
3. Recent dysuria, stranguria, diarrhea, or tenesmus
B. Physical examination
1. Perform thorough examination.
a) Auscultation and percussion of chest
b) Close scrutiny of abdominal wall, especially near contusions or wounds
d) Abdominal palpation
e) Rectal examination
C. Radiography
1. Diaphragmatic hernias
a) Plain radiography of chest and abdomen

Note:

(1) Alteration of the diaphragmatic outline

(2) Increased soft tissue density in chest and loss of cardiac silhouette

(3) Demonstration of loops of bowel within the chest

(4) Absence of abdominal viscera

If thoracic detail is obscurred by fluid within the chest, remove as much fluid as possible via thoracentesis and repeat the plain films.

b) Consider contrast radiography to confirm rupture of diaphragm:

(1) Barium swallow—outlines displacement of gastrointestinal tract

(2) Pneumoperitoneography—helps delineate small tears in the diaphragm

2. Body wall hernias

a) Plain radiography

(1) Will help to differentiate subcutaneous hematomas and emphysema from true hernias.

(2) Gas-filled loops of bowel, gravid uterus may be seen.

b) Contrast radiography

Positive contrast cystogram is helpful in locating bladder if it is suspected of being trapped within the hernia.

V. Treatment

A. Objectives:

1. Combat shock.
2. Relieve other life threatening injuries.
3. Stabilize the animal.
4. Prepare for surgery.
5. See Table 7-7.

B. Insert IV catheter.

Begin rapid fluid therapy, ± glucocorticoids.

C. Assess other injuries.

1. Ensure patent airway.

TABLE 7-7. PROTOCOL FOR THE TREATMENT OF HERNIAS

1. Ensure patent airway, administer O_2.
2. Insert IV catheter.
   Begin fluid therapy for shock.
3. Assess other injuries.
   a. Handle carefully.
   b. Control any hemorrhage.
   c. Perform thorough examination.
   d. Wrap open thoracic or abdominal wounds.
   e. Record ECG.
4. Begin supportive care.
   a. Continued fluid therapy
   b. O_2
   c. ± Bicarbonate
   d. Antibiotics
   e. Antiarrhythmic medications
   f. Remove free thoracic fluid and air.
5. Attempt manual reduction of body wall hernia.
   Empty bladder.
6. Perform diagnostic tests.
   a. Draw laboratory samples.
   b. Plain radiography—chest, abdomen
   c. ± Contrast radiography
7. Stabilize animal
   a. Delay surgery until animal is stable.
   b. Perform emergency surgery for persistent respiratory distress.

2. Handle gently. Reduced tidal volumes with diaphragmatic hernias leaves the animal extremely susceptible to stress.
3. Administer O_2.
4. Arrest any active hemorrhaging.
5. Wrap or bandage open thoracic or abdominal wounds.
6. Perform thorough physical examination.
7. Record ECG. Arrhythmias are common following thoracic and abdominal trauma.

D. Begin supportive care.
   1. Continue fluid therapy.
   2. Oxygen
   3. ± Sodium bicarbonate

4. Antibiotics for contaminated wounds
5. Antiarrhythmic drugs as needed
6. Remove free thoracic fluid via thoracentesis or indwelling chest tube.

E. Attempt manual reduction of body wall hernias.
   1. Apply belly wrap to prevent reherniation.
   2. Empty bladder before reducing hernia.
      a) Catheterize if possible.
      b) Perform cystocentesis if bladder is incarcerated in the hernia.

F. Diagnostic tests
   1. Draw laboratory samples.
      a) Complete blood count
      b) Blood gases
      c) Biochemical organ profile
      d) Urinalysis
   2. Plain radiography of chest, abdomen
   3. Consider contrast radiography.

G. Stabilize animal.
   1. Immediate surgical repair of most hernias is not desirable or necessary.
   2. It is preferrable to delay surgery until:
      a) The animal is hemodynamically stable.
      b) The extent of all other injuries are assessed and stabilized.
      c) All arrhythmias are under control.

H. Prepare for surgery.
   1. Diaphragmatic hernias
      a) Surgery should be performed immediately if respiratory distress cannot be relieved any other means.
      b) The need for emergency surgery warrants a guarded prognosis as the mortality rate under these circumstances is high.
      c) Withhold all food.
      d) Induction of anesthesia must be done very carefully. Positive pressure ventilation is begun immediately because the normal bellows action of

the diaphragm does not occur efficiently when it is torn.

e) Perform cranial midline abdominal approach.

2. Body wall hernias
   a) Withhold all food.
   b) Delay surgery until precipitating factors or complicating diseases are under control.

VI. Patient monitoring
   A. Monitor shock therapy with measurements of:
      1. Packed cell volume, TS
      2. Central venous pressure
      3. Heart, pulse rate
      4. Urine output
   B. Respiration, mucous membrane color
   C. Body temperature
   D. Abdominal pain
   E. Ability to void urine, bladder size
   F. Onset of vomiting, diarrhea

BIBLIOGRAPHY

Crane SW: Evaluation and management of abdominal trauma in the dog and cat. Vet Clin N Am 10(3):655, 1980

Crowe DT: Autotransfusion in the trauma patient. Vet Clin N Am 10(3):581, 1980

Crowe DT, Rawlings CA: The acute abdomen. Proceed Am Animal Hosp Assoc: 19, 1983

DeHoff WD, Greene RW, Greiner TP: Surgical Management of abdominal emergencies. Vet Clin N Am 2(2):301, 1972

Easley JC: Intestinal obstruction. p. 739. In Kirk RW (ed.): Current Veterinary Therapy. Vol. 6. WB Saunders, Philadelphia, 1974

Hunt CA: Diagnostic peritoneal paracentesis and lavage. Compend Contin Ed Pract Vet 2(6):449, 1980

Kleine LJ: Radiology of acute abdominal disorders in the dog and cat (Part I). Compend Contin Ed Pract Vet 1(7):520, 1979

Kleine LJ: Radiology of acute abdominal disorders in the dog and cat (Part II). Compend Contin Ed Pract Vet 1(8):614, 1979

Kleine LJ: Clinical and radiographic aspects of acute pancreatitis in the dog. Compend Contin Ed Pract Vet 2(4):295, 1980

Kolata RJ: Abdominal trauma. Compend Contin Ed Pract Vet 1(6):445, 1979

Lantz GC: The pathophysiology of acute mechanical small bowel obstruction. Compend Cont Ed Pract Vet 3(19):910, 1981

Lantz GC, Cantwell HD, Van Vleet JF, et al: Pharyngostomy tube induced esophagitis in the dog: an experimental study. JAAHA 19(2):207, 1983

Lipowitz AJ: Diagnosis of blunt abdominal trauma. Region I AAHA Symposium, November 1975

Morgan RV: Surgical emergencies. p. 239. In Tracy DL, Warren RG (eds.): Small Animal Surgical Nursing. CV Mosby, St. Louis, 1983

Mulnix JA, Severin GA: Medical emergencies of the digestive tract. Vet Clin N Am 2(2):293, 1972

Mulvany MH, Feinberg CK, Tilso DL: Clinical characterization of acute necrotizing pancreatitis. Compend Contin Ed Pract Vet 4(5):394, 1982

Root CR: Interpretation of abdominal survey radiographs. Vet Clin N Am 4(4):763, 1974

Strombeck DR: Small Animal Gastroenterology. Stonegate Publishing, Davis, CA, 1979

Toomey A, Bojrab MJ: Traumatic diaphragmatic hernias. Compend Contin Ed Pract Vet 2(2):866, 1980

Twedt DC, Grauer GF: Fluid therapy for gastrointestinal, pancreatic, and hepatic disorders. Vet Clin N Am 12(3):463, 1982

8

Acute Gastric Dilatation—Volvulus

I. Definition

Acute gastric dilatation (AGD) is a sudden and abnormal distention of the stomach with gas, fluid, or ingesta with impairment of gastric outflow. Gastric volvulus is the twisting of this distended stomach on its mesenteric axis with partial or complete occlusion of the esophagus. Acute gastric dilatation—volvulus complex is a very complex medical and surgical emergency associated with high morbidity and mortality. It occurs in many animal species and humans, but in veterinary medicine affects primarily large, deep-chested breeds of dogs, such as Great Danes, Irish setters, Saint Bernards, German shepherds, Doberman pinschers, Irish wolfhounds, and boxers.

II. Pathophysiology

- A. The etiology is not well understood and no causal agent has been determined. Factors that contribute to the development of AGD include:
  1. Ingestion of large amounts of processed cereal foods
  2. Ingestion of large quantities of water
  3. Active exercise after eating
  4. Stress may play a role
  5. Genetic factors are suspected
- B. Gas accumulation is necessary for dilatation to occur, and may develop from:
  1. Aerophagia
  2. Chemical diffusions from the bloodstream

3. Bacterial fermentation of carbohydrates
4. Gastric acid-bicarbonate reactions

C. Fluid accumulation in the distended stomach is attributed to:
   1. Ingesta
   2. Gastric, pancreatic, and small bowel secretions
   3. Transudate from venous occlusion

D. Proposed mechanisms of gastric outflow obstruction include:
   1. Lack of eructation may occur because antireflex mechanisms are anatomically exaggerated in deep-chested dogs.
   2. Mechanical obstruction of the pylorus is rare but may be seen with pyloric stenosis, neoplasia, or foreign material.
   3. Hypotonia of gastric and pyloric musculature may result from eating infrequent, large meals.
   4. This hypotonia coupled with failure of the pylorus to open after gastric contraction may explain the development of AGD in many dogs.
   5. With progressive dilatation the duodenum becomes compressed against the body wall, and this further occludes the gastric exit.
   6. Reflex inhibition of gastric motility and drugs that delay gastric emptying may contribute to AGD, especially following:
      a) General anesthesia
      b) Blunt abdominal trauma
      c) Prolonged recumbency
      d) Lengthy surgical procedures
      e) Spinal cord injuries

E. The basic sequence of events is similar in all cases of AGD, but the degree of severity may differ:
   1. Dilatation begins with an accumulation of gas and/or fluid in the stomach (Fig. 8-1).
   2. Normal means of relief such as vomiting, eructation, or pyloric emptying fail to take place.
   3. Continuous enlargement of the stomach and pas-

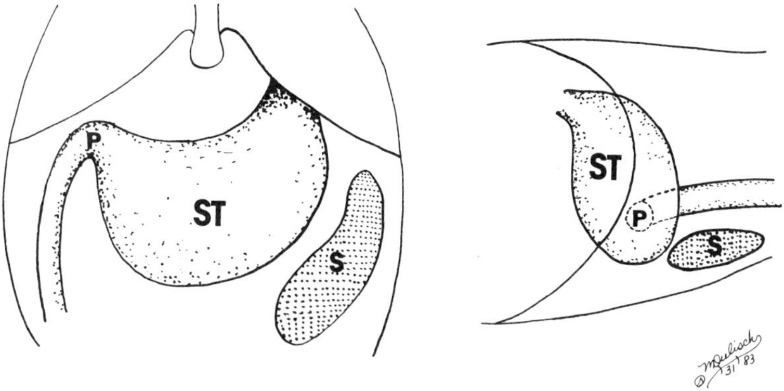

Fig. 8-1. The normal anatomic relationships of the pylorus (P) of the stomach (ST) and spleen as they appear on the ventrodorsal view (left) and the lateral view (right).

sive movement of the spleen allows the stomach to rotate on its axis (Fig. 8-2).

4. The spleen remains on the left side of the stomach and the duodenum is minimally displaced with a simple dilatation.

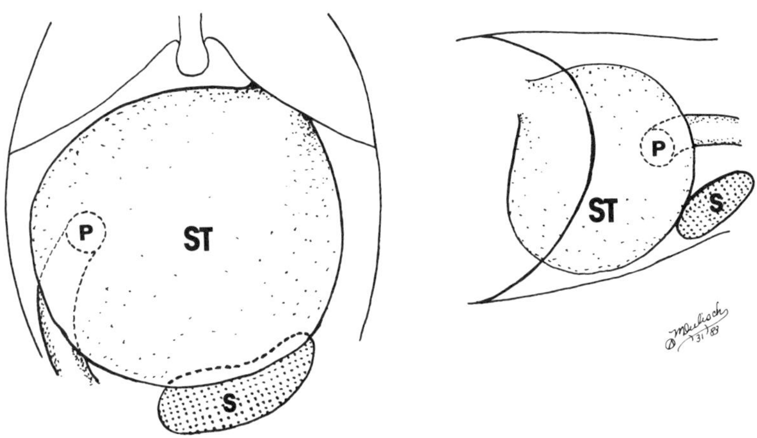

Fig. 8-2. The stomach (ST) has dilated and begun to rotate on its axis in a clockwise direction. The spleen (S) has moved ventrally and to the right. The pylorus (P) is now displaced cranially and ventrally.

5. During volvulus the esophagus acts as a "stem" and the stomach rotates 90–360° in a clockwise direction (viewed ventrodorsally). The spleen moves to the right and ventrally, coming to rest between the stomach and the liver or diaphragm (Fig. 8-3).
6. With volvulus the distal esophagus is twisted and compression of the duodenum entirely occludes the stomach.

III. Hemodynamic changes
   A. Normal venous return to the heart is decreased by:
      1. Compression of caudal vena cava
      2. Compression of portal veins by gastric distention
   B. Hypovolemic shock may occur with decreased:
      1. Central venous pressure
      2. Cardiac output and stroke volume
      3. Mean arterial pressure
   C. Multiple organ dysfunction develops from hypovolemia and vascular stasis with alterations in:
      1. Serum potassium, phosphorus

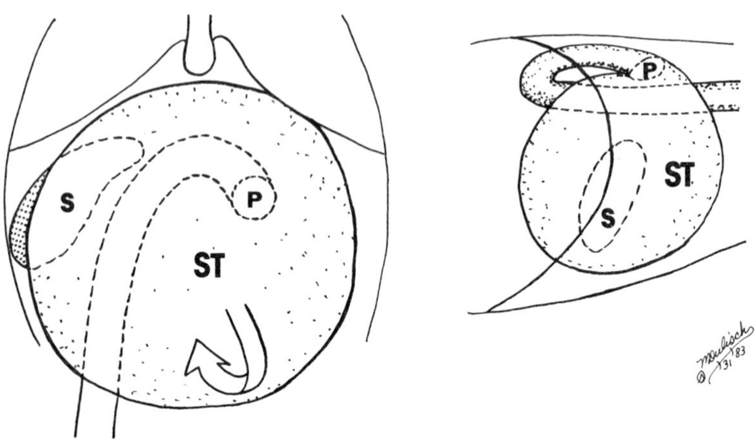

Fig. 8-3. A 270° volvulus of the stomach (ST). The pylorus (P) is now located dorsal to the stomach and to the left of the midline. The spleen (S) lies between the stomach and the liver and diaphragm.

2. Serum aspartate aminotransferase (SGOT)
3. Serum alanine aminotransferase (SGPT)
4. Serum lactic acid

D. Acid-base changes most commonly reveal metabolic acidosis, but metabolic alkalosis may also occur.
E. Hemoconcentration with sequestration of fluid in the stomach develops.
F. Microvascular changes result in endotoxemia and DIC.
G. Myocardial ischemia, hypoxia, and release of myocardial depressant factor from the hypoxic pancreas result in cardiac dysrhythmias.

IV. Clinical signs
   A. Distended, tympanic abdomen
   B. Excessive salivation
   C. Unsuccessful efforts to vomit and repeated retching
   D. Pallor, weak femoral pulses
   E. Dyspnea, cyanosis, mental dullness

V. Diagnosis
   A. Typical clinical signs and physical findings allow immediate recognition of a gastric dilatation.
   B. Gastric decompression and correction of shock should take precedence over all other diagnostic measures!
   C. Volvulus may be suspected with inability to pass a stomach tube.
   D. Perform radiography of abdomen when animal is stable. Routine views usually allow accurate assessment of rotation of the stomach (Figs. 8-2 and 8-3).
   E. Rarely, volvulus is diagnosed only at exploratory laparotomy.

VI. Treatment
   A. Objectives:
      1. Immediate decompression of stomach
      2. Correction of circulatory collapse
   B. Pass stomach tube.
      1. Measure a rigid stomach tube from the point of nose to xyphoid.
      2. Attempt to pass tube in a variety of positions.

3. Resistance met before entire length of tube is passed may be due to incorrect intubation of trachea or closure of cardia of stomach from volvulus.
4. Sedation to facilitate passage of the tube must be done with great caution (see Table 8-1).

TABLE 8-1. PROTOCOL FOR ACUTE GASTRIC DILATATION–VOLVULUS

1. Pass stomach tube
   a. First measure tube
   b. Sedation: meperidine HCl—0.5 mg/kg IM or fentanyl-droperidol—0.3–0.5 ml/55 kg IV
2. Insert IV catheter
   a. Rapid infusion: multiple electrolyte solution with 5% dextrose or saline and dextrose—80–100 ml/kg in 1–2 h
   b. Sodium bicarbonate
   c. Corticosteroids
   d. Oxygen
   e. See treatment protocol for shock
3. If unable to pass stomach tube
   a. Use 18-gauge needle trocars
   b. Temporary gastrostomy
   c. Temporary tube gastrostomy
4. Empty stomach and lavage with 3–6 L warm saline
5. Start supportive care
   a. Antibiotics
   b. Antiarrhythmic drugs
   c. Antacid-simethicone preparations
6. Radiograph when stable
7. Prevent recurrence while awaiting surgery
   a. Temporary gastrostomy
   b. Pharyngostomy
8. Prepare for surgery
   a. Anesthesia
      i. Preanesthetize with atropine
      ii. Fentanyl-droperidol—1 ml/15 kg diluted in 20 ml saline given IV slowly followed by gas anesthesia, ± succinylcholine choloride
      iii. Thiobarbiturate—slow IV administration followed by gas anesthesia
   b. Decompression, correction of volvulus
   c. Splenectomy if needed
   d. Preventive measure

5. Evacuate stomach, lavage with 3–6 L warm saline.
6. If surgery is needed but is to be delayed, insert pharyngostomy tube to prevent recurrence of dilatation.

C. Treat shock.
1. Insert large-gauge IV catheter in one or more veins.
2. Consider corticosteroids.
3. Administer O_2 for cyanosis and dyspnea.
4. Obtain blood samples for blood gas analysis and biochemical organ profile.

D. Inability to pass stomach tube
1. Trocharize stomach with several 18-gauge needles percutaneously to temporarily relieve gaseous distension.
2. Perform temporary gastrostomy:
   a) Clip and prepare right paracostal region.
   b) Anesthetize area with "L" block of locally infiltrated xylocaine.
   c) Incise skin over area of greatest distention.
   d) Bluntly dissect through abdominal musculature until stomach is exposed.
   e) Place two stay sutures into stomach at either end of incision.
   f) Suture stomach to skin with simple continuous pattern.
   g) Incise stomach wall, evacuate stomach contents, and lavage stomach.
   h) Oversew cut edges of stomach to control bleeding.
   i) This procedure is also useful to allow time for stabilizing patient in anticipation of surgery or referral to another hospital.
3. Perform temporary tube gastrostomy.
   a) Approach the stomach in the manner outlined in the above steps.

   b) Once the stomach has been opened and evacuated insert a 24- to 26-Fr Foley catheter in the stomach and anchor it in place with two pursestring sutures.
   c) Oversew the stomach for a short distance, creating a tunnel for the Foley catheter. This will prevent leakage of stomach contents into the abdomen.
   d) Allow the stomach to return to a free position in the abdomen.
   e) Suture the paracostal incision closed, anchoring the Foley catheter in the incision.

E. Start supportive care.
   1. Systemic antibiotics
   2. Antacid-simethicone preparations may be administered per os or via stomach tube.
   3. ± IV sodium bicarbonate
   4. ± IV potassium supplementation
   5. Antiarrhythmic drugs—ventricular dysrhythmias are common.

F. Attempt radiography—when patient is stable.

G. Prepare for surgery.
   1. Indications:
      a) When distention cannot be relieved by other means
      b) To examine stomach and spleen
      c) To determine presence of volvulus
      d) To reposition stomach
      e) To undertake preventative measures since the incidence of recurrent AGD is high
   2. Anesthesia must be undertaken with great care because these patients are rarely stable cardiovascularly.
      a) Narcotics or balance anesthetic regimens with muscle relaxants—for compromised patients
      b) Short-acting thiobarbiturate induction—for

stable animals only (barbiturates depress the myocardium)

c) Nitrous oxide increases gasesous distention and is contraindicated.

3. Close temporary gastrostomy.

H. Ventral midline celiotomy
   1. Decompress stomach if still distended.
   2. Reposition stomach—find pylorus near the cardia and elevate it with the right hand while depressing the fundus with the left hand.
   3. Examine and rerotate spleen.
   4. Perform splenectomy if necrotic or if circulation is compromised.
   5. Examine stomach for evidence of necrosis:
      a) Avulsion of vessels from greater curvature may necessitate partial gastrectomy.
      b) Areas that fail to become perfused with rerotation of the stomach may need resection.
      c) Mortality increases when partial or total gastrectomies are required.

I. Surgical prophylactic measures
   1. Remove any cause of outflow obstruction.
   2. Facilitate outflow with pylorplasty or pyloromyotomy as needed.
   3. Perform tube gastrostomy.
      a) A stab incision is made through the abdominal wall to the right of the ventral midline 4–5 cm caudal to the last rib.
      b) A 24- to 26-Fr Foley catheter is passed through the incision into the abdomen (see Table 8-2).
      c) The Foley catheter is then passed through several layers of greater omentum.
      d) A purse string suture is preplaced in the antrum of the stomach.
      e) The stomach wall is incised in the center of the purse string; the tip of the Foley catheter

TABLE 8-2. COMMERCIAL PRODUCTS USED IN ACUTE GASTRIC DILATATION

Antacids-simethicone preparations Mylanta, Stuart Pharmaceuticals, Wilmington, DE 19897 Gelusil-II, Parke-Davis, Morris Plains, NJ 07950
Foley catheter—Imex Foley catheter, Iminmed, New York, NY 10016
Meperidine HCl—Demerol, Winthrop Laboratories, New York, NY 10016
Fentanyl-droperidol—Innovar-Vet, Pitman-Moore, Washington Crossing, NJ 08560
Succinylcholine chloride—Sucostrin, ER Squibb, Princeton, NJ 08540
Lidocaine—Xylocaine, Astra Pharmaceutical Products, Worcester, MA 01606
Procainamide—Pronestyl, ER Squibb, Princeton, NJ 08540

is inserted into the stomach and the bulb is inflated with 5 cc of air.

f) The stomach is oversewn around the Foley catheter, creating a tunnel-like effect.
g) The stomach is drawn to the body wall by traction on the catheter.
h) A gastropexy is completed by suturing stomach wall to body wall adjacent to the tube.
i) The gastrostomy tube is secured to the body wall with tacking sutures and a body bandage is applied.
j) The tube is left in place for 5–7 days allowing a gastric fistula to form which will enhance adhesion formation.
k) Decompression of the stomach can also be accomplished via the gastrostomy tube if dilatation recurs.
l) The tube is removed by deflating the retaining bulb; the secondary fistula is treated as an open wound.

4. Lavage abdomen with saline.
5. Consider installation of antibiotics in abdomen if contaminated with ingesta.
6. Close abdomen in routine fashion.

Note: Many surgical techniques have been described and performed as prophylactic measures. No single technique has been found to completely prevent recurrence of dilatation or volvulus. In the author's experience the tube gastrostomy has provided the most consistent and most prolonged means of fixing the stomach to the body wall and provides a mechanism for allowing easy postoperative evacuation of the stomach when needed. A relatively new procedure described as the rib gastropexy technique (see Fallah, Bibliography) is currently becoming popular and will need some long-term evaluation.

VII. Postoperative care
  A. Three major complications are common:
    1. Circulatory collapse or hemodynamic abnormalities

TABLE 8-3. POSTOPERATIVE CARE FOR ACUTE GASTRIC DILATATION

1. Fluid therapy—multiple electrolyte solution or 5% D/W IV—5 to 10 ml/kg q6–8h
2. Monitor
   a. Mucous membrane color and CRT
   b. PCV, CVP, urine output
   c. Electrolytes, blood gases
   d. ECG
3. Treat ventricular arrhythmias
   a. Lidocaine—2 mg/kg IV bolus; or 1 g in 500 ml 5% D/W drip
   b. Procainamide—500 mg in 500 ml 5% D/W drip at 3–25 ml/min, 6–20 mg/kg IM q4–6h, or 6–20 mg/kg PO q8–12h
4. Prevent recurrent gastric distention
   a. Measure abdominal girth
   b. Suction gastric tube q3–4h for 3–4 days
   c. Nothing PO for 1–2 days
5. Oral intake
   a. Start water on day 2 or 3
   b. Start gruel on day 3 or 4
   c. Decrease suction of gastric tube on day 3 or 4
   d. Start solid food on day 4–6
   e. Remove gastric tube on day 7–10

2. Ventricular arrhythmias
3. Recurrent gastric distention

(See Table 8-3.)

B. Fluid therapy is continued until the patient is able to retain liquids and food.

Monitor:
1. Mucous membrane color and refill
2. Pulse strength
3. Hematocrit (PCV)
4. Central venous pressure
5. Urine output
6. Serum electrolytes
7. Blood gases

C. Ventricular arrhythmias, particularly premature ventricular contractions (PVC), slow ventricular rhythms, paroxysmal ventricular tachycardia, and ventricular tachycardia are common within the first 48 h postoperatively.

Monitor:
1. Electrocardiogram
2. Heart rate versus pulse rate
3. Mucous membrane color and refill
4. Respirations

D. Isolated PVCs may require no treatment.

E. Paroxysmal or continuous ventricular tachycardia should be treated vigorously:
1. Lidocaine as an IV bolus may convert arrhythmia to normal sinus rhythm.
2. Lidocaine and procainamide as continuous IV infusions are good for long-term control of arrhythmias. (See protocol for ventricular arrhythmias in Chapter 2.)

F. Abdominal distention may recur within the first 2–3 days postoperatively.

Monitor:
1. Measure abdominal girth behind last rib with animal standing, every 3–4 h.
2. Consider suctioning of gastric tube (compensate

for the amount of fluid removed by increasing the amount of fluid therapy).

3. Keep animal NPO (nothing per os) for 48 h.

G. Introduce food slowly

1. Start water and/or gruel on day 2, 3, or 4. Decrease frequency of gastric suctioning.
2. Gastric motility usually begins to improve by day 3.
3. Start solid food on day 4–6
4. Remove gastric tube day 7–10.
5. Treat gastric fistula as an open wound until it granulates closed.

VIII. Prophylactic advice

Although there are no guaranteed measures that are certain to prevent recurrence of AGD, the owner should be educated to avoid situations that may predispose to bloat. The following are instructions that may be given to the owner:

A. Food

1. Avoid single, large meals; feed two to three small meals per day.
2. Avoid processed carbohydrate food; feed canned, meaty food.
3. Feed a variety of foods.
4. If the owner insists upon feeding it, soak all dry food with warm water for 20 min prior to feeding.

B. Water

Avoid the intake of large quantities of water at a single time.

C. Exercise

Avoid exercise for 1 h after animal has eaten.

D. Symptomatic therapy

With onset of excessive eructation or signs of colic, 4-8 oz of an antacid-simethicone preparation may be given orally.

E. Kennel manager or owners with numerous high-risk dogs may be taught to intubate the stomach with a commercial stomach tube or appropriately sized vinyl garden hose. These owners, particularly if they are some distance from a veterinarian, can be instructed to pass the tube at the first sign of bloat with the dog in a sitting position with the head extended. Immediately after initial decompression or if intubation cannot be achieved, veterinary attention should be sought.

F. Much research needs to be done to delineate the cause of AGD and a means of preventing it. Emergency clinicans should make every attempt to keep abreast of new developments in the study of this disease.

BIBLIOGRAPHY

Andrews AH: A study of ten cases of gastric torsion in the bloodhound. Vet Rec 86:689, 1970

Berg P: Gastric torsion. p. 538. In Kirk RW (ed.): Current Veterinary Therapy. Vol. 4. WB Saunders, Philadelphia, 1971

Betts CW, Kneller SK, Rosin E: Recurring gastric volvulus in a dog. J Small Anim Pract 16:433, 1975

Betts CW, Wingfield WE, Greene RW: A retrospective study of gastric dilatation-torsion in the dog. J Small Anim Pract 15:727, 1974

Betts CW, Windfield WE, Rosin E: Permanent gastropexy as a prophylactic measure against gastric volvulus. JAAHA 12:177, 1976

Boothe HW, Ackerman N: Partial gastric torsion in two dogs. JAAHA 12:27, 1976

Caywood D, Teague HD, Jackson DA, et al: Gastric gas analysis in the canine gastric dilatation-volvulus syndromes. JAAHA 13:459, 1977

Christie TR, Smith CW: Gastropexy for prevention of recurrent gastric volvulus. JAAHA 12:173, 1976

Crane SW: Placement and maintenance of a temporary feeding tube gastrostomy in the dog and cat. Compend Contin Ed Pract Vet 2(10):770, 1980

Dann JR: Medical and surgical treatment of canine acute gastric-dilatation. JAAHA 12:17, 1976

Dingwall JS, Eger CE: Management of acute gastric dilatation with torsion and rupture: a case report. JAAHA 12:23, 1974

Fallah AM, Lumb WV, Nelson AW, et al: Circumcostal gastropexy in the dog—a preliminary study. Vet Surg 11(1):9, 1982

Funkquist B: Gastric torsion in the dog. Non-surgical reposition. J Small Anim Pract 10:507, 1969

Funkquist B, Garner L: Pathogenic and therapeutic aspects of torsion of the canine stomach. J Small Anim Pract 8:523, 1967

Kagan KG, Schaer M: Gastric dilatation and volvulus in a dog—a case justifying electrolyte and acid-base assessment. J Am Vet Med Assoc 182(7):703, 1983

Kneller SK: Radiographic interpretation of the gastric-dilatation-volvulus complex in the dog. JAAHA 12:154, 1976

Lees GE, Leighton RL, Hart R: Management of gastric dilatation-volvulus and disseminated intravascular coagulation in the dog. J Small Anim Pract 15:735, 1974

Merkley DF, Howard DR, Eyster GE, et al: Experimentally induced acute gastric dilatation in the dog: cardiopulmonary effects. JAAHA 12:143, 1976

Merkley DF, Howard DR, Eyster GE, et al: Experimentally induced acute gastric dilatation in the dog: clinicopathologic findings. JAAHA 12:149, 1976

Muir WW, Lipowitz AJ: Cardiac dysrhythmias associated with gastric dilatation-volvulus in the dog. J Am Vet Med Assoc 172(6):683, 1978

Parks JL, Green RW: Tube gastrostomy for the treatment of gastric volvulus. JAAHA 12:168, 1976

Pass, MA, Johnston DE: Treatment of gastric dilatation and torsion in the dog. Gastric decompression by gastrostomy under local analgesia. J Small Anim Pract 14:131, 1973

Pritchard D: Prevention of acute gastric dilatation by gastrojejunostomy. Canine Pract 1:51, 1977

Rawlings CA, Wingfield, WE, Betts CW: Shock therapy and anesthetic management in gastric dilatation-volvulus. JAAHA 12:158, 1976

Stockner PK: Acute gastric dilatation-volvulus: a breeder's point of view. JAAHA 12:134, 1976

Strombeck DR: Acute gastric dilatation-volvulus. p. 896. In Kirk RW (ed.): Current Veterinary Therapy. Vol. 7. WB Saunders, Philadelphia, 1980

Todoroff RJ: Gastric dilatation-volvulus. Compend Contin Ed Pract Vet 1(2):142, 1979

Van Kruningen HJ, Gregoire K, Meuten DJ: Acute gastric dilation: a review of comparative aspects, by species and a study in dogs and monkeys. JAAHA 10:294, 1974

Walshaw R, Johnston DE: Treatment of gastric dilatation-volvulus by gastric decompression and patient stabilization before major surgery. JAAHA 12:162, 1976

Wingfield WE, Betts CW, Greene RW: Operative techniques and recurrence rates associated with gastric volvulus in the dog. J Small Anim Pract 16:427, 1975

Wingfield WE, Betts CW, Rawlings CA: Pathophysiology associated with gastric dilatation-volvulus in the dog. JAAHA 12:136, 1976

Wingfield WE, Cornelius LM, DeYoung DW: Experimental acute gastric dilation and torsion in the dog. 1. Change in biochemical and acid-base parameters. J Small Anim Pract 15:41, 1974

Wingfield WE, Cornelius LM, DeYoung DW: Experimental acute gastric dilatation and torsion in the dog with venous angiographic alterations seen in gastric dilatation. J Small Anim Pract 15:55, 1974

Wingfield WE, Cornelius LM, DeYoung DW: Pathophysiology of the gastric dilatation-torsion complex in the dog. J Small Anim Pract 15:735, 1974

9

Endocrine and Metabolic Emergencies

DIABETIC KETOACIDOSIS

I. Definition

Diabetic ketoacidosis (DKA) is a metabolic state characterized by hyperglycemia, ketonemia, volume depletion, and metabolic acidosis. It most commonly results from alterations in carbohydrate, fat, and protein metabolism following prolonged insulin deficiency.

II. Pathophysiology

- A. Altered glucose metabolism with hyperglycemia
  1. Insulin
     - a) Potent regulator of anabolic reactions involving:
       - (1) Carbohydrates
       - (2) Fats
       - (3) Protein
       - (4) Nucleic acids

         (See Table 9-1.)
     - b) Required by most tissues for glucose uptake
     - c) Regulates gluconeogenesis in liver
     - d) Insulin deficiency results in decreased cellular uptake and utilization of glucose with subsequent hyperglycemia.
  2. Counter-regulatory hormones
     - a) Aid in counteracting hypoglycemia.
     - b) Include:
       - (1) Epinephrine

TABLE 9-1. METABOLIC EFFECTS OF INSULIN DEFICIENCY

Carbohydrates	
	Decreased uptake of glucose, especially in muscles and fat
	Loss of control of gluconeogenesis in liver
	Resultant hyperglycemia with osmotic diuresis
Protein	
	Catabolism of muscle as potential energy source
	Protein synthesis inhibited
	Resultant muscle wasting
Fat	
	Production of acetylcoenzyme A and ketone bodies as a potential energy source
	Regulation of lipolysis inhibited
	Resultant accumulation of ketone bodies with osmotic diuresis and acidosis

(2) Cortisols
(3) Growth hormone

c) Are often increased during DKA secondary to other physiologic changes.
d) Diabetic ketoacidosis patients often exhibit increased sensitivity to their effects.
e) Contribute to hyperglycemic state

B. Ketonemia
1. Insulin deficiency makes glucose unavailable as source of energy, therefore body turns to metabolism of protein and fats.
2. Ketoacids (acetoacetate, β-hydroxybutyrate) accumulate in plasma due to:
   a) Increased synthesis in liver
   b) Lack of normal insulin control of lipolysis
   c) Fixed utilization in peripheral tissues

C. Systemic effects
1. Hyperglycemia leads to osmotic diuresis with volume depletion and dehydration.
2. Accelerated ketogenesis leads to metabolic acidosis.
3. Circulatory collapse with shock, renal failure, coma, and death may result.

III. Clinical signs
   A. Suspicious history
      1. Polydipsia (PD), polyuria (PU)
      2. Weight loss despite polyphagia
      3. Rapid onset of cataracts
      4. Sex predisposition to diabetes mellitus:
         a) Female dogs
         b) Male cats
   B. Physical findings
      1. Vomiting
      2. Dehydration
      3. Weakness, collapse, mental dullness
      4. Kussmaul's respiration—rate and depth are increased
      5. Sweet acetone odor to breath
      6. Cataracts
      7. Hepatomegaly
      8. Muscle wasting
      9. ± Abdominal pain
   C. Accompanying or precipitating systemic disorders
      1. Obesity
      2. Infections
      3. Pyometra
      4. Acute pancreatitis
      5. Renal or cardiac disease
      6. Hyperadrenocorticism
      7. Exogenous steroid or progesterone therapy

IV. Diagnosis
   A. History
   B. Physical examination
   C. Laboratory tests
      1. Urinalysis
         a) Positive for glucose and ketones
         b) ± Evidence of infection
      2. Blood glucose >250 mg/dl with ketonemia
      3. Electrolytes
         a) Na^+

(1) May be normal or low
(2) Lowered by losses from vomiting and osmotic effects of hyperglycemia

b) K^+
(1) Initial plasma concentration is often high from metabolic acidosis.
(2) Total body stores are usually depleted.

c) PO_4^-
(1) Initial values may be low, normal, or high.
(2) Total body depletion is often severe.

d) Cl^-
May be low initially due to losses from vomiting.

4. Blood urea nitrogen, creatinine are usually elevated from decreased peripheral perfusion and dehydration or other systemic illnesses.
5. Blood gas analysis usually reflects metabolic acidosis.
6. Serum alkaline phosphatase (SAP) is elevated with fatty infiltration of liver or steroid hepatopathy.
7. Serum amylase and lipase are elevated with concurrent pancreatitis.
8. Serum osmolality is usually increased from osmolar effects of hyperglycemia, elevated BUN, and volume depletion.

V. Treatment

A. Primary objectives:
1. Return blood glucose to normal.
2. Correct dehydration and electrolyte abnormalities.
3. Correct acidosis.
4. Identify and treat concurrent diseases.

B. Perform thorough physical examination.
1. Estimate extent of dehydration.
2. Identify systemic illnesses.

C. Collect laboratory samples.
1. Draw blood.
2. Collect urine by cystocentesis or transient catheterization.

D. Fluid therapy
   1. Insert IV catheter.
   2. Begin rapid infusion of normal saline or multiple electrolyte solution.
   3. Calculate therapy needed to correct for shock, dehydration, and losses from vomiting and diarrhea:

      Replacement = % dehydration × body weight (kg) × 1 L plus losses

   4. Calculate maintenance requirements:

      Maintenance = 10–15 ml × body weight (kg)

   5. Maximum fluid administration rate in first hour is:
      a) Dog: 90 ml/kg
      b) Cat: 150 ml
   6. Try to replace or correct 80% of total need in first 24 h.

E. Insulin therapy
   1. Regular (crystalline) insulin is chosen:
      a) Rapid onset of action
      b) Short half-life
   2. Insulin protocols utilized during DKA are currently changing in veterinary medicine. Some clinicians believe that decreased peripheral perfusion and inherent insulin resistance at the peak of DKA necessitate high doses of IV insulin. Other clinicians support the use of low-dose IM insulin. Below are two different protocols which have been used successfully in animal patients. (See Table 9-2.)
   3. *Intravenous/subcutaneous insulin*
      a) With severe dehydration give 1–2 U/kg IV. With adequate peripheral perfusion give $\frac{1}{2}$ U/kg IV and $\frac{1}{2}$–1 U/kg SQ.
      b) Monitor blood glucose every 3 h. *Note:* glucose oxidase strips are useful to detect extreme variations in blood sugar (<50 mg/dl, >250 mg/dl),

TABLE 9-2. PROTOCOL FOR DIABETIC KETOACIDOSIS

1. Perform thorough physical examination.
2. Collect blood and urine samples.
3. Insert IV catheter.
   a. Fluids of choice: normal saline, or multiple electrolyte solution
   b. Rapid infusion—approximate need: 20 ml/kg IV q6h
      i. Correct dehydration and losses
      ii. Provide maintenance
4. Institute regular insulin.
   a. IV/SQ insulin protocol:
      i. Initial dose:
         Dog—1 U/kg IV
         Cat—0.5 U/kg IV
      ii. Monitor blood glucose q3h.
         If blood glucose > 250 mg/dl at 3 hours → repeat 1–2 U/kg insulin IV.
         If blood glucose < 250 mg/dl at 3 h → withhold insulin until blood glucose begins to rise again.
   b. Low-dose IM insulin protocol
      i. Initial dose:
         <10 Kg body weight—2 U IM
         >10 Kg body weight—0.25 U/kg IM
      ii. Monitor blood glucose q1h, repeat following dose until blood sugar < 250 mg/dl:
         <10 kg—1 U IM
         >10 kg—0.1 U/Kg IM
5. Start supportive care.
   a. Antibiotics
   b. KCl: add 30 mEq/L fluids; maximum infusion 0.5 mEq/kg/h
   c. Antiemetics
   d. Bicarbonate if needed
6. Patient monitoring
   a. Blood glucose
   b. Urine
      i. Amount of output
      ii. Presence of sugar, ketones q6–12h
   c. Hematocrit (PCV) and total solids q6–8h
   d. Electrolytes and BUN q4h until normal
   e. Blood gases
   f. CVP
   g. ECG
   h. Serum osmolality
7. Diagnose and treat concurrent diseases.

but are not very accurate in monitoring small changes in blood glucose levels.

(1) If at 3 h the glucose >250 mg/dl, then repeat 1–2 U/kg insulin IV.

(2) If at 3 h the glucose <250 mg/dl, then withhold insulin.

(3) If at 6 h the glucose remains >250 mg/dl, repeat 1–2 U/kg insulin IV.

(4) Insulin may be given SQ once dehydration is corrected.

c) *Caution:* Repeated administration of IV insulin and slow absorption of SQ insulin with delayed peak activity may result in hypoglycemia hours later.

4. *Low-dose intramuscular insulin*

a) Initial insulin dose

(1) <10 kg body weight—2U IM

(2) >10 kg body weight—0.25 U/kg IM

b) Monitor blood glucose hourly.

c) Until the blood sugar falls below 250 mg/dl repeat the following doses hourly:

(1) <10 kg body weight—1 U IM

(2) >10 kg body weight—0.1 U/kg IM

Usually the blood sugar falls below 250 mg/dl within 4 h.

d) Low-dose IM insulin is not known to cause delayed hypoglycemia but requires more frequent monitoring.

5. Replacement therapy with isophane or protamine zinc insulin is instituted when hyperglycemia and ketonemia are diminished, metabolic acidosis is corrected, and the patient is stable.

(See Table 9-3.)

F. Potassium supplementation

1. Hypokalemia tends to develop 2–4 hours after therapy is begun.

This occurs when potassium returns to the cells as acidosis is corrected.

TABLE 9-3. COMMERCIAL PRODUCTS USED IN DIABETIC KETOACIDOSIS

Regular insulin—Insulin injection USP, ER Squibb, Princeton, NJ 08540
Glucose oxidase strips
Chemstrips BG, Bio-Dyamics, Indianapolis, IN 46250
Dextrostix, Ames Division, Miles Laboratories, Elkhart, IN 46515
Isophane insulin—NPH insulin, ER Squibb, Princeton, NJ 08540
Protamine zinc insulin—PZI insulin, ER Squibb, Princeton, NJ 08540

2. Potassium supplementation should be started at the onset of therapy if the initial serum potassium is low or normal.
3. Potassium is otherwise begun 2–4 h into therapy or when serum glucose begins to fall.
   (See Table 9-2.)

G. Bicarbonate supplementation
   1. Metabolic acidosis is usually corrected with insulin and fluid therapy alone.
   2. Use only for persistent acidosis as demonstrated by blood gas analysis.
   3. Correct acidosis slowly over 24–48 h.
   4. Rapid bicarbonate supplementation may lead to CNS depression and stupor from paradoxical cerebrospinal fluid acidosis.

H. Supportive care
   1. Maintain normal body temperature with heat.
   2. Antibiotics
   3. Antiemetics

VI. Patient monitoring
   A. Blood glucose
      1. Monitor as outlined in Table 9-2.
      2. Try to keep blood sugar in range of 100–250 mg/dl.
      3. Blood glucose may decline rapidly following insulin therapy. Use IV infusion of 5% D/W as needed to maintain blood sugar ≥ 100 mg/dl.
   B. Urine output

1. Amount of output is useful in determining adequacy of fluid therapy.
2. Monitor urine sugar and ketones frequently.

C. Packed cell volume and TS

May be used to evaluate level of dehydration and response to fluid therapy.

D. Electrolytes
1. When laboratory analysis is unavailable the ECG can be used to crudely estimate presence of hyperkalemia.
2. Electrocardiographic changes with hyperkalemia:
   a) Spiked T waves
   b) Prolongation of P-R interval
   c) Prolongation QRS complex
   d) Depressed P waves
   e) Heart block
3. Electrocardiographic changes with hypokalemia:
   a) Small T waves
   b) ST segment depression
   c) Appearance of U waves

E. BUN, creatinine

F. Blood gases

G. Central venous pressure
1. Measurements of CVP allow an accurate assessment of fluid replacement.
2. Is an important tool for monitoring patients with concomitant cardiac disease.

H. Serum ketones

I. Serum osmolality
1. Stupor or coma may occur in hyperglycemic, nonketotic patients from severe hyperosmolality.
2. Signs referable to serum hypertonicity occur with osmolalities >375 mOsm/kg (normal = 300 mOsm/kg).
3. Failure of osmolality to return to normal with conventional fluid therapy necessitates institution of half-strength saline infusion.

J. Body temperature
   1. Body temperature initially may be low, especially if the animal is comatose.
   2. Because infections are common in diabetic patients, continue to monitor temperature throughout hospitalization.

ADRENAL CORTICAL INSUFFICIENCY

I. Definition

Adrenal cortical insufficiency or hypoadrenocorticism is a deficiency of aldosterone and/or glucocorticoids which results from dysfunction of the adrenal cortex. Anatomically and functionally the adrenal gland has three zones. The inner zone, the zona reticularis, secretes small amounts of glucocorticoids and sex hormones. The middle zone, the zona fasciculata, produces glucocorticoids. The outer zone, the zona glomerulosa, secretes the mineralocorticoids, particularly aldosterone. Although adrenal cortical insufficiency has not been found to arise with dysfunction of the zona reticularis alone, hypoadrenocorticism may develop with failure of either or both of the outer zones.

II. Causes of hypoadrenocorticism

A. Diseases or destruction of adrenal glands

Usually produce deficiency of both mineralocorticoids and glucocorticoids.

1. Idiopathic necrosis
   a) Most common cause in the dog
   b) May be immune mediated
   c) Involves all three zones of cortex
2. Systemic mycoses
3. Tuberculosis
4. Metastatic tumors
5. Canine distemper
6. Hemorrhagic infarction
7. Amyloidosis

8. O, p-DDD therapy (Lysodren)
   a) Produces selective deficiency of glucocorticoids from destruction of the zona fasciculata.
   b) Used in the medical therapy of hyperadrenocorticism

B. Decreased corticotropin secretion
   1. Hypothalamic lesions

      Cause decreased secretion of corticotropin releasing factor (CRF) which in turn causes decreased release of ACTH.
   2. Pituitary lesions
      a) Result in decreased secretion of ACTH. Adrenocorticotropic hormone stimulates the adrenal cortex to produce glucocorticoids.
      b) Examples of pituitary lesions:
         (1) Infection
         (2) Degenerative diseases
         (3) Tumors
   3. Exogenous corticosteroid therapy
      a) Produces a decrease in ACTH secretion from prolonged negative feedback.

      Note: Because mineralocorticoid (aldosterone) secretion is independent of corticotropin, disorders of ACTH secretion selectively cause glucocorticoid deficiencies.

III. Pathophysiology
   A. Glucocorticoids
      1. Function:
         a) Stimulate gluconeogenesis
         b) Mobilize fat from adipose tissue
         c) Enhance extravascular fluid movement to the vascular compartment
         d) Stabilize lysosomal enzymes
         e) Counteract the effects of stress
      2. Deficiency results in:
         a) Impaired water excretion through the kidneys
         b) Impaired energy metabolism

- c) Diminished stress tolerance
- d) Electrolyte abnormalities are rare.

B. Aldosterone

1. The major effects of this hormone occur in the distal renal tubules.
2. Function:
   - a) Stimulates absorption of Na^+
   - b) Facilitates excretion of K^+
   - c) Secondarily increases chloride and water absorption
3. Deficiency results in:
   - a) Hyponatremia
     - (1) Concomitant renal water loss
     - (2) Lethargy, nausea
     - (3) Impaired cardiac output
     - (4) Poor renal perfusion
     - (5) Hypotension, hypovolemia
   - b) Hyperkalemia
     - (1) Muscle weakness
     - (2) Decreased cardiac conduction
     - (3) Decreased cardiac excitability

IV. Clinical signs

- A. Anorexia
- B. Vomiting, diarrhea
- C. Lethargy, muscle weakness
- D. Dehydration
- E. Bradycardia even in the face of hypotension
- F. Intolerance to stress

V. Diagnosis

- A. History, clinical signs
- B. Physical examination
- C. Laboratory analysis
  1. Hypoaldosteronism
     - a) Na^+ often <135 mEq/L
     - b) K^+ often >5.5 mEq/L
     - c) Na/K ratio $<25:1$
       (normal Na/K ratio $= 33:1$)

2. Glucocorticoid deficiency
    a) Resting plasma cortisol usually <10 ng/ml
    b) Plasma cortisols do not respond to exogenous ACTH, that is, there is little or no change in cortisol 2 h following IM injection of 0.5 U/kg ACTH

       Note: Replacement glucocorticoid therapy must be withheld while the ACTH response test is being performed.
3. Complete blood count
    a) Elevated PCV and TS reflect dehydration.
    b) Peripheral eosinophilia and lymphocytosis may occur from diminished cortisol influence.
4. Biochemical organ profile

   Elevated BUN, creatinine
    a) Prerenal uremia
    b) Onset of renal failure

D. Electrocardiogram

The ECG may reflect changes compatible with hyperkalemia (see discussion of patient monitoring during DKA).

E. Radiography

Thoracic radiographs may reveal a small heart from hypovolemia.

VI. Treatment

A. Primary objectives:
1. Correct dehydration and hypovolemic shock.
2. Return kidney function to normal.
3. Correct electrolyte imbalances.
4. Supplement glucocorticoids.

B. Perform thorough physical examination.

C. Draw blood samples
1. Complete blood count
2. Biochemical profile
3. Resting plasma cortisol

D. Fluid therapy
1. Insert large-gauge IV catheter.

2. Begin rapid infusion of normal saline
Twenty to 90 ml/kg within first hour for shock. (See Table 9-4.)

E. Glucocorticoid supplementation
1. Withhold steroids unless animal is in shock, until ACTH response test is completed.
2. For shock, use rapid-onset corticosteroids:
   a) Hydrocortisone sodium succinate
   b) Prednisolone sodium succinate
3. Other, slower-onset corticosteroids are used for supplementation:
   a) Dexamethasone
   b) Prednisolone acetate

TABLE 9-4. PROTOCOL FOR ADRENAL CORTICAL INSUFFICIENCY

1. Insert IV catheter.
   a. Draw laboratory samples.
   b. Fluid therapy—normal saline ± 10% dextrose
      i. First hour: 20–90 ml/kg
      ii. Maintenance: 20 ml/kg q6h
2. Record ECG.
3. Perform ACTH response test: 0.5 U/kg ACTH IM, take resting and 2-h sample.
4. Glucocorticoid supplementation
   a. Hydrocortisone sodium succinate, 8–20 mg/kg IV
   b. Prednisolone sodium succinate, 11–25 mg/kg IV
   c. Dexamethasone, 2–4 mg/kg IV or SQ
   d. Prednisolone acetate, 0.1–0.2 mg/kg IM q8–12h
   e. Hydrocortisone acetate 0.1–0.2 mg/kg IM q8–12h
5. Supportive care
   a. Heat
   b. Antibiotics
   c. Sodium bicarbonate—2–4 mEq/kg in IV fluids in first 24 h
6. Mineralocorticoid supplementation
   a. Desoxycorticosterone acetate, 1–5 mg IM q24h
   b. Fludrocortisone, 0.1–0.6 mg PO q24h
7. Patient monitoring
   a. ECG q6h
   b. Electrolytes q4–8h
   c. Hematocrit, TS, and urine output
   d. CVP
   e. Blood gases

c) Hydrocortisone acetate
(See Table 9-5.)

F. Combat hyperkalemia
1. Add 10% dextrose to IV fluids. Dextrose promotes potassium uptake by cells.
2. Correction of acidosis with sodium bicarbonate and adequate fluid therapy will also lower serum K^+.

G. Mineralocorticoid supplementation
Begin once electrolyte abnormalities are confirmed:
1. Desoxycorticosterone acetate in oil
2. Fludrocortisone

H. Supportive care
1. Heat
2. ± Antibiotics
3. Padded bedding

I. Maintenance therapy
1. When the patient is stabilized, begin slow conversion to maintenance drugs.

TABLE 9-5. COMMERCIAL PRODUCTS FOR USE IN HYPOADRENOCORTICISM

Hydrocortisone sodium succinate—Solu-Cortef, Upjohn, Kalamazoo, MI 49001
Prednisolone sodium succinate—Solu-Delta-Cortef, Upjohn, Kalamazoo, MI 49001
Dexamethasone Azium, Schering, Kenilworth, NJ 07033 Dexate-SP, Burns Biotec Laboratories, Omaha, NB 68103
Prednisolone acetate—DepPredalone, O'Neal, Jones and Feldman Pharmaceuticals, Maryland Heights, MO 63043
Hydrocortisone acetate—Hydrocortone acetate, Merck, Sharp and Dohme, West Point, PA 19486
Desoxycorticosterone acetate—DOCA, Organon Pharmaceuticals, West Orange, NJ 07052
Fludrocortisone—Florinef acetate, ER Squibb, Princeton, NJ 08540
Desoxycorticosterone pivalate—Percorten pivalate, CIBA Pharmaceutical, Summit, NJ 07901
Desoxycorticosterone acetate pellets—Percorten acetate, CIBA Pharmaceutical, Summit, NJ 07901

TABLE 9-6. MAINTENANCE THERAPY FOR ADRENAL CORTICOL INSUFFICIENCY

Mineralocorticoids

1. Fludrocortisone
   Small dogs: 0.1–0.2 mg/day PO
   Medium dogs: 0.2–0.3 mg/day PO
   Large dogs: 0.4–0.6 mg/day PO
   Giant breeds: 0.6–1.2 mg/day PO
2. Desoxycorticosterone pivalate (DOCP)—25 mg = 1 mg/day of active desoxycorticosterone acetate released for 25 days
3. DOCP pellets—125-mg pellet releases 0.5 mg/day of active desoxycorticosterone acetate for approximately 6 months

Glucocorticoids

Prednisolone—0.05 mg/kg/daily or QOD; increase if stressed

2. Mineralocorticoids are often necessary for life:
   a) Fludrocortisone
   b) Desoxycorticosterone pivalate
   c) Desoxycorticosterone acetate pellets
3. Glucocorticoid supplementation at low levels may also be necessary indefinitely. Oral prednisolone may be given daily or every other day and increased during times of stress.
4. Add salt to the diet to provide continuous source of sodium.
   (See Table 9-6.)

HYPOGLYCEMIA

I. Definition

Hypoglycemia is defined as any blood glucose level less than 50 mg/dl. Normal resting blood glucose in dogs is 120–180 mg/dl and in cats is 120–200 mg/dl. Normal fasting blood sugar is 75–110 mg/dl. Normal glucose regulation is a complex process involving intestinal absorption, hepatic production, and peripheral utilization. Hypoglycemia usually follows a disruption of one or more of these processes.

II. Causes
- A. Increased glucose removal or utilization
  - 1. Excessive insulin
    - a) Overdose of exogenous therapy (insulin shock)
    - b) Functional β-cell tumors (insulinomas) of the pancreas
    - c) Ingestion of hypoglycemia drugs such as sulfonylurea and biquanide compounds (rare in animals)
  - 2. Renal glycosuria
- B. Decreased glucose production
  - 1. Glycogen storage diseases
  - 2. Functional hypoglycemia
  - 3. Starvation
  - 4. Malabsorption
  - 5. Liver disease
  - 6. Severe adrenal cortical insufficiency

III. Pathophysiology
- A. Excessive insulin
  - 1. Insulin, which is produced by the β-cells of the pancreas, stimulates glucose uptake and utilization by most tissues. As insulin levels increase, blood glucose falls.
  - 2. Sources of excess insulin include:
    - a) Overdosage with exogenous insulin during therapy of diabetes mellitus.
    - b) Stimulation of β-cells with certain drugs.
    - c) Production of excessive levels of endogenous insulin by tumors of the β-cells.
- B. Renal loss of glucose

  Renal glucosuria is a defect of tubular absorption. Despite normal or low blood sugar levels, glucose is still lost in the urine. This condition is rare in the dog.
- C. Glycogen storage diseases
  - 1. Cause recurrent hypoglycemia in juveniles.
  - 2. Type I or von Gierke's disease is a deficiency of glucose 6-phosphatase which prevents conversion of glucose 6-phosphate to free glucose in the liver.

3. Other types of glycogen storage diseases may also be found to exist in the dog.

D. Functional hypoglycemia
   1. Hypoglycemia develops easily in the young because their:
      a) Glucose requirements are high.
      b) Gluconeogenic enzymes are immature.
      c) Feedback mechanisms between plasma glucose and hepatic production are poorly developed.
   2. Hypoglycemia occurs in neonates following stress or hypothermia.
   3. Hypoglycemia occurs in young toy breed dogs with:
      a) Systemic diseases
      b) Hypothermia
      c) Starvation
      d) Stress of shipping

E. Starvation

   Hepatic reserves of glycogen are depleted, therefore conversion of glycogen to free glucose is minimal.

F. Malabsorption

   Absorption of glucose is impaired and liver glycogen stores are depleted.

G. Liver disease
   1. If the enzyme systems of the liver that are responsible for glycolysis and storage of glycogen are affected, hypoglycemia may develop.
   2. It is rare for hypoglycemia to develop alone, without other signs of liver disease.

H. Severe hypoadrenocorticism

   Both gluconeogenesis and glycogenolysis are impaired with prolonged glucocorticoid deficiency.

IV. Clinical signs

A. Glucose is the primary energy source of the brain. The clinical signs associated with hypoglycemia result from CNS dysfunction. The severity of the clinical signs depends on the rate of decline and duration of low blood sugar rather than the final numerical value reached.

B. Signs include:
  1. Incoordination, weakness, collapse
  2. Confusion, personality changes
  3. Muscle tremors
  4. Seizures—must be included in differential diagnosis of status epilepticus
C. Signs may be episodic and recurrent with:
  1. Hyperinsulinism
  2. Glycogen storage diseases

V. Diagnosis
  A. History
    1. Known administration of exogenous insulin
    2. Exposure to hypoglycemic drugs
    3. Recurrent, episodic symptoms
    4. Recent stress from shipping, exposure to cold, other illnesses (young dogs)
    5. Poorly regulated hypoadrenocorticism
  B. Classic clinical signs
  C. Laboratory confirmation of hypoglycemia
  D. Determining the cause of hyperglycemia may require extensive diagnostic testing:
    1. Overdosage of insulin
       Suspect in any diabetic animal found weak, confused, collapsed, or in a coma.
    2. Insulinoma
      a) High serum immunoreactive insulin
      b) Abnormal amended insulin glucose ratio:
        (1) $$\frac{\text{Serum insulin } (\mu\text{U/ml}) \times 100}{\text{Plasma glucose (mg/dl)} - 30}$$
        (2) Normal $<$30 mg/dl
      c) Surgical exploration of abdomen
    3. Hypoglycemic drugs
       Known exposure or ingestion of sulfonylurea and biquanide compounds
    4. Renal glycosuria
       Demonstration of persistent glycosuria with a low or normal blood glucose

5. Defects in gluconeogenic enzymes
    a) Suspicious age group, breed
        (1) Six to 12 weeks—toy breeds, Lapland terrier
        (2) Adults—hunting dogs, German shepherd
    b) Recurrent nature
    c) Assays of plasma pyruvate and alanine, blood ketones
6. Functional hypoglycemia
    a) Neonates recently stressed
    b) Juvenile toy breeds recently stressed
7. Malabsorption
    a) Biochemical organ profile, fecal examination
    b) Intestinal absorption studies
    c) Surgical biopsies of intestine and liver
8. Liver disease
    a) Biochemical organ profile
    b) Sulfobromophthalein (BSP) excretion
    c) Glucose tolerance test
    d) Surgical biopsy
9. Severe hypoadrenocorticism
    a) Abnormal electrolytes
    b) Low plasma glucocorticoid levels

VI. Treatment
- A. Primary objectives:
    1. Return blood glucose to normal.
    2. Confirm hypoglycemia.
    3. Determine and treat cause.
- B. Initial considerations
    1. Insert an IV catheter.
    2. Draw laboratory samples (see Table 9-7).
    3. Prevent self-trauma during major motor seizures.
    4. Ensure patent airway if comatose.
- C. Glucose therapy
    1. Most seizures subside and patients become alert with supplemental glucose.
    2. Administer 50% dextrose IV slowly if patient is large enough for vena puncture.

TABLE 9-7. PROTOCOL FOR HYPOGLYCEMIA

1. Insert IV catheter.
2. Draw laboratory samples for :
   a. Quantitative blood glucose
   b. Semiquantitative blood glucose
   c. Serum immunoreactive insulin
   d. Biochemical profile
   e. CBC
3. Institute glucose therapy.
   a. 50% dextrose:
      0.5–2.0 ml/kg IV slowly (20 ml maximum)
      1–2 ml via stomach tube in neonate
   b. 5% D/W—10–20 ml/kg IV q6–8h
   c. Maintain blood glucose ≥ 90 mg/dl
4. Start supportive care.
   a. IV fluid therapy:
      5% D/W, saline/dextrose, or lactated Ringer's with 5% dextrose
   b. Diazepam for refractory seizures
      Dog: 5–40 mg IV
      Cat: 2.5–5.0 mg IV
   c. Heat for hypothermia
   d. Consider dexamethasone and mannitol for persistent CNS signs.
5. Diagnose and treat cause.

3. Administer 50% dextrose orally in neonates or small animals.
4. Maintain blood sugar levels ≥90 mg/dl with continuous IV 5% D/W or repeated oral glucose.
5. Avoid supplementation with large quantities of dextrose in patients with insulinomas. The supplemental glucose may stimulate further release of insulin, producing profound hypoglycemia 1–3 h later.

D. Supportive care
   1. Diazepam—for refractory seizures
   2. Heat
   3. Consider dexamethasone and mannitol for persistent CNS signs.
      (See Table 9-8.)

E. Diagnose and correct cause.

The author would refer the reader to the Bibliography at the end of the chapter for a detailed discussion of

TABLE 9-8. COMMERCIAL PRODUCTS AVAILABLE FOR USE IN HYPOGLYCEMIA AND HYPOCALCEMIA

50% Dextrose—50% dextrose injection, USP, Invenex Laboratories, Orlando, FL 32809

Diazepam—Valium, Roche Laboratories, Nutley, NJ 07110

Dexamethasone
  Azium, Schering, Kenilworth, NJ 07033
  Dexate-SP, Burns Biotec Laboratories, Omaha, NB 68103

20% Mannitol—20% Mannitol injection, USP, Cutter Laboratories, Berkeley, CA 94700

10% calcium gluconate—Calcium gluconate injection, USP, Upjohn, Kalamazoo, MI 49001

Oral calcium gluconate—Calcet, Mission Pharmaceutical, San Antonio, TX 78210

Oral calcium carbonate—Titralac, Riker Laboratories, Northridge, CA 91324

Oral calcium lactate—Calcium lactate, Eli Lilly, Indianapolis, IN 46285

Vitamin D_2—Drisdol, Winthrop Laboratories, New York, NY 10016

Dihydrotachysterol—Hytakeral, Winthrop Laboratories, New York, NY 10016

1,25-dihydroxy-vitamin D_3—Rocaltrol, Roche Laboratories, Nutley, NJ 07110

long-term medical and surgical remedies for the causes of hypoglycemia.

VII. Patient monitoring
  A. Vital signs, especially neurologic status
    See Chapter 3, section on Status Epicepticus.
  B. Body temperature, ambient temperatures
  C. Blood sugar
    Maintain ≥90 mg/dl.
  D. Resume normal nutrition, glucose intake.
  E. Minimize stress.

HYPOCALCEMIA

I. Definition

Clinical signs of *hypocalcemia* develop with calcium levels less than 6–7 mg/dl. Normal serum calcium is 9–11 mg/dl.

II. Causes
   A. Lactation
      1. Hypocalcemia in lactating animals is known as eclampsia or puerperal tetany.
      2. Most frequently occurs in small, nervous breeds of dogs.
      3. Often arises 7–21 days postpartum.
      4. Thought to result from failure of normal calcium homeostatic mechanisms to compensate for peak calcium demands
      5. Much more common in the bitch than the queen
   B. Hypoparathyroidism
      1. Parathormone (PTH) is the major hormone responsible for maintenance of normal serum calcium.
      2. Any disorder of the parathyroids may result in abnormal PTH secretion with subsequent hypocalcemia.
      3. Causes of parathyroid disorders include:
         a) Injury or inadvertent removal during surgery, especially accompanying thyroidectomies. This is a common cause of hypocalcemia in cats and arises 6–72 h postoperatively.
         b) Destruction by primary or metastatic neoplasms
         c) Primary lymphocytic parathyroiditis is a recognized disease of dogs.
         d) Congenital agenesis
   C. Others
      Although these conditions rarely cause significant neurologic signs, hypocalcemia may develop with:
      1. Pancreatitis
      2. Chronic diarrhea, malabsorption
      3. Renal failure
      4. Hypoproteinemia
      5. Nutritional secondary hyperparathyroidism
III. Clinical signs
   A. Hyperactivity
   B. Hyperventilation with dilated pupils

C. Flared nostrils
D. Ataxia, weakness
E. Muscle tremors, tonic-clonic spasms
F. Tetanic seizures
G. Mild to severe hyperthermia
H. Hypocalcemic tetany should be included in the differential diagnosis of seizure disorders.

IV. Diagnosis
A. History may allow a presumptive diagnosis in the lactating animal.
B. Clinical signs
C. Laboratory confirmation of hypocalcemia
D. Alterations of serum phosphorous
1. Usually low with eclampsia.
2. Often elevated with hypoparathyroidism
E. Tests that aid in the diagnosis of hypoparathyroidism:
1. Serum immunoreactive PTH
2. Urine and plasma cyclic adenosine monophosphate (cAMP) assays
3. Urinary excretion of calcium
4. Urinary tubular resorption of phosphorus
5. Parathyroid biopsy

V. Treatment
A. Objectives:
1. Return serum calcium to normal.
2. Diagnose and correct the cause.
B. Obtain complete history.
Note date of parturition or previous surgery.
C. Perform thorough physical examination.
1. Note evidence of lactation.
2. Note any surgical incisions in the ventral neck area.
3. Note other systemic abnormalities.
D. Confirm hypocalcemia.
1. Draw laboratory samples.
2. Perform ECG.
Low calcium may produce:
a) Q-T interval prolongation
b) ST segment prolongation

3. Response to therapy

In the event that no diagnostic aids are available, and the seizure is unresponsive to both diazepam and 50% dextrose IV, calcium may be given cautiously IV. Cessation of the seizure in response to calcium supplementation allows a presumptive diagnosis of hypocalcemia (see section on status epilepticus, Chapter 3).

E. Provide supplemental calcium.
   1. Begin slow IV administration of 2–10 ml of 10% calcium gluconate.
      (See Table 9-9.)
   2. Monitor heart rate closely.
   3. Halt administration of calcium if:
      a) Heart rate increases
      b) Arrhythmias occur
      c) Animal appears nauseated
   4. With sufficient calcium supplementation, muscle spasms, panting, abnormal behavior, and seizures subside.

F. Supportive therapy
   1. Intravenous fluids may be instituted as needed.

TABLE 9-9. PROTOCOL FOR HYPOCALCEMIA

1. Confirm hypocalcemia.
   a. Draw blood for serum calcium.
   b. Take ECG.
   c. Response to therapy.
   d. Draw laboratory samples for other diagnostic tests.

2. Supply calcium.
   10% calcium gluconate—slow IV injection
   Dog: 2–10 ml
   Cat: 0.5–4.0 ml

3. Start supportive care.
   a. IV fluids—add 10% Ca gluconate PRN
   b. Diazepam for refractory seizures
   c. Cool water bath for hyperthermia
   d. Consider mannitol and dexamethasone for cerebral edema.

4. Diagnose and treat cause.

2. Give diazepam for refractory seizures.
3. Monitor body temperature closely.
   For animals with temperatures >41°C (106°F), institute cool water compresses or baths until their temperatures fall to 39.5°C (103°F).
4. Use mannitol and dexamethasone for cerebral edema from seizures.
5. Corticosteroids may be indicated for lymphocytic parathyroiditis.

G. Maintenance therapy
   Begin when the calcium has returned to normal and the patient is stable.
   1. Calcium
      a) Ca gluconate—150–250 mg/kg IM, PO q6–8 h
      b) Ca carbonate—150–200 mg/kg PO q6–8h
      c) Ca lactate—150–200 mg/kg PO q8h
   2. Vitamin D
      a) Vitamin D_2—12,000–25,000 U/day
      b) Dihydrotachysterol—0.01–0.02 mg/kg/day
      c) 1,25 $(OH)_2$Vitamin D_3—0.03–0.06 μg/kg/day

VI. Patient monitoring
   A. Serum calcium
      Maintain between 8 and 11 mg/dl.
   B. Body temperature
      Avoid overzealous lowering of temperature following a seizure because hypothermia may occur.
   C. Remove all pups and kittens from the mother. Hand-rear all offspring not yet weaned.
   D. Warn owner of possible recurrences with future pregnancies and lactation.

HEPATIC ENCEPHALOPATHY

I. Definition
   Hepatic encephalopathy (HE) is a metabolic disorder of the CNS which arises from abnormal liver function. The liver is normally responsible for removing potential neurotoxins

that are produced by the intestinal microflora and are absorbed into the circulation through the gut. If blood is shunted away from the liver or if severe hepatic insufficiency exists, these chemicals will remain in the circulation and accumulate in the brain where they exert a neurotoxic effect.

II. Causes
  A. Congenital portal vein anomalies
  B. Acquired portosystemic shunts
  C. Severe parenchymal diseases of the liver
    1. Cirrhosis
    2. Acute, toxic liver failure
    3. Extensive neoplasia
  D. Congenital urea cycle enzyme deficiencies
    1. Arginosuccinate synthetase
    2. Carbamyl phosphate synthetase I

III. Pathophysiology
  A. Several biochemical abnormalities are believed to occur.
    1. Toxins that are proposed to be involved in the development of hepatic encephalopathy include:
      a) Ammonia
      b) Mercaptans (methanethiol)
      c) Short-chain fatty acids
    2. Decrease in branched-chain amino acids
      a) Valine
      b) Leucine
      c) Isoleucine
      d) Alanine
      e) Taurine
      f) Threonine
    3. Increase in aromatic amino acids:
      a) Tyrosine
      b) Phenylalanine
      c) Glutamic acid
      d) Serine
      e) Tryptophan (indoles, skatoles)
    4. Decrease in normal neurotransmitters
  B. The biochemical mechanisms by which these chemicals

produce altered CNS function is not well understood. Proposed effects include:
   1. Interference with nerve cell membrane function
   2. Altered cellular energy metabolism
   3. Altered neurotransmission
C. Ammonia is considered one of the most significant toxins involved in hepatic encephalopathy. Serum ammonia is almost always elevated during episodes of HE, although the magnitude of hyperammonemia may not be correlative with the severity of the clinical signs.
D. Certain events that increase the production of nitrogenous toxins in the gut or alter intestinal pH, and therefore alter absorption of toxins, or compromise either liver or brain function may precipitate an acute episode of HE. Such contributing conditions are:
   1. Gastrointestinal bleeding
   2. Hypovolemic shock
   3. Increased protein consumption
   4. Alkalosis, hypokalemia
   5. Uremia
   6. Infections
   7. Exposure to CNS depressant drugs

IV. Clinical signs
A. Neurologic signs
   1. Behavioral abnormalities
      a) Hysteria
      b) Viciousness
      c) Dementia
   2. Listlessness, depression, coma
   3. Weakness, ataxia
   4. Head pressing
   5. Circling, pacing
   6. Blindness
   7. Seizures
B. Accompanying signs of liver disease
   1. Stunted growth
   2. Weight loss

3. Polyuria, PD
4. Anorexia
5. Vomiting, diarrhea
6. Ascites
7. Panting, shaking

V. Diagnosis
  A. History
    1. Congenital shunts produce signs in young dogs (<6 mo).
    2. Chronic parenchymal diseases usually occur in older dogs.
    3. Acute toxic liver failure may occur at any age.
    4. Clinical signs may be worse after eating.
    5. Exposure to precipitating factors should be determined.
  B. Physical examination
    Suspicious clinical signs and physical findings
  C. Laboratory analysis
    1. Evidence of advanced liver disease
      a) Increased:
        (1) Serum alanine aminotransferase (SGPT)
        (2) Serum aspartate aminotransferase (SGOT)
        (3) Serum glutamyl transpeptidase (SGGT)
        (4) Serum alkaline phosphatase (SAP)
        (5) Abnormal BSP retention, often >12–15%
      b) Decreased:
        (1) Serum albumin
        (2) Blood urea nitrogen
        (3) Prothrombin activity
    2. Blood ammonia
      a) Fasting blood ammonia
        (1) Normal $\leq$120–150 μg/dl
        (2) May be normal or high
      b) Ammonia tolerance test
        (1) Measure fasting blood ammonia
        (2) Give NH_4Cl 100 mg/kg PO (Maximum dose = 3 gm)

(3) Take 30-min sample
(4) Normal post-NH_4Cl value <200–250 μg/dl

3. Altered plasma amino acid concentrations
   a) Increased aromatic amino acids
   b) Decreased branched-chain amino acids
4. Urinalysis
   May demonstrate ammonium biurate crystals
5. Serum bile acid assay (Center)
   a) Fasting level
      (1) Normal ≤ 5.0 μM/L
      (2) May be normal or high
   b) Post prandial level
      (1) Feed high protein diet (PD).
      (2) Take 2 h sample.
      (3) Normal ≤ 15.5 μM/L
6. Altered glucagon tolerance test (Macy)
   a) Fast animal for 12 h.
   b) Give glucagon 0.03 mg/kg IV.
   c) Take 0, 15, 30, 60 min samples for blood glucose assay.
   d) Glucose curve remains flat in HE dogs.
   e) Glucose curve often returns to normal with surgical correction of portal caval shunts.

D. Radiography
   1. Plain—small liver
   2. Contrast angiography of the portal venous system is necessary to document and define a portal shunt.

E. Neurologic examination
   1. Abnormal neurologic findings are symmetrical.
   2. Cerebrospinal fluid analysis is normal.
   3. Electroencephalogram demonstrates bilateral, synchronous, symmetrical high-voltage slow waves compatible with a nonspecific metabolic disorder.

F. Liver biopsy
   1. Will diagnose parenchymal changes.
   2. May be normal or show only hepatocyte atrophy in presence of congenital portal vein anomaly.

3. Perform enzyme assay on biopsied tissue to determine congenital deficiency of urea cycle enzymes.

VI. Treatment
- A. Objectives:
  1. Remove toxic agents, reverse neurologic signs.
  2. Provide supportive care.
  3. Diagnose and treat precipitating cause.
- B. Initial therapy when collapsed or in coma
  1. Ensure patent airway, administer O_2.
  2. Draw laboratory samples.
     - a) Complete blood count
     - b) Biochemical organ profile
     - c) Blood ammonia
     - d) Plasma amino acids, serum bile acids
     - e) Blood gases
     - f) Urinalysis
  3. Insert IV catheter.
     - a) Treat shock if present.
     - b) Correct:
       - (1) Dehydration, azotemia
       - (2) Alkalosis
       - (3) Hypokalemia
       - (4) Administer glucose to decrease amino acid breakdown.
  4. Peritoneal dialysis
     Rapidly lowers blood ammonia
- C. Reduce intestinal ammonia production.
  1. Withhold all food, especially dietary protein.
  2. Cleanse the bowel.
     - a) Cathartic
     - b) Enemas
       - (1) Vinegar and water (1:10 dilution)
       - (2) 10% povidone-iodine
       - (3) Soapy water
  3. Alter gastrointestinal microflora.
     - a) Neomycin—20 mg/kg PO q8–12h
     - b) Kanamycin—1.2 mg/kg PO q8–12h

c) Gentamycin—0.25–0.5 mg/kg PO q8–12h
d) Vancomycin—3 mg/kg PO q8–12h
e) Rectal neomycin as an enema

D. Decrease absorption of ammonia.
1. Laxatives
Decrease contact time of stool with colonic mucosa.
2. Lactulose
a) Nonabsorbable synthetic disaccharide
b) Mechanisms of action:
(1) Cathartic
(2) Hydrolyzes colonic bacteria to acids which:
i) Change NH_3 to NH_4^+ which is less diffusable across gut mucosa

TABLE 9-10. PROTOCOL FOR HEPATIC ENCEPHALOPATHY

1. Ensure patent airway.
   Administer O_2 for hypoxia.
2. Draw laboratory samples.
3. Insert IV catheter.
   a. Treat shock—multiple electrolyte solution with dextrose
   b. Correct:
      Dehydration
      Alkalosis—0.45% saline with 5% dextrose, ± bicarbonate
      Hypokalemia—add 20–40 mEq KCl/L
4. Consider peritoneal dialysis.
5. Reduce ammonia production, absorption.
   a. Withhold food.
   b. Cathartics, enemas
   c. Oral antibiotics
   d. Oral lactulose
6. Start supportive care.
   a. Maintain body temperature.
   b. Systemic antibiotics.
   c. Withdraw offensive drugs.
   d. Stop blood transfusions.
   e. Stop parenteral hyperalimentation.
   f. Stop gastrointestinal bleeding.
7. Consider surgery for congenital shunts.

TABLE 9-11. COMMERCIAL PRODUCTS FOR USE IN HEPATIC ENCEPHALOPATHY

Neomycin SO_4—Biosol liquid, Upjohn, Kalamazoo, MI 49001
Kanamycin—Kantrim injection, Bristol Laboratories, Syracuse, NY 13201
Gentamycin SO_4—Gentocin, Schering, Kenilworth, NJ 07033
Vancomycin—Vancocin HCl, Eli Lilly, Indianapolis, IN 46206
Lactulose Cephulac syrup, Merrill-National Laboratories, Cincinnati, OH 45215 Duphulac syrup, Philips Roxane Laboratory, Columbus, OH 43216

ii) Promote growth of non-urease-producing bacteria

(3) Synergistic with neomycin

c) Five to 30 ml PO q6–8h until stools are soft (See Tables 9-10 and 9-11.)

E. Treat precipitating cause.

1. Terminate use of offending drugs.
   a) Tranquilizers, depressants
   b) Diuretics
   c) Oral methionine
   d) Anticonvulsants
   e) Organophosphates
2. Diagnosis and control gastrointestinal bleeding.
3. Stop transfusions of stored blood and parenteral hyperalimentation due to high ammonia content.
4. Treat any infections with systemic antibiotics.
5. Correct hypovolemia, alkalosis, and hypokalemia with adequate fluid therapy.

F. Prepare for surgery.

Partial surgical closure of congenital portal caval shunts may be indicated.

VII. Patient monitoring

A. Body temperature

B. Central nervous system signs

C. Blood gases

D. Serum electrolytes

E. Blood glucose
F. Blood ammonia
G. Urine output
H. Number, consistency of bowel movements
I. Body weight

HEAT PROSTRATION

I. Definition

Heat stroke or *heat prostration* is a polysystemic emergency which develops with acute elevations of body temperature above 41°C (106°F). Heat stroke occurs when the heat load on an animal's body greatly exceeds the capacity of the panting mechanism to dissipate heat.

II. Causes
   A. Confinement in overheated enclosures and exposure to hot humid environments are the most common causes.
   B. Probability of heat stroke depends on:
      1. Amount of heat
      2. Length of exposure to heat
      3. Amount of air circulation
      4. Humidity
      5. Anxiety of the animal
      6. Breed of dog
      7. Preexisting medical problems, especially upper airway and cardiovascular diseases

III. Pathophysiology
   A. Adverse effects develop from cellular necrosis following hyperthermia and results in alterations in all organ systems.
   B. See Table 9-12.
   C. Body temperatures of 42–43°C (107–109°F) are tolerated for only a few minutes before cellular destruction occurs.

IV. Clinical signs
   A. Clinical signs depend on the systemic organs affected. Their severity is proportional to the amount and duration of exposure to heat.

TABLE 9-12. SYSTEMIC EFFECTS OF HEAT STROKE

Cardiovascular
- Increased metabolic rate leads to increased O_2 demand.
- Myocardial degeneration and necrosis
- Hypoxia leads to hypotension and hemoconcentration.
- Hypovolemic shock

Acid-base balance, electrolytes
- Panting leads to respiratory alkalosis.
- Muscle activity and shock lead to metabolic acidosis.
- Hypercalcemia, hypophosphatemia
- Terminal hypocalcemia

Musculoskeletal
- Rhabdomyolysis, myoglobinemia

Renal
- Acute tubular necrosis
- ARF

Gastrointestinal
- Necrosis of mucosa with hemorrhagic vomiting, diarrhea

Neurologic
- Neuronal degeneration, gliosis of brain
- Cerebral edema

Coagulation
- DIC

B. Listed in increasing severity:
1. Panting, excitement
2. Brick red mucous membranes
3. Tachycardia
4. Hyperthermia
5. Severe respiratory distress, cyanosis
6. Hemoconcentration with poor peripheral circulation
7. Stupor
8. Hemorrhagic vomiting, diarrhea
9. Generalized petechiae
10. Anuria
11. Seizures, coma
12. Respiratory arrest

V. Diagnosis
- A. Recognition of clinical signs
- B. Suspicious history

C. Demonstration of elevated temperature upon physical examination

VI. Treatment

A. Objectives:
1. Immediate reversal of hyperthermia
2. Correction of shock and cerebral edema
3. Detection and treatment of delayed complications, for instance, renal failure, gastrointestinal necrosis
4. Removal of predisposing factors

B. Ensure patent airway.
1. Intubate if comatose.
2. Administer O_2 if cyanotic
3. For animals with upper respiratory disease:
a) Sedate
b) Anesthesize and intubate
c) Perform tracheostomy
(see section on Airway Obstruction, Chapter 12.)

C. Insert IV catheter.
Treat for shock as needed

D. Rapidly reduce body temperature.
1. The body temperature is lowered to 39.5°C (103°F) within the first 10 min.
2. Once the body temperature reaches 103°F, moderate treatment and lower temperature further by 1°/h.
Note: Once body temperature begins to fall, it may do so precipitously, therefore resulting in hypothermia.
3. Use ice baths and cold water enemas for unresponsive hyperthermia *only*.
See Table 9-13.

E. Supportive care
1. Corticosteroids for shock
2. Sodium bicarbonate for metabolic acidosis
3. Diazepam for seizures, and muscle tremors
4. Antibiotics for evidence of infection
(See Table 9-8 for commercial products.)

TABLE 9-13. PROTOCOL FOR HYPERTHERMIA

1. Ensure patent airway.
   a. O_2 therapy
   b. Sedation, intubation, tracheostomy
2. Insert IV catheter.
   a. Fluid of choice is multiple electrolyte solution.
   b. Treat for shock.
3. Rapid reduction of body temperature
   a. Immerse in cool water.
   b. Alcohol bath
   c. Cold water enema
   d. Lower temperature to 39.5°C in 10 min.
4. Start supportive care.
   a. Antibiotics
   b. Corticosteroids
   c. Diazepam
   d. Sodium bicarbonate
5. Patient monitoring
   a. Body temperature
      i. Moderate treatment when 39.5°C is reached
      ii. Avoid hypothermia
   b. Urine output
      Insert urinary catheter
   c. Hematocrit, TS
   d. Blood urea nitrogen, creatinine
   e. Evidence of DIC
   f. Level of consciousness, neurologic signs
6. Institute therapy for renal failure
   a. Forced diuresis
      i. Diuretics—furosemide
      ii. 10% D/W
      iii. Mannitol
   b. Peritoneal dialysis

VII. Patient monitoring
   A. Hospitalize in an air-conditioned, low-humidity environment.
   B. Body temperature
      1. Avoid hypothermia
      2. If hypothermia occurs, warm IV solutions and apply heat.
   C. Urine output
      1. Assess adequacy of fluid therapy.

2. If anuria or oliguria occurs, institute therapy for renal failure:
   a) Forced diuresis
      (1) Furosemide
      (2) Ten percent D/W
      (3) Twenty percent mannitol
   b) Peritoneal dialysis

D. Packed cell volume, TS
   1. Maintain PCV <45%.
   2. Note hemolysis.

E. Blood urea nitrogen, creatinine
   Watch for ARF.

F. Blood gases
   Measure frequently if respiratory distress persists.

G. Serum electrolytes

H. Evidence of DIC
   1. Petechiae, ecchymoses
   2. Protracted bleeding
   3. Abnormal clotting survey

I. Level of consciousness, neurologic symptoms
   1. Institute mannitol for cerebral edema.
   2. *Note:* The use of mannitol is contraindicated in the presence of DIC or hemoconcentration.

J. Prepare for surgery if correction of upper airway problems is required.

HYPOTHERMIA AND FROSTBITE

I. Definition

Hypothermia is any profound decrease in body temperature. *Frostbite* or cold injury is actual freezing of body tissue. Both conditions are rare in animals because they can withstand cold temperatures due to their long-haired coats and will instinctively seek shelter from inclement weather. Hypothermia and frostbite are obviously more common in temperate climates.

II. Causes
  A. Accidental hypothermia
    1. Deep cooling from exposure to environmental cold
      a) Animal can not seek shelter:
        (1) Unconscious
        (2) Injured, unhealthy
        (3) Immobile (caught in traps)
        (4) Negligence on part of owner
      b) Animal has increased susceptibility to cold:
        (1) Injured, unhealthy
        (2) Aged
        (3) Unacclimated to new, cold environment
    2. Failure of normal thermoregulatory mechanisms
      a) Anesthetics
      b) Sedatives
      c) Prolonged exposure of body cavity to room temperature during surgery
    3. Iatrogenic
      Detention of animals in storage lockers, freezers, refrigerators
  B. Frostbite
    1. Exposure to cold or chilling air
    2. Contact with cold metal, glass, liquids
    3. Iatrogenic freezing with cryogens

III. Pathophysiology
  A. Hypothermia
    1. As body core temperature decreases, metabolic processes begin to slow.
    2. Blood is shunted from surface areas and extremities by extreme vasoconstriction.
    3. Cardiac rate and output fall.
    4. Renal perfusion decreases.
    5. Mental awareness and neurologic processes diminish.
    6. Terminally, ventricular fibrillation occurs.
    7. Mild hypothermia
      a) Body temperature = 30–32°C (86–90°F)
      b) May be withstood for 24–36 h

8. Moderate hypothermia
    a) Body temperature = 22–25°C (72–77°F)
    b) Animals may survive for 4–24 h.
9. Severe hypothermia
    a) Body temperature ≤15°C (60°F)
    b) Maximum survival time = 5–6 h
    c) Survival time may only be 1–2 h if complicated by other systemic diseases.

B. Frostbite
1. When frostbite accompanies hypothermia, body temperatures below 34°C (93°F) result in decreased blood flood to the skin and extremities.
2. Avascular necrosis may also occur with simple freezing of any exposed body surface area.
3. Tissue necrosis is increased if subsequent refreezing occurs after an affected part has been thawed.
4. Commonly affected areas:
    a) Cats
        (1) Pinnae of ears
        (2) Tail
        (3) Footpads
    b) Dogs
        (1) External genitalia
        (2) Footpads

IV. Clinical signs
A. Diminished consciousness
B. Low blood pressure—weak or absent pulses
C. Bradycardia
D. Shallow, infrequent respirations
E. Dilated pupils
F. Delayed, diminished reflexes
G. Shivering
H. Increased muscle tone without shivering occurs at body temperatures below 32°C (90°F).
I. Cyanotic or pale appearance of frozen part
J. Anesthesia of frozen part

V. Diagnosis
A. History of exposure to cold
B. Recognition of clinical signs

C. Demonstration of low body temperature
D. Standard thermometers record body temperatures above 34.4°C (94°F)
E. Hypothermic thermometers are available that record body temperatures to 27.8°C (82°F).

VI. Treatment
- A. Objectives:
  1. Return core body temperature to normal.
  2. Correct shock.
  3. Reverse life-threatening arrhythmias.
  4. Thaw and protect frozen tissue.
- B. Ensure a patent airway
  1. Intubate if collapsed.
  2. Administer O_2.
     (See Table 9-14.)
- C. Insert an IV catheter.
  1. Begin rapid infusion of multiple electrolyte solution or normal saline.
  2. Warm solutions to 40–43°C (104–109°F) in water bath or incubator.
  3. Solutions can also be warmed in the IV line by passing the tubing through a warm water bath.
- D. Rewarm animal.
  1. External or surface warming
     - a) Passive methods
       - (1) Remove animal from source of cold.
       - (2) Wrap animal in blankets.
       - (3) Is easy and safe
       - (4) Effective for mild hypothermia
     - b) Active methods
       - (1) Warm water bottles
       - (2) Water or electric heating pads
       - (3) Immersion in warm water
       - (4) May cause peripheral vasodilation with resultant "after-drop" of core temperature.
       - (5) May cause local thermal burns if not monitored closely
  2. Internal or core warming

TABLE 9-14. PROTOCOL FOR HYPOTHERMIA

1. Ensure patent airway, O_2
2. Begin IV fluid therapy
   a. Fluids of choice:
      Normal saline
      Multiple electrolyte solution
   b. Consider warming fluids
   c. Correct shock
3. Rewarm animals
   a. Mild hypothermia:
      Remove from cold
      Wrap with blankets
      Warm water bottles
   b. Moderate hypothermia:
      Warm water bottles
      Water or electric heating pads
      ± Immersion in water
      ± Peritoneal dialysis
   c. Profound hypothermia:
      Continuous warmed IV solutions
      Warm peritoneal dialysis
      ± Warm colonic lavage
      ± Warm gastric lavage
   d. Frostbitten area:
      Remove from cold
      Apply warm compresses
      Immerse in warm water
      Prevent refreezing
4. Start supportive care.
   a. Combat arrhythmias.
   b. Draw laboratory samples.
   c. Provide analgesia.
   d. Prevent self-trauma.
   e. Consider Dextran-40 for frostbite.
   f. Begin local care of cold-injured areas.
   g. Consider systemic antibiotics.

a) Administration of warmed IV solutions
b) Peritoneal dialysis
   (1) Warm dialysate to 43° C (109°F).
   (2) Infuse rapidly.
   (3) Remove immediately.
   (4) Repeat procedure until body temperature >36°C (96°F).
   (5) Six to 8 infusions may be necessary.

(6) Advantages:
  i) Easy to perform
  ii) Rapidly raises temperature
  iii) Improves cardiac output

c) Colonic lavage with warm saline
d) Gastric lavage with warm saline

Note: Core warming should be reserved for body temperatures <32°C (90°F) or prolonged hypothermia.

3. Thaw frozen part
   a) Remove from source of cold.
   b) Apply warm compresses.
   c) Immerse frozen part in warm water (40–43°C, 102–104°F).
   d) Prevent refreezing.

   Intravenous infusion of low-molecular-weight dextran may prevent peripheral sludging: 20–40 ml/kg/day in 5% D/W

E. Start supportive care.
   1. Monitor and treat any cardiac arrhythmia.
      a) Atrial fibrillation and ventricular tachycardia are common.
      b) Many drugs have reduced effectiveness when the heart is cold and may also exhibit delayed metabolism.
      c) See section on Arrhythmias, Chapter 2.
   2. Draw laboratory samples.
      a) Blood gases
      b) Serum electrolytes
      c) Correct any abnormalities.
   3. Analgesia
      a) As thawing of frozen tissue occurs, severe pain may arise.
      b) Consider use of analgesics in the awake and hemodynamically stable patient:
         (1) Morphine SO_4—0.2–0.5 mg/kg IM
         (2) Meperidine HC1—3–5 mg/kg IM
         (3) Pentazocine lactate—0.2–0.5 mg/kg IM

         (See Table 9-15.)

TABLE 9-15. COMMERCIAL PRODUCTS FOR USE IN COLD INJURY

Dextran 40—Rheomacrodex, Pharmacia Laboratories, Piscataway, NJ 08854
Morphine sulfate—Morphine sulfate Carpuject, Winthrop Laboratories, New York, NY 10016
Meperidine HCl—Demerol HCl, Winthrop Laboratories, New York, NY 10016
Pentazocine lactate—Talwin lactate, Winthrop Laboratories, New York, NY 10016

4. Prevent self-trauma to cold-injured areas.
   a) Elizabethan collar
   b) Wet dressings to gangrenous areas
   c) Leave warm, erythematous, or edematous areas exposed to the air.
5. Consider antibiotics for infection.

VII. Patient monitoring

A. Body temperature
1. Once body temperature has reached 36°C (96.8°F), moderate therapy.
2. Maintain temperature above 38°C (100°F) until thermoregulatory mechanisms return to normal.

B. Electrocardiogram
1. Monitor continuously for first 24–36 h.
2. Monitor every 4–6 h for first 4 days or until arrhythmias cease.

C. Urine output
Watch for anuria.

D. Serum electrolytes, BUN, creatinine
Monitor q24–48 h.

E. Packed cell volume, TS
1. Maintain normal hydration.
2. Avoid overhydration because it may aggravate edema at sites of frostbite.

F. Thoracic radiography
Pneumonia is a frequent complication of hypothermia.

G. Cold-injured areas
1. Rapid return of warmth, sensation, and erythema are favorable signs.

2. Persistent cold, pale, anesthetic skin warrants a guarded prognosis for the affected area.
3. Delay debridement.

   Demarcation begins in 4–7 days and may take 15–20 days to outline nonviable tissue.

H. Body weight
1. Institute high-protein, high-caloric diet.
2. Supplement vitamins.

BIBLIOGRAPHY

Bardens JW: Glycogen storage disease in puppies. VM/SAC 61:1174, 1966

Barrett RE: Canine hepatic encephalopathy. p. 822. In Kirk RW (ed.): Current Veterinary Therapy. Vol. 7. WB Saunders, Philadelphia, 1980

Capen CC, Belshaw BE, Martin SL: Endocrine disorders. p. 1424. In Ettinger SJ (ed.): Textbook of Veterinary Internal Medicine. WB Saunders, Philadelphia, 1975

Capen CC, Martin SL: Calcium metabolism and disorders of the parathyroid glands. Vet Clin N Am 7(3):513, 1977

Caywood DD, Wilson JW: Functional pancreatic islet cell adenocarcinoma in the dog. p. 1020. In Kirk RW (ed.): Current Veterinary Therapy. Vol. 7. WB Saunders, Philadelphia, 1980

Caywood DD, Wilson JW, Hardy RM, Shull RM: Pancreatic islet cell adenocarcinoma: clinical and diagnostic features in six cases. J Am Vet Med Assoc 174(7):714, 1979

Center SA: Bile acids in diagnosis of hepatic disease in the dog. Sci Pro Acvim: 102, 1984

Chastain CB, Nichols CE: Low-dose intramuscular insulin therapy for diabetic ketoacidosis in dogs. J Am Vet Med Assoc 178(6):561, 1981

Cotten RB, Cornelius LM, Theran P: Diabetes mellitus in the dog: a clinicopathologic study. J Am Vet Med Assoc 159:863, 1971

Dietrich RA: Cold injury. p. 199. In Kirk RW (ed.): Current Veterinary Therapy. Vol. 7. WB Saunders, Philadelphia, 1980

Feldman EC: Diabetic ketoacidosis in dogs. Compend Contin Ed Pract Vet 2(6):456, 1980

Feldman EC, Ettinger SJ: The electrocardiographic changes associated with electrolyte distubances. p. 385. In Kirk RW (ed.): Current Veterinary Therapy. Vol. 7. WB Saunders, Philadelphia, 1980

Feldman EC, Tyrrell JB: Hypoadrenocorticism. Vet Clin N Am 7(3):555, 1977

Foster DW, McGarry JD: The metabolic derangements and treatment of diabetic ketoacidosis. N Engl J Med 309(3):159, 1983

Johnson KE: Pathophysiology of heat stroke. Compend Contin Educ Pract Vet 4(2):141, 1982

Johnson RK: Insulinoma in the dog. Vet Clin N Am 7(3):629, 1977

Johnson RK, Atkins CE: Non-neoplastic causes of canine hypoglycemia. p. 1023. In Kirk RW (ed.): Current Veterinary Therapy. Vol. 7. WB Saunders, Philadelphia, 1980

Kornegay JN, Greene CE, Martin C, et al: Idiopathic hypocalcemia in four dogs. JAAHA 16(5):723, 1980

Krum SH, Osborne CA: Heatstroke in the dog: a polysystemic disorder. J Am Vet Med Assoc 170(5):531, 1977

Ling CV, Lowenstine LJ, Pulley LT, Kaneko JJ: Diabetes mellitus in dogs: a review of initial evaluation, immediate and long-term management, and outcome. J Am Vet Med Assoc 170(5):521, 1977

Lorenz MD: Metabolic emergencies. Vet Clin N Am 2(2):331, 1972

Lorenz MD: Hypoadrenocorticism—diagnosis and treatment. Compend Contin Ed Pract Vet 1(8):634, 1979

Macy DM: Alterations in glucagon tolerance test in dogs with portal caval shunts. Unpublished data.

Martin SL, Capen CC: Puerpural tetany. p. 1027. In Kirk RW (ed.): Current Veterinary Therapy. Vol. 7. WB Saunders, Philadelphia, 1980

Moise NS, Reimers TJ: Insulin therapy in cats with diabetes mellitus. J Am Vet Med Assoc 182(2):158, 1983

Oliver JE, Knecht CD: Diseases of the brain. p. 394. In Ettinger SJ (ed.): Textbook of Veterinary Internal Medicine. WB Saunders, Philadelphia, 1975

Patterson DF: A catalog of genetic disorders of the dog. p. 82. In Kirk RW (ed.): Current Veterinary Therapy. Vol. 7. WB Saunders, Philadelphia, 1980

Peterson ME: Treatment of canine and feline hypoparathyroidism. J Am Vet Med Assoc 181(11):1434, 1982

Richardson RC: Diseases of the growing puppy. Vet Clin N Am 8(1):101, 1978

Schaer M: A clinical survey of thirty cats with diabetes mellitus. JAAHA 13(1):23, 1977

Schaer M: Hypoadrenocorticism. p. 983. In Kirk RW (ed.): Current Veterinary Therapy. Vol. 7. WB Saunders, Philadelphia, 1980

Schaer M, Scott R, Wilkins R, et al: Hyperosmolar syndrome in the non-ketoacidotic dog. JAAHA 10(4):357, 1974

Schall WD: Heat stroke. p. 195. In Kirk RW (ed.): Current Veterinary Therapy. Vol. 7. WB Saunders, Philadelphia, 1980

Schall WD, Cornelius LM: Diabetes mellitus. Vet Clin N Am 7(3):613, 1977

Sherding RG: Hepatic encephalopathy in the dog. Compend Contin Ed Pract Vet 1(1):55, 1979

Sherding RG, Meuten DJ: Primary hypoparathyroidism in the dog. J Am Vet Med Assoc 176(5):439, 1980

Siegel ET: Endocrine Diseases of the Dog. Lea & Febinger, Philadelphia, 1977

Steinberg HS: Insulin secreting pancreatic tumors in the dog. JAAHA 16(5):695, 1980

Strombeck DR: Small Animal Gastroenterology. Stonegate Publishing, Davis, Ca, 1979

Strombeck DR, Roger Q, Freedland R, McEwan LC: Fasting hypoglycemia in a puppy. J Am Vet Med Assoc 173(3):299, 1978

Swaim SF: Trauma to the skin and subcutaneous tissues of dogs and cats. Vet Clin N Am 10(3):599, 1980

Thornhill JA: Peritoneal dialysis in the dog and cat: an update. Compend Contin Ed Pract Vet 3(1):20, 1981

Twedt DC: Jaundice, hepatic trauma and hepatic encephalopathy. Vet Clin N Am 11(1):121, 1981

Wilson JW, Caywood DD: Functional tumors of the pancreatic beta cells. Compend Contin Educ Pract Vet 3(5):458, 1981

Wood PA: Metabolic complications of diabetes mellitus. Compend Contin Ed Pract Vet 3(3):218, 1981

Zenoble RD: Accidental hypothermia. p. 197. In Kirk RW (ed.): Current Veterinary Therapy. Vol. 7. WB Saunders, Philadelphia, 1980

10

Urogenital Emergencies

URINARY TRACT TRAUMA

I. Introduction

Urinary tract injuries may result from automobile accidents, blunt blows to the abdomen, falls, and penetrating wounds. All animals with evidence of external abdominal trauma, spinal or pelvic injuries, and injury to other intraabdominal organs should be evaluated carefully for urinary tract trauma. Clinical signs associated with urinary injuries include shock, abdominal pain, depression, vomiting, an enlarging abdominal mass, abdominal distention with fluid, stranguria, hematuria, oliguria, and anuria. An accurate history and thorough physical examination are essential to accurately diagnose trauma to the urinary tract. Figure 10-1 is a schematic flow chart than can help in the localization of urinary injuries. Specific injuries to the kidneys, ureters, bladder, and urethra are discussed below.

II. Renal trauma

- A. Classification of injuries
  1. Serious renal trauma is uncommon.
     - a) The kidneys are well protected by vertebrae, lumbar muscles, and ribs.
     - b) They are also covered by a tough fibrous capsule and are not fixed in a rigid position.
  2. Types of injury include:
     - a) Parenchymal contusions
     - b) Subcapsular hematomas

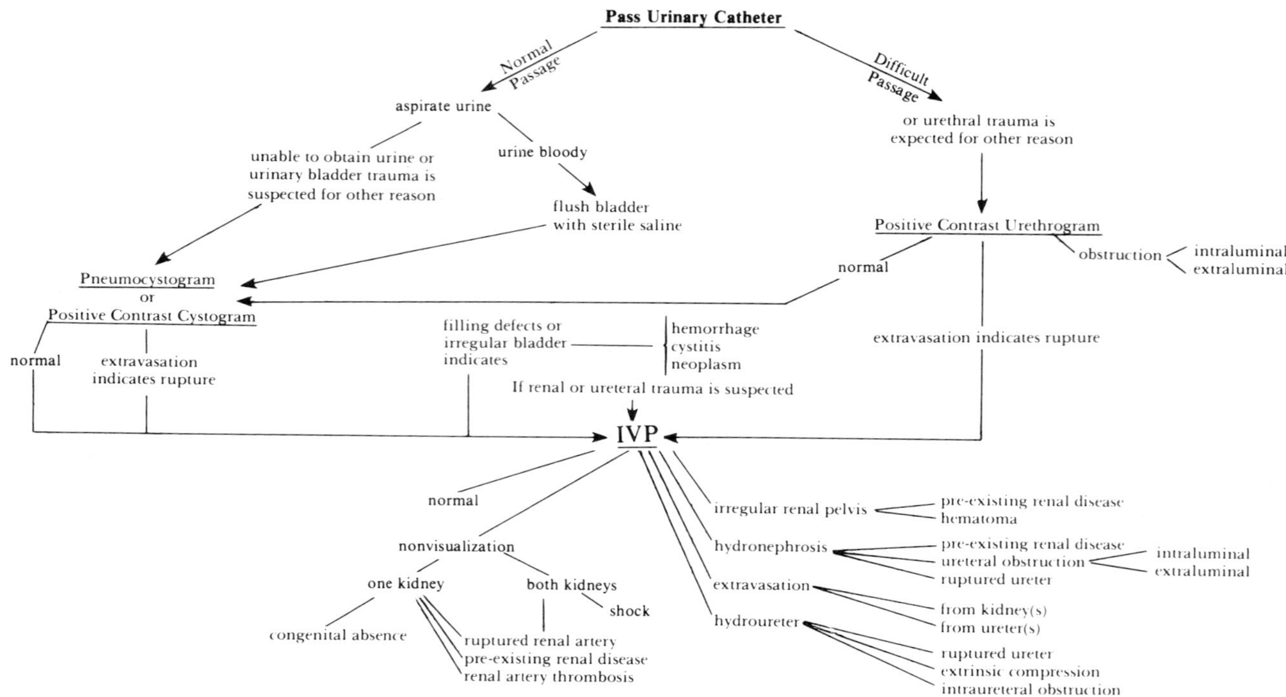

Fig. 10–1. Schematic flow chart for radiographic localization of urinary tract trauma. (Kleine LJ: Radiographic diagnosis of urinary tract trauma in the dog and cat. Small Anim Vet Med Update Series 7:2, 1978.)

c) Laceration with rupture of the capsule
d) Avulsion of renal vasculature

B. Clinical signs
1. Parenchymal contusions and subcapsular hematomas may produce no clinical signs. Red blood cell casts and microscopic hematuria may be noted.
2. Lacerations of parenchyma with rupture of the capsule produce:
   a) Pain
   b) Enlarging sublumbar mass
   c) ± Free abdominal fluid
   d) Gross and microscopic hematuria
   e) ± Red blood cell casts in urine
3. Avulsion of renal artery and vein often cause:
   a) Massive hemorrhage into the abdominal cavity or retroperitoneal space
   b) Hypovolemic shock
   c) Animal may die prior to reaching the emergency clinic.

C. Diagnosis

Diagnosis of renal trauma is not always easy.
1. Urinalysis
   a) Microscopic hematuria
   b) Proteinuria
   c) Does not localize the lesion(s).
2. Blood urea nitrogen, creatinine
   a) May reflect prerenal azotemia from hypovolemic shock
   b) May be normal, especially if the trauma is unilateral
3. Abdominal fluid analysis
   a) Perform abdominal paracentesis and/or peritoneal lavage if free abdominal fluid is noted.
   b) Analyze fluid for:
      (1) Red blood cells
      (2) Urea
      (3) Creatinine
      (4) Bacteria
      (5) White blood cells

(6) Foreign material, that is, ingesta

Note: Peritoneal fluids with creatinine levels greater than serum creatinine indicates urinary tract rupture.

4. Radiography of abdomen
   a) Plain radiographs may reveal:
      (1) Displacement, assymetry, or nonvisualization of one or both kidneys
      (2) Increased and irregular density in the sublumbar area
      (3) Loss of intraabdominal contrast
   b) Intravenous pyelography should be performed if:
      (1) Kidney silhouette is displaced or not visualized.
      (2) Sublumbar area appears abnormal.
      (3) Analysis of abdominal fluid reflects urinary tract rupture and the bladder is intact.
      (4) Clinical signs are suspicious of renal trauma.
   c) Possible findings:
      (1) Extravasation of contrast media: rupture
      (2) Nonvisualization of kidney:
         i) Avulsion of renal vasculature
         ii) Preexisting renal disease
         iii) Anomalous absence of kidney
         iv) Renal artery thrombosis
      (3) Irregular renal pelvis:
         i) Preexisting renal disease
         ii) Hematoma
      (4) Hydronephrosis:
         i) Ureteral obstruction
         ii) Ruptured ureter
         iii) Preexisting renal, ureteral, or bladder disease
   d) Renal arteriography

      Should be considered if an IVP fails to visualize one or both kidneys.

D. Treatment
  1. Primary objectives:
    a) Control hemorrhage.
    b) Combat shock.
    c) Maintain adequate kidney function.
    d) Repair structural damage to the kidney(s).
  (see Table 10-1.)
  2. Combat shock.
    a) Insert IV catheter.
    b) Begin rapid IV fluid administration.
    c) See protocol for shock, Chapter 1.
    d) Consider whole blood transfusion for active intraabdominal bleeding.

TABLE 10-1. PROTOCOL FOR THE TREATMENT OF URINARY TRACT TRAUMA

1. Treat for shock; evaluate systemic injuries.
2. Insert urinary catheter.
   a. Establish patency of lower urinary tract.
   b. Collect samples for urinalysis, culture, and bacterial sensitivity.
3. Diagnostic procedures
   a. Radiography
      i. Survey abdominal films
      ii. Excretory urography
      iii. Positive contrast cystography
      iv. Retrograde urethrography
   b. Complete blood count, BUN, serum creatinine, electrolytes
   c. Abdominal paracentesis, peritoneal lavage
4. Supportive care
   a. Treat other injuries.
   b. Fluid therapy with multiple electrolyte solutions
   c. Antibiotics
   d. Sodium bicarbonate
5. Surgical repair
6. Patient monitoring
   a. Urine output
   b. BUN, serum creatinine
   c. Electrolytes
   d. Temperature, WBC
   e. Follow-up radiography
      i. Excretory urography
      ii. Urethrography

3. Perform thorough physical examination.
   a) Assess other injuries.
   b) Note any evidence of abdominal trauma such as exterior bruises, tire track marks, and fractures of the pelvis.
4. Stabilize the animal.
   a) Correct any life-threatening injuries.
   b) Begin diagnostic procedures:
      (1) Catheterize bladder.
      (2) Paracentese abdomen.
      (3) Begin radiography.
   c) Define type of injury.
5. Institute appropriate remedies for specific renal injuries:
   a) Contusions, subcapsular hemotomas:
      (1) Do not usually require surgical intervention.
      (2) Continue IV therapy.
      (3) Monitor urine output, urinalysis, BUN, creatinine.
      (4) Repeat IVP in 2–3 weeks.
   b) Lacerations of parenchyma and capsule: Surgically debride and suture.
   c) Localized severe trauma to parenchyma: Perform partial nephrectomy.
   d) Generalized severe trauma:
      (1) Examples:
         i) Maceration of ≥50% of the kidney
         ii) Avulsion of vasculature
         iii) Uncontrollable hemorrhage
      (2) Perform total nephrectomy.
         Note: Normal function of the contralateral kidney must be ensured before a nephrectomy is undertaken.

E. Postoperative monitoring
   1. Continue fluid therapy.
   2. Consider use of antibiotics.

3. Monitor:
    a) Urine output
    b) Persistence of abdominal pain or distention
    c) Blood urea nitrogen, creatinine
    d) Body temperature
    e) Microscopic or gross hematuria
4. Repeat excretory urogram (IVP) in 10–21 days to evaluate surgical results.

III. Ureteral injury

A. Causes of injury
1. Trauma
2. Obstruction with calculi
3. Poor surgical technique, especially at the time of ovariohysterectomy
4. Neoplasms of the ureter

B. Clinical signs
1. May arise suddenly and mimic those of renal trauma.
2. May develop over several days as retroperitonitis or peritonitis occurs from leakage of urine.
3. Signs accompanying hydronephrosis may not become obvious for several days to weeks.
4. Suspect ureteral trauma in patients with a history of recent abdominal trauma or surgery exhibiting any of the following signs:
    a) Sublumbar, abdominal pain
    b) Abdominal distention
    c) Enlargement of one or more kidneys
    d) Pyrexia, depression
    e) Anorexia, vomiting
    f) ± Hematuria, pollakuria, stranguria

C. Diagnosis
1. Urinalysis
    Microscopic hematuria is common.
2. Blood urea nitrogen, creatinine
    Usually elevated with extravasation of urine into the abdomen or prolonged hydronephrosis.

3. White blood cell count

   Leukocytosis (>25,000/mm^3) is common with peritonitis.
4. Abdominal paracentesis

   May reveal presence of free urine in the abdomen.
5. Radiography
   a) Survey radiographs may show:
      (1) Loss of abdominal contrast
      (2) Irregular, streaking sublumbar density
      (3) Enlargement of one or more kidneys
   b) Intravenous pyelogram
      (1) Is usually necessary to confirm ureteral injuries
      (2) May demonstrate:
         i) Extravasation of contrast media: rupture
         ii) Hydronephrosis:
            (*A*) Obstruction of ureter
            (*B*) Rupture of ureter
         iii) Hydroureter:
            (*A*) Rupture
            (*B*) Extrinsic compression
            (*C*) Intraureteral compression
   c) Avulsion of the ureter away from the bladder is sometimes discovered with positive contrast cystography.

D. Treatment
   1. Therapeutic objectives are the same as those applied to renal trauma.

      (See Table 10-1.)
   2. Specific remedies
      a) Most ureteral injuries require surgical intervention.
      b) The location of the rupture or obstruction dictates the type of repair undertaken:
         (1) Injuries near the bladder—transplant the ureter into a healthy area of the bladder.
         (2) Incomplete tears along the length of the

ureter—attempt minimal debridement and suturing.

(3) Transecting lacerations—attempt anastomosis around an indwelling polyethylene catheter that is passed through the bladder and out the urethra.

(4) Severe ureteral damage, extensive involvement of renal pelvis or hydronephrosis—total nephrectomy.

E. Postoperative monitoring
   1. Continue fluid therapy.
   2. Consider antibiotics.
   3. Maintain all polyethylene stents for 7–10 days.
   4. Monitor:
      a) Urine output
      b) Presence of hematuria
      c) Persistence of abdominal pain or distention
      d) Blood urea nitrogen, creatinine
      e) Electrolytes
      f) White blood cell count
      g) Body temperature
   5. Repeat IVP in 10–21 days to assess success of surgery.
   6. Common complications of ureteral rupture:
      a) Stricture
      b) Hydronephrosis

IV. Bladder trauma
   A. Causes
      1. Blunt abdominal trauma
         a) Automobile accidents
         b) Falls
      2. Urethral obstruction
      3. Overzealous palpation
      4. Poor catheterization techniques

Note: Rupture of the bladder is the most common traumatic injury of the urinary tract. It is likely to occur when the bladder is full prior to injury, and most tears occur in the fundus.

B. Clinical signs
  1. Traumatic rupture:
    a) Shock
    b) Abdominal pain
    c) Free abdominal fluid
    d) Hematuria
    e) ± Anuria
  2. Nontraumatic rupture:
    a) Symptoms are delayed until peritonitis and uremia develop.
    b) Depression
    c) Abdominal distention
    d) Pain
    e) ± Pyrexia
    f) ± Hypothermia
    g) Vomiting

    Note: In the event of rupture of the bladder, the ability to pass urine is variable. Death may occur within 48–72 h if the ruptured bladder is not repaired.

C. Diagnosis
  1. Physical examination
    a) Suspicious clinical signs
    b) Bladder is small or not palpable.
  2. Catheterization of bladder

    Note: The presence of urine upon catheterization of the bladder and the continuous passage of urine through the catheter does not preclude a bladder rupture.
  3. Urinalysis
    a) Findings are nonspecific
    b) ± Hematuria, proteinuria, pyuria
  4. Blood urea nitrogen, creatinine

    Elevated with prolonged leakage of urine or presence of hypovolemic shock.
  5. White blood cell count

    Elevated with peritonitis

6. Abdominal paracentesis, lavage
   Reveals free urine in abdomen
7. Radiography
   a) Plain radiographs may reveal
      (1) Poor delineation of bladder
      (2) ± Greatly contracted bladder
      (3) Decreased abdominal contrast
   b) Positive contrast cystography
      (1) Is the most accurate and reliable method of diagnosing a rupture.
      (2) Preferred over pneumocystography
      (3) Use water-soluble organic iodide (Hypaque) contrast media. (See Table 10-2.)

TABLE 10-2. COMMERCIAL PRODUCTS FOR USE IN URINARY TRACT TRAUMA AND ACUTE RENAL FAILURE

Hypaque meglumine 60%—Winthrop Laboratories, New York, NY 10016

Indwelling urinary catheter—Argyle suction catheter, Division of Sherwood Medical, St. Louis, MO 63103

20% mannitol—20% Mannitol injection, Abbott Laboratories, N. Chicago, IL 60064

Furosemide—Lasix, American Hoechst, Somerville, NJ 08876

10% calcium gluconate—Calcium gluconate injection, Invenex Laboratories, Orlando, FL 32809

Sodium polystyrene sulfonate—Kayexalate, Breon Laboratories, New York, NY 10016

Nandrolone decanoate—Deca-Durabolin, Organon Pharmaceuticals, West Orange, NJ 07052

Stanozolol—Winstrol-V, Winthrop Laboratories, New York, NY 10016

Oxymetholone—Anadrol suspension, Syntex Laboratories, Palo Alto, CA 94304

Aluminum hydroxide
- ALternaGEL liquid, Stuart Pharmaceuticals, Wilmington, DE 19897
- Amphojel suspension, Wyeth Laboratories, Philadelphia, PA 19109
- Creamalin, Winthrop Laboratories, New York, NY 10016

Cimetidine—Tagamet, Smith, Kline and French Laboratories, Philadelphia, PA 19101

Chlorpromazine—Thorazine, Smith, Kline and French Laboratories, Philadelphia, PA 19101

8. Other laboratory data
    a) Electrolyte abnormalities are common:
        (1) Hyponatremia
        (2) Hypochloremia
        (3) Hyperkalemia
    b) Metabolic acidosis frequently occurs.

D. Treatment
1. Therapeutic objectives are the same as those applied to renal trauma.
   (See Table 10-1.)
2. Institute IV therapy.
    a) Correct fluid deficits.
    b) Improve electrolyte abnormalities and uremia.
    c) Correct metabolic acidosis.
3. Insert indwelling urinary catheter to minimize leakage of urine into the abdomen.
4. Stabilize the animal.
    a) Treat other life-threatening injuries.
    b) Consider peritoneal dialysis in those animals with severe uremia or septic peritonitis.
    c) Perform diagnostic procedures.
5. Prepare for exploratory laparotomy.
    a) Surgically repair bladder.
    b) Examine all other organs closely.
    c) Lavage peritoneal cavity generously with physiologic saline.

E. Postoperative monitoring
1. Continue fluid therapy.
2. Consider antibiotics.
3. Monitor urine output.
    a) Indwelling urinary catheters are not commonly advised postoperatively.
    b) If they are used, they should be soft and pliable. (See Table 10-2.)
4. Monitor
    a) Presence of hematuria
    b) Blood urea nitrogen, creatinine
    c) Electrolytes

d) White blood cell count
e) Body temperature
f) Persistence or return of abdominal pain or distention
g) Appetite

5. If postoperative dehiscence of the repaired bladder wall occurs, it is most likely to happen within 48–72 h after the surgery. The animal should remain hospitalized until this period has successfully passed.

V. Urethral injuries
A. Causes
1. Fractures of pelvis
2. Bite wounds
3. Poor catheterization techniques
4. Urethral obstructions
a) Calculi
b) Neoplasms
c) Soft tissue injuries or disease
5. Fractures of the os penis
B. Clinical signs
1. Proximal injuries produce clinical symptoms similar to those of a ruptured bladder.
2. Tears in the distal urethra induce:
a) Soft tissue cellulitis
b) Pain
c) Dysuria
d) ± Hematuria
C. Diagnosis
1. Suspicious history and clinical signs
2. Urinalysis
a) Nonspecific findings
b) ± Hematuria
c) ± Pyuria
3. Catheterization of the urethra
a) May be unremarkable.
b) May occur with resistance.
c) May not be possible.

4. Positive contrast radiography
   Retrograde urethrography will confirm the diagnosis.
5. Others
   a) Blood urea nitrogen, creatinine are often normal.
   b) Hemogram is often normal.
   c) Plain radiographs may reveal:
      (1) Fractures of pelvis
      (2) Radiopaque calculi in the urethra
      (3) Fractures of the os penis

D. Treatment
1. Assess and treat any other serious injuries.
   (See Table 10-1.)
2. Catheterize or empty bladder via cystocentesis.
3. Stabilize the animal.
   a) Assess renal function.
   b) Consider institution of IV fluid therapy.
   c) Assess seriousness of precipitating cause of rupture.
   d) Prepare for surgery.
4. Specific types of therapy
   a) Small tears in distal urethra
      Place indwelling urinary catheter for 14–21 days.
   b) Ruptures caused by fracture of os penis
      (1) Surgical stabilization of the os, placement of an indwelling urinary catheter
      (2) Urethrostomy proximal to the fracture
   (c) Tears in pelvic urethra
      (1) Anastomosis via pelvic symphysiotomy is preferred—an indwelling catheter is also placed at the time of surgery.
      (2) Prepubic urethrostomy
   d) Severe damage to the perineal urethra
      Permanent perineal urethrostomy

E. Postoperative monitoring
1. Continue any fluid therapy already instituted.
2. Consider antibiotics.

3. Maintain urethral patency with an indwelling catheter.
   a) The catheter should remain 7–21 days.
   b) Prevent premature removal of the catheter:
      (1) Elizabethan collar
      (2) Tranquilizers
      (3) Hobbles
4. Monitor
   a) Urine output
   b) Ease of urination
   c) Hematuria
   d) Soft tissue swelling, necrosis
   e) Body temperature

ACUTE RENAL FAILURE

I. Definition

Acute renal failure is a rapidly developing disease which occurs when at least three fourths of the parenchyma of both kidneys has been destroyed. Although ARF may be precipitated by prerenal disease and postrenal obstructions and ruptures, this discussion will be limited to intrinsic renal disease. Renal parenchymal disease should be suspected in any severely azotemic animal with an intact and patent lower urinary tract.

II. Causes of acute intrinsic renal failure
   A. Infections
      1. Leptospirosis
      2. Diffuse bacterial pyelonephritis
   B. Ischemia

      Hypovolemia resulting from surgery, burns, or trauma with hemorrhage.
   C. Vascular abnormalities
      1. Embolism
      2. Thrombosis
   D. Hypersensitivity reactions
      1. Anaphylaxis
      2. Vasculitis

- E. Nephrotoxins
  - 1. Drugs
    - a) Aminoglycosides
    - b) Sulfonamides
    - c) Amphotericin
    - d) Methoxyflurane
  - 2. Organic compounds
    - a) Ethylene glycol
    - b) Carbon tetrachloride
    - c) Trichloroethylene
  - 3. Heavy metals
    - a) Bismuth
    - b) Uranium
    - c) Arsenic
    - d) Lead
    - e) Silicone
    - f) Mercury
  - 4. Pigments
    - a) Myoglobin
    - b) Hemoglobin
  - 5. Others
    - a) Iodides
    - b) Hypercalcemia

III. Clinical signs
- A. Weakness
- B. Depression
- C. Anorexia
- D. Vomiting
- E. Uremic odor to breath
- F. Uremic frost or ulcers in mouth
- G. Anuria or oliguria with fixed urine specific gravity

IV. Diagnosis
- A. Obtain an accurate history.

  Attempt to document potential exposure to:
  - 1. Nephrotoxins
  - 2. Infectious diseases
  - 3. Trauma
  - 4. Preexisting systemic diseases
  - 5. Allergies

B. Laboratory data
  1. The following are classically very elevated:
     a) Blood urea nitrogen
     b) Creatinine
     c) Serum phosphorous
     d) Serum potassium
  2. Serum calcium
     a) Elevated during calcium nephropathy
     b) May be normal or reduced in other forms of renal failure
  3. Metabolic acidosis is common
  4. Urinalysis
     a) Isothenuria
     b) ± Proteinuria
     c) Granular and/or cellular casts are common.
     d) Calcium oxalate crystals in urine sediment are very suggestive of ethylene glycol toxicity.
     e) Urine sodium concentration is often high (>40 mEq/L).
     f) Urinary creatinine/plasma ratio is low (<10 : 1).

C. Define cause of renal failure.
  1. History
  2. Serology
  3. Bacterial culturing of urine
  4. Dark-field examination of the urine
  5. Biopsy of kidney
     a) Examination under polarized light for calcium oxalate crystals
     b) Histopathology
     c) Electron microscopy
     d) Culture and sensitivity

D. Differentiate from chronic renal failure
  1. Many forms of ARF are potentially reversible. Chronic renal failure is usually progressive and irreversible.
  2. In contrast to ARF, chronic renal failure is usually characterized by:
     a) Polyuria, polydipsia
     b) Weight loss

c) Nonregenerative anemia
d) Osteomalacia
e) Small, irregular kidneys

V. Treatment
A. Primary objectives:
1. Correct dehydration.
2. Correct acid-base and electrolyte abnormalities.
3. Remove or reverse the cause.
4. Maintain improved renal function while repair processes begin.

B. Treat shock and other life-threatening problems.
1. Control hemorrhage.
2. Combat anaphylaxis.
3. Withdraw all nephrotoxic drugs and chemicals.
4. Insert IV catheter.
5. Collect all diagnostic blood samples.

C. Ensure patent urinary tract.
1. Catheterize if necessary.
2. Collect urine for analysis and culture.

D. Begin fluid therapy.
1. Calculate volume deficits:
Need (L) = % dehydration × body weight (kg) × 1 liter + losses from vomiting and diarrhea
2. Fluids of choice:
a) Normal saline—if K^+ or Ca^{+2} are increased
b) Multiple electrolyte solution—if electrolytes are normal
3. Replace need within first 4–6 h.
4. Watch for evidence of improved hydration and adequate fluid replacement:
a) Improved skin turgor
b) Packed cell volume and TS return to normal.
c) Central venous pressure is normalized.
(See Table 10-3.)

E. Consider use of osmotic diurectics.
1. Indications
a) As a prophylactic measure prior to onset of ARF in patients with anuria

TABLE 10-3. PROTOCOL FOR THE TREATMENT OF ACUTE RENAL FAILURE

1. Assure patent urinary tract.
   a. Insert urinary catheter.
   b. Collect urine for urinalysis, culture, and bacterial sensitivity.
2. Insert IV catheter
   a. Treat shock.
   b. Correct volume deficits—multiple electrolyte solutions or normal saline, 10–20 ml/kg IV q2–4h.
3. Collect diagnostic samples.
   a. Complete blood count, biochemical profile
   b. Blood gas determinations
   c. Leptospirosis titer
4. Consider ECG and survey radiographs of abdomen and chest.
5. Start diuresis
   a. 10% D/W
   b. 20% mannitol
   c. Furosemide
6. Treat or remove specific cause.
   a. Ethyl alcohol for ethylene glycol poisoning
   b. BAL (dimercaprol) for arsenic poisoning
   c. Calcium versenate for lead poisoning
7. Start supportive care.
   a. Hyperkalemia
      i. IV fluids with dextrose
      ii. Sodium bicarbonate
      iii. 10% calcium gluconate
      iv. Sodium polystyrene sulfonate
   b. Metabolic acidosis—sodium bicarbonate
   c. Hypocalcemia associated with ethylene glycol toxicity—10% calcium gluconate
   d. General supportive care
      i. Antibiotics
      ii. High-caloric foods
      iii. Anabolic steroids
      iv. Oral phosphate binders
      v. Antiemetics
8. Complete diagnostic workup
   a. Excretory urography
   b. Renal biopsy
9. Patient monitoring
   a. Urine output
   b. PCV, TS
   c. BUN, serum creatinine, and electrolytes
   d. CVP
   e. Blood gases
   f. ECG
10. Consider peritoneal dialysis in case of
   a. Anuria
   b. Severe hyperkalemia
   c. Patient unresponsive to IV therapy

b) As an adjunct therapy to improve renal function in animals with oliguric or polyuric ARF
c) Use with caution in oliguric patients because hypervolemia with secondary pulmonary edema may arise.

2. Types of diuretics
   a) Ten percent D/W
      (1) Diuretic of choice
      (2) Also supplies source of calories
      (3) Combats hyperkalemia by inducting release of endogenous insulin
   b) Twenty percent mannitol
   c) Furosemide
      (See Table 10-2.)
3. Discontinue osmotic diuretic if evidence of overhydration occurs:
   a) Pulmonary edema
   b) Weight gain
   c) Elevated CVP

F. Consider peritoneal dialysis.
   1. Indicated for animals that fail to improve with standard fluid therapy.
   2. Often requires referral to institutional practice.
   3. See work by Thornhill in chapter Bibliography for discussion of current dialysis techniques.

G. Combat hyperkalemia.
   1. Diagnosis
      a) Found on laboratory analysis
      b) Suspect in those animals with:
         (1) Bradycardia
         (2) Significant electrocardiographic changes:
            i) Peaked T waves
            ii) P-R interval prolongation
            iii) Diminished P-wave amplitude
            iv) Absent P waves
            v) Second-degree heart block
   2. Therapy
      a) Mild hyperkalemia (4.8–6.0 mEq/L)

(1) Replacement fluid therapy
(2) Sodium bicarbonate supplementation

b) Severe hyperkalemia (6–8.0 mEq/L)
(1) Begin hypertonic glucose IV.
(2) Start slow IV infusion of 10% calcium gluconate to combat cardiac depression.
(3) Consider peritoneal dialysis.

c) Prolonged control of hyperkalemia
Administer an ion exchange resin, sodium polystyrene sulfonate, orally or by high enema.

H. Start supportive measures.
1. Sodium bicarbonate
2. Consider antibiotics.
Avoid potentially nephrotoxic antibiotics that is, cephalosporins, aminoglycosides, sulfonamides.
3. Begin antidotes to specific nephrotoxins.
See Chapter 15 for specific therapy of ethylene glycol, arsenic, and lead poisoning.
4. Combat protein catabolism
a) Consider anabolic steroids.
Examples:
(1) Nandrolone decanoate
(2) Stanozolol
(3) Oxymetholone
(See Table 10-2.)
b) Forced exercise
5. Combat hyperphosphotemia.
Administer oral phosphate binders such as aluminum hydroxide.
6. Consider antiemetics.
a) Cimetidine effectively lowers serum gastrin levels and decreases vomition.
b) Central antiemetics such as the phenothiazine derivatives (chlorpromazine) may also be considered.
(See Table 10-4 for drug dosages used in ARF.)
7. Institute high-caloric and protein-restricted diet.

TABLE 10-4. DRUG DOSAGES USED IN THE TREATMENT OF ACUTE RENAL FAILURE

Drug	Dosage
10% D/W	20 ml/kg alternated with 20 ml/kg normal saline or lactated Ringer's solutions IV q6–8h
20% mannitol	5–10 ml/kg over 30 min; single dose only
Furosemide	Initial dose: 2–4 mg/kg IV. If no response (second and third doses): 4–8 mg/kg IV
Sodium bicarbonate	1–2 mEq/kg IV q12–24h
10% calcium gluconate	0.5 ml/kg IV slowly
Sodium polystyrene sulfonate	Dog: 8–15 g PO q8h
Nandrolone decanoate	5 mg/kg/week IM with maximum dose of 200 mg
Stanozolol	Dog: 2–10 mg PO or IM q12h Cat: 1–2 mg/PO q12h
Oxymetholone	1 mg/kg PO q24h
Aluminum hydroxide	Dog: 5–15 ml with each meal Cat: 1–5 ml with each meal
Cimetidine	1.5–2.0 mg/kg IV, PO, SQ q6h
Chlorpromazine	0.1–0.15 mg/kg SQ q12h

VI. Patient monitoring
  A. Urine output—continuously.
  B. Packed cell volume and TS—q8–12h
  C. Central venous pressure—q6–12h.
  D. Serum electrolytes—q24–48h
  E. Arterial blood gases q12–24h
  F. Blood urea nitrogen, creatinine q24–48h.
  G. Electrocardiogram

For crude evaluation of serum electrolytes record as often as needed.

Note: The prognosis for recovery from acute renal failure varies with the cause and severity of the lesion. Diseases such as leptospirosis are usually responsive to therapy, whereas ethylene glycol poisoning is routinely fatal. Although the prognosis for primary oliguric renal failure is guarded, therapy may achieve a compensated state that is compatible with life.

URETHRAL OBSTRUCTION SYNDROME

I. Definition

Acute *urethral obstruction* most often affects the male animal. Anatomically, the urethra of the male is narrower than that of the female and at certain points along its course, is surrounded by rigid or fixed tissue which limits its distensibility. In some instances, such as urate and silicate urolithiasis, males may also be predisposed to development of calculi which are potentially obstructive.

II. Causes

- A. Most common causes are gelatinous urethral plugs and uroliths.
- B. Other causes in the male:
  1. Prostatic diseases
  2. Prostatic neoplasia
  3. Trauma to the urethra, pelvis, os penis
- C. Other causes in the female:
  1. Trauma to the pelvis, urethra
  2. Urethral neoplasia
  3. Obstructive urethritis
  4. Complication of dystocia

III. Pathogenesis of urolithiasis

- A. The most common sites of urolith obstruction are the penile urethra of the cat and the urethra just proximal to the os penis of the dog.
- B. Clinical data on urolithiasis are summarized in Table 10-5.
- C. For a more complete discussion on the pathogenesis of urolithiasis, see the Bibliography at the end of the chapter.

TABLE 10-5. UROLITHIASIS

Type	Pathogenesis	Breeds Affected	Radiopacity
Magnesium ammonium phosphate $NH_4MgPO_4 \cdot 6H_2O$	Bacterial urinary infections Genetic factors Alkaline urine	Miniature schnauzer Welsh corgi Dachshund Poodle Beagle Mixed breeds	Usually radiopaque
Urate	Inherited defect of uric acid transport in liver and kidney	Dalmation	Usually radiolucent
	Abnormal urate and ammonia metabolism secondary to hepatic insufficiency	Boxer Dachshund Fox terrier Welsh corgi Chihuahua Mixed breeds	
	Inherited uricase enzyme deficiency		
Cystine	Inherited disorder of renal tubular transport of cystine and other amino acids	Dachshund Other breeds reported sporadically	Variable
Calcium oxalate	Etiology not well understood	More common in Europe than in United States	Radiopaque
	Oxalate is a product of glyoxylic and ascorbic acid metabolism. Hyperuricosuria may predispose to oxalate urolithiasis.		
Silicate	Diets high in silica may be causative factor.	German shepherd Native Kenyan dogs	Radiopaque
Feline struvite	Etiology not well understood. Viral factors Dietary factors Bacterial infections probably play a minor role.	All breeds	Usually radiolucent

IV. Clinical signs
   A. The most common symptoms are:
      1. Stranguria
      2. Inability to urinate
      3. Anxiety, pacing
      4. Licking at penis
      5. Abdominal pain
   B. The owner may mistake these signs for constipation.
   C. Progressive postrenal uremia, metabolic acidosis, and hyperkalemia may produce:
      1. Depression
      2. Anorexia, vomiting
      3. Bradycardia
      4. Weakness, coma
      5. Dehydration
      6. Hyperventilation
      7. Hypothermia
   D. Extreme distention of the bladder may result in necrosis and eventual rupture. (See section above on Bladder Trauma.)
   E. Death may occur within 3–5 days if the obstruction is not alleviated.

V. Diagnosis
   A. History
      1. Repeated, unsuccessful attempts to urinate
      2. Suspicious clinical signs
      3. Any previous obstructions should be noted.
   B. Physical examination
      1. Bladder is large, taut, and cannot be manually expressed.
      2. Uroliths may be visible or palpable in the penile urethra.
      3. It may be difficult or impossible to pass a urinary catheter.
   C. Radiography
      1. Plain radiography
         a) Will locate radiopaque uroliths
         b) Confirms presence of dystocia
         c) Confirms enlargement of prostate

2. Positive contrast radiography
   a) Retrograde urethrogram
      Will locate radiolucent uroliths and periurethral soft tissue disease
   b) Double-contrast cystogram
      (1) Will confirm prostate disease
      (2) Will localize radiolucent cystic calculi
      (3) Will confirm masses and trauma of bladder neck and proximal urethra

D. Laboratory data
   1. Urinalysis
   2. Urine culture and sensitivity
   3. Biochemical organ profile
   4. Consider arterial blood gases if metabolic acidosis suspected.

VI. Treatment

A. Primary objectives:
   1. Relieve or bypass obstruction.
   2. Correct fluid and electrolyte abnormalities.
   3. Maintain patency of urethra.
   4. Remove or institute therapy for cause of obstruction.
      (See Table 10-6.)

B. Treat any life-threatening conditions.
   1. Separate animal from owner.
   2. Handle patient gently and minimize stress.
   3. Avoid overzealous palpation of the bladder.
   4. Combat severe hyperkalemia:
      a) Intubate if comatose.
      b) Insert IV catheter.
      c) Begin calcium gluconate IV slowly to reverse cardiac depression.
      d) See Section above on ARF.

C. Relieve urinary obstruction
   1. Attempt hydropulsion of calculi out of the urethra or into the bladder. Is routinely successful in cats. Is frequently successful in dogs.
      a) Technique: A large urinary catheter or cannula is inserted into the penile urethra and the pen-

TABLE 10-6. PROTOCOL FOR THE TREATMENT OF URETHRAL OBSTRUCTION

1. Establish patency of lower urinary tract.
   a. Insert urinary catheter past obstruction.
   b. Use hydropulsion to relieve obstruction.
      i. Sedate if necessary.
      ii. Backflush with normal saline.
   c. Suture catheter in place.
   d. If unable to relieve obstruction, perform cystocentesis.
2. Collect diagnostic sample
   a. Urine—analysis and culture
   b. Blood—PCV, TS, biochemical profile, and blood gases
   c. Uroliths—qualitative and quantitative analysis
3. Institute fluid therapy.
   a. SQ—multiple electrolyte solutions, 5 ml/kg SQ q8–12h
   b. IV
      i. Correct volume deficits—multiple electrolyte solutions and normal saline.
         Need (L) = % dehydration × body weight (kg) × 1 liter
      ii. Institute diuresis—see renal failure protocol; multiple electrolyte solutions and 10% D/W 10–20 ml/kg IV q6–8h
4. Start supportive care.
   a. Hyperkalemia
      i. Sodium bicarbonate in normal saline IV
      ii. Hypertonic dextrose IV
      iii. 10% calcium gluconate
   b. Metabolic acidosis—sodium bicarbonate
   c. Antibiotics
5. Monitor
   a. Urine output—watch for post-obstructive diuresis
   b. PCV, TS, BUN, electrolytes, serum creatinine
   c. ECG
6. Perform emergency surgical procedures.
   a. Cat—perineal urethrostomy
   b. Dog—prescrotal urethrostomy or tube cystotomy
7. Perform further diagnostic workup.
   a. Plain radiography
   b. Contrast radiography
8. Stabilize patient and prepare for elective surgery.

ile urethra is co. ʼpressed manually. Saline is injected into the c. heter in an attempt to flush the grit or uroliths back toward the bladder. In the canine patient, an assistant simultaneously inserts a finger into the rectum and compresses the urethra against the pelvic floor. Saline is injected to distend the urethra and the catheter is quickly removed while digital pressure is released. Small calculi may be forcefully expelled from the distal urethra and large calculi may be retropulsed into the bladder.

b) Successful hydropulsion usually allows passage of a catheter beyond the obstruction, even if some uroliths still remain in the urethra.

2. Sedation may be required to attempt hydropulsion
    a) Use all sedatives cautiously in uremic animals.
    b) Narcotic agents are preferred because their effect is reversible with commercial antagonists.

TABLE 10-7. COMMON DRUG DOSAGES USED IN URETHRAL OBSTRUCTION

Oxymorphone—Dog: 0.1–0.2 mg/kg IV	
Fentanyl-droperidol—Dog: 0.3–0.5 ml/55 kg IV	
Acepromazine HCl	
Dog: 0.025 mg/kg (1 mg/20 lb) IV	
Cat: 0.05 mg/kg (1 mg per cat) IV	
Promazine HCl—Dog: 1.1–2.2 mg/kg IV, IM	
Cocktails for use in cats	
Oxymorphone—0.02–0.04 mg/kg Promazine HCl—0.4–0.8 mg/kg Atropine—0.22 mg/kg	IM
Acepromazine—1 mg Ketamine HCl—5–10 mg Atropine—0.05 mg	IV
Narcotic antagonists	
Naloxone HCl	
Dog: 0.02 mg/kg IV	
Cat: 0.02–0.03 mg/kg IV	
Levallorphan tartrate	
Dog: 0.02–0.2 mg/kg IV	
Cat: 0.22–0.45 mg/kg IV	
Sodium bicarbonate—1–2 mEq/kg q12–24h PRN	
10% calcium gluconate 0.5 ml/kg IV slowly up to 10 ml	

Examples:
(1) Oxymorphone
(2) Fentanyl-droperidol
(See Tables 10-7 and 10-8.)

c) Promazine tranquilizers may be used if the animal is not hypotensive.
d) Avoid barbiturates in depressed animals.
e) Agents such as ketamine that are excreted in the urine should also be avoided unless patency of the urethra is achieved and the animal is not uremic.

3. Emergency surgical procedures
    a) May be undertaken if hydropulsion fails to relieve the obstruction.
    b) Empty bladder via cystocentesis as often as necessary while preparing for surgery.
    c) Stabilize the animal medically with fluid therapy.
    d) Emergency procedures to consider:
        (1) Cat—perineal urethrostomy
        (2) Dog
            i) Prescrotal urethrostomy
            ii) Tube cystotomy
4. Collect urine sample for analysis and culture.

D. Maintain patency of urethra.
    1. Suture urinary catheter in place.

TABLE 10-8. COMMERCIAL PRODUCTS FOR USE IN URETHRAL OBSTRUCTIONS

Oxymorphone—Numorphan, Endo Laboratories, Garden City, NY 11530
Fentanyl-droperidol—Innovar Vet, Pitman-Moore, Washington Crossing, NJ 08560
Acepromazine HCl—Acepromazine, Fort Dodge Laboratories, Fort Dodge, IA 50501
Promazine HCl—Sparine, Wyeth Laboratories, Philadelphia, PA 19101
Ketamine—Vetalar, Parke-Davis, Morris Plains, NJ 07950
Naloxone HCl—Narcan, Endo Laboratories, Garden City, NY 11530
Levallorphan tartrate—Lorfan, Roche Laboratories, Nutley, NJ 07110

2. Controversy exists concerning the use of open indwelling catheters in male cats (see Lees et al., works in Bibliography).
3. Indwelling catheters should be reserved for cats with poor urine streams or repeated obstructions. In the author's experience, it is often necessary to resort to their use.

E. Begin medical therapy.
   1. Collect all laboratory samples.
   2. Institute SQ fluids in the alert and minimally dehydrated animal.
   3. Begin IV fluid therapy in uremic animals.
      a) Use multiple electrolyte solutions or normal saline to correct dehydration.
      b) Consider osmotic diuretics once the animal is rehydrated, especially if ARF is present.
   4. Combat hyperkalemia as discussed in ARF section of this chapter.
   5. Consider sodium bicarbonate supplementation for severe metabolic acidosis.
   6. Consider antibiotic therapy.

F. Perform further diagnostic tests.
   1. Delay diagnostic tests until the animal is stable.
   2. Examples:
      a) Plain radiography
      b) Contrast radiography

G. Stabilize the patient and prepare for elective, corrective surgery.

VII. Patient monitoring

A. Urine output
   1. Monitor continuously
   2. Record measurements of output q2–4h
   3. Watch carefully for onset of postobstructive diuresis that often develops within 1–2 days following relief of any severe obstruction. This solute diuresis occurs from retained metabolites and transient renal tubular disorders. It may precipitate

electrolyte abnormalities and dehydration (See Jaenike reference, Bibliography).

B. Packed cell volume, TS q6–12h.
C. Serum electrolytes q12–48h
D. Blood urea nitrogen, creatinine q24–48h
E. Electrocardiogram
   1. Allows crude assessment of electrolytes.
   2. Record as often as necessary.
F. Body temperature
G. Hematuria

MALE GENITAL EMERGENCIES

I. Definition

Paraphimosis and trauma to the prepuce, penis, scrotum, and testes are the most commonly encountered emergencies of the male genital tract. Although these conditions are not usually life threatening, they demand immediate attention and prompt treatment. If left unattended, each may produce serious sequelae requiring surgical intervention to maintain normal urogenital functions.

II. Paraphimosis

A. Definition

Paraphimosis is protrusion of the semierect penis beyond the prepuce. Constriction proximal to the glans of the penis by the retracted prepuce prevents normal replacement of the penis.

B. Causes
   1. Most frequently develops following coitus
      Occurs in young dogs at sexual maturity.
   2. Strangulation of penis by rubber bands, string, ribbon, and so forth
   3. Self-trauma stimulated by chronic balanoposthitis
   4. Lacerations of penis, prepuce
   5. Chronic priapism
   6. Phimosis may also predispose the animal to paraphimosis.

   7. Occurs rarely in cat; secondary to the stranguria of feline urologic syndrome.

C. Clinical signs
   1. Protrusion of the penis beyond the prepuce
   2. Discomfort
   3. Excessive licking of penis
   4. Stranguria
   5. Reluctance to urinate
   6. Obvious engorgement of penis
   7. Secondary signs from injury to penis:
      a) Mild drying
      b) Edema, excoriation
      c) Gangrene
      d) Necrosis

D. Diagnosis
   1. Classic clinical signs and physical findings
   2. History

E. Treatment
   1. Objectives:
      a) Control hemorrhage.
      b) Examine for systemic injuries.
      c) Sedate animal and replace penis.
      d) Maintain patency of lower urinary tract.
      e) Remove the cause, prevent recurrence.
   2. Control hemorrhage.
      a) Apply pressure and/or cold compresses to bleeding penis or prepuce.
      b) Combat shock if present.
   3. Perform thorough physical examination.
      a) Note trauma to other external genitalia.
      b) Determine patency of urinary tract.
      c) Determine underlying cause(s) of paraphimosis.
   4. Sedate or anesthetize animal.
      a) Wash penis with mild surgical soap and lukewarm water.
      b) Manually replace penis into prepuce.

   c) If necessary, incise the prepuce to enlarge the orifice, then replace the penis. (See Table 10-9.)

5. Maintain urethral patency.
   a) If the penis is severely traumatized:
      (1) Debride necrotic tissue.
      (2) Insert and suture urinary catheter in place.
      (3) Replace penis.
   b) If the urethra is damaged:
      (1) Perform partial amputation of penis.
      (2) Reconstruct urethral opening.
      (3) Insert and suture urinary catheter in place.

TABLE 10-9. PROTOCOL FOR THE TREATMENT OF MALE GENITAL EMERGENCIES

1. Sedate or anesthetize animal.
2. Control hemorrhage; examine for systemic injuries; treat for shock.
3. Clean affected area(s) well with mild surgical soap; keep all exposed areas moist.
4. Once the animal is stable, perform surgery.
   a. Replace prolapsed penis.
      i. Manual replacement with or without incision of prepuce.
      ii. Insert pursestring suture at prepucial orifice.
      iii. Consider debridement and amputation of necrotic tissue.
   b. Suture lacerations.
   c. Explore, debride, and drain puncture wounds.
   d. Perform castration for injuries to testicular parenchyma.
   e. Consider scrotal ablation for severe scrotal injuries.
   f. Consider amputation of penis for fractures of os penis or necrosis following protracted paraphimosis.
5. Establish patency of lower urinary tract.
   a. Indwelling urinary catheter
   b. Urethrostomy
6. Supportive care
   a. Antibiotics
   b. Sedation
      i. To prevent erection of penis
      ii. To prevent self-trauma
   c. Elizabethan collar

6. Prevent recurrence.
   a) If the prepuce was incised, close the incision in two layers.
   b) To combat phimosis and to enlarge the preputial opening, suture the prepuce closed in one layer, by suturing mucosa to epithelium.
   c) To prevent recurrent prolapse, place a pursestring suture at the end of the prepuce.
   d) Prevent erection of the penis with castration and tranquilizers.

F. Postoperative care
1. Start systemic antibiotics.
2. Monitor daily for:
   a) Purulent discharge from prepuce
   b) Evidence of necrosis of penis
   c) Ability to urinate
3. Consider amputation of the penis or reconstruction of penis and prepuce if:
   a) Severe gangrene of the penis develops
   b) Edema and inflammation of penis and prepuce fail to improve within 48 h.

III. Trauma to external genitalia

A. Classification of injuries
1. Contusions
   a) Automobile accidents
   b) Blunt trauma
   c) Bite wounds
2. Lacerations
   a) Jumping over fences
   b) Bite wounds
   c) Malicious injuries induced by humans
3. Chemical irritation
   a) Household cleaners
   b) Industrial solutions and chemicals
   c) Road or rock salt

B. Clinical signs
1. Vary with the cause and type of injury
2. Pain

3. Dysuria
4. Extensive hemorrhage, shock
5. Soft tissue swelling, necrosis
6. Urethral obstruction with stranguria
7. Superficial inflammation, excoriation, edema
8. Reluctance to lie down
9. Lethargy, malaise
10. Pyrexia
11. May seek out cool, smooth places

C. Diagnosis
   1. History
   2. Physical findings

D. Treatment
   1. Objectives:
      a) Control hemorrhage.
      b) Establish patency of lower urinary tract.
      c) Surgically repair injuries.
   2. Control hemorrhage.
      a) Apply pressure and cold compresses.
      b) Combat shock if present.
         (See Table 10-9.)
   3. Establish patency of urinary tract.
      a) If rupture of penile urethra is suspected, insert and suture urinary catheter in place.
      b) Suture all lacerations of the urethra.
      c) Perform urethrostomy proximal to site of injury if the urethra is macerated or irreversibly damaged.
      d) Fractures of the os penis may require amputation of the penis or permanent urethrostomy.
   4. Repair any injuries.
      a) Contusions
         Usually require only gentle cleansing and prevention of self-trauma.
      b) Lacerations
         (1) Debride and suture
         (2) Provide drainage if contaminated

c) Wounds into parenchyma of testes
   Perform castration.

d) Severe trauma to scrotum
   (1) Castration
   (2) Scrotal ablation

e) Chemical irritation
   (1) Lavage, cleanse site.
   (2) Apply warm compresses.
   (3) Consider use of topical antibiotic/steroid preparations.

E. Postoperative care
1. Consider use of systemic antibiotics.
2. Continue warm compresses, topical care of wounds.
3. Prevent self-trauma with Elizabethan collars and tranquilization if needed.
4. Monitor:
   a) Ability to urinate
   b) Viability of soft tissue
   c) Healing of all sutured areas
   d) Body temperature

FEMALE GENITAL EMERGENCIES

I. Definition

Trauma to the female genital tract is rare. The ovaries and uterus lie well protected within the abdomen, and the vulva is neither as prominent nor as exposed as the genitalia of the male. Four types of genital emergencies that are commonly encountered in the female are vaginal hyperplasia and prolapse, uterine prolapse, pyometritis, and dystocia.

II. Vaginal hyperplasia

A. Definition

Vaginal hyperplasia is an edematous enlargement of the floor of the vagina that occurs during estrus in young large-breed dogs. Vaginal hyperplasia may progress to prolapse or eversion of the vaginal canal through the vulva; it is prolapse of the vagina that causes most owners to seek emergency care for the dog.

B. Cause

Although the cause of vaginal hyperplasia is not well understood, the condition is believed to be a heightened response to the increased levels of estrogen that are produced during proestrus and estrus. Vaginal hyperplasia will often subside during metestrus and recur with subsequent heat cycles.

C. Clinical signs

1. Large reddish mass protruding from vulva
2. Excessive licking at area, matting of hair
3. Drying, edema, necrosis of prolapsed tissue
4. Stranguria, anuria

D. Diagnosis

1. History of recent onset of proestrus or estrus
2. Finding a large mass protruding from vulva on physical examination.
3. Vaginal cytology may help define stage of estrous cycle.
4. Be sure to differentiate from vaginal leiomyoma.
   a) Vaginal hyperplasia
      (1) Soft, pliable, begins cranial to urethral orifice, and can often be reduced.
      (2) Prolapses in a cylindrical manner, therefore often assumes a doughnut shape.
      (3) Is associated with estrus
      (4) Usually occurs in young bitches
      (5) Often spontaneously regresses in metestrus
   b) Leiomyoma
      (1) Firm, sessile mass which may be attached anywhere in vagina
      (2) Cannot be reduced
      (3) Is not associated with estrus
      (4) Usually occurs in older bitches
      (5) Does not spontaneously regress

E. Treatment
   1. Objectives:
      a) Replacement or amputation of exposed tissue
      b) Interruption of estrus
      c) Maintenance of urinary tract patency
   2. Treat exposed tissue.
      a) Mild prolapse
         (1) Anesthetize the animal.
         (2) Clean edematous tissue.
         (3) Coat tissue with lubricants.
         (4) Prevent self-trauma with Elizabethan collar.
         (5) Wait for regression.
            (See Table 10-10.)
      b) Large prolapses
         (1) Clean, lubricate, and manually reduce exposed tissue.

TABLE 10-10. PROTOCOL FOR THE TREATMENT OF VAGINAL AND UTERINE PROLAPSE

1. Perform thorough physical examination; obtain complete history.
2. Stabilize animal; treat for shock; control hemorrhage.
3. Clean and lubricate prolapse.
4. Anesthetize animal.
   a. Manually reduce prolapse; follow with temporary retention sutures.
   b. Amputate prolapse.
   c. Perform ovariohysterectomy.
5. Supportive care
   a. Systemic antibiotics
   b. Oxytocin, 5–15 U IM to hasten subinvolution of uterus following uterine prolapse.
   c. Avoid estrogens and progesterones in vaginal hyperplasia.
   d. Sedation; Elizabethan collars to prevent self-trauma
6. Monitor patient for
   a. Ability to urinate
   b. Persistence of abdominal pain
   c. Development of abdominal effusion
   d. Fever
7. Warn owner of likelihood of recurrence.

(2) Place temporary retention sutures in the vulva.

c) Necrotic prolapses

Perform surgical amputation.

3. Interrupt estrus.

a) Ovariohysterectomy

Indicated for all nonbreeding animals

b) Hormonal therapy

(1) Mibolerone is ineffective in interrupting estrus after the onset of proestrus and is not indicated in this disease.

(2) Megesterol acetate is usually ineffective this late in the estrous cycle and may cause worsening of the hyperplasia since all progesterones tend to induce cystic endometrial hyperplasia in the estrogen-primed genital tract (see Rushmer work, Bibliography).

(3) Use of human chorionic gonadotropin and gonadotropin-releasing hormone has had only limited success.

4. Maintain urinary tract patency.

a) If the urethra if obstructed secondary to the prolapse, empty the bladder via cystocentesis until the prolapse is corrected.

b) Consider insertion of indwelling catheter at time of surgical amputation of the prolapse to identify urethra.

c) Consider insertion of a urinary catheter following reduction of the prolapse until the tissue has reduced in size.

F. Monitor

1. Ability to urinate
2. Signs of reprolapse of vaginal tissue
3. Evidence of persistent necrosis, onset of gangrene
4. Body temperature
5. Warn owner of likelihood of recurrence during subsequent estrus periods.

III. Prolapse of the uterus

A. Definition

Prolapse of the uterus is a rare condition which occurs postpartum while the cervix is still dilated. It is seen in both the queen and the bitch.

B. Cause

The cause has not been determined.

C. Clinical signs

1. Partial prolapse of one horn or uterine body into cranial vagina may produce vague signs:
   a) Abdominal straining
   b) Pain
   c) Restlessness, anxiety
   d) Abnormal postures
2. Complete prolapse will cause:
   Protruding mass seen at the vulva
3. Rupture of uterine vessels may result in:
   a) Intraabdominal bleeding
   b) Hypovolemic shock
   c) Peritonitis
4. Necrosis of exposed uterine tissue may produce:
   a) Malaise, fever
   b) Peritonitis
   c) Septicemia

D. Diagnosis

1. History of recent parturition
2. Physical findings of protrusion of one horn or body of uterus from vulva.
3. Vaginal examination
   a) To diagnose partial prolapse of uterus
   b) To assess extent of injury to uterus, uterine vessels, broad ligament
4. Radiography of abdomen
   a) To delineate position of uterus
   b) To determine position of bladder
   c) To detect presence of retained fetuses
5. Others
   a) Laparoscopy
   b) Complete blood count

c) Biochemical organ profile
d) Abdominal paracentesis
e) To evaluate secondary complications and detect presence of peritonitis

E. Treatment
1. Objectives:
a) Control hemorrhage, treat shock.
b) Replace or amputate prolapsed tissue.
c) Treat complications.
d) Prevent recurrence.
2. Control hemorrhage.
a) Apply pressure, cold compresses to bleeding uterine prolapse.
b) Insert IV catheter and institute fluid therapy for shock.
c) Consider whole blood transfusions for active intraabdominal bleeding.
d) Assess secondary complications and perform further diagnostic tests.
e) Stabilize the animal. (See Table 10-10.)
3. Treat prolapsed uterus.
a) Partial prolapse
(1) Anesthetize the animal.
(2) Clean and lubricate exposed tissue.
(3) Replace prolapse.
b) Complete prolapse
(1) Attempt replacement
(2) Consider amputation if tissue is necrotic or if prolapse cannot be reduced.
4. Consider exploratory laparotomy.
a) If active hemorrhage is present
b) If extensive damage to uterus is found
c) If peritonitis is suspected
5. Prevent recurrence.
a) Ovariohysterectomy is advised
b) Hysteropexy or suturing the vagina should be attempted if ovariohysterectomy is not performed.
c) Administration of oxytocin (Pitocin, Parke-

Davis, Morris Plains, NJ 17950) will hasten involution of the uterus.

F. Postoperative monitoring
   1. Recurrence of prolapse
   2. Development of abdominal pain or effusion
   3. Signs of systemic infection
      a) Fever
      b) Malaise
      c) Leukocytosis

IV. Pyometritis

A. Definition

Pyometritis (pyometra) is most often a disease of the middle-aged or aged bitch and queen. Spontaneous pyometritis develops during metestrus and is a complication of cystic endometrial hyperplasia that arises from the complex interaction of estrogen, luteal progesterone, and bacterial organisms. Pyometritis may occur in a closed form with no vaginal discharge or the cervix may remain open, in which case purulent discharge is readily noted.

B. Clinical signs

Two clinical syndromes are recognized:

1. Slowly progressive, insidious disease

   Nonspecific signs:
   a) Polyuria
   b) Polydipsia
   c) Nocturia
   d) Anorexia
   e) Lethargy
   f) Uterine enlargement
   g) ± Vaginal discharge
2. Acutely ill and toxic crisis
   a) Often occurs late in the course of insidious disease
   b) Signs:
      (1) Vomiting
      (2) Weakness
      (3) Depression
      (4) Collapse, coma

(5) Dehydration, azotemia
(6) Hypo- or hyperthermia

C. Diagnosis
1. History
a) Suspicious signs
b) Estrus occurred 30–60 days earlier
c) Previous administration of estrogens, mismating injections, or other hormones
2. Physical examination
a) ± Purulent vaginal discharge
b) Palpably enlarged uterus
3. Abdominal radiography
a) Usually reveals homogeneous tubular enlargement of both horns of the uterus.
b) *Note:* The normal uterus is not often visualized on radiography. The gravid uterus produces a silhouette with numerous sacculations.
4. Complete blood count
White blood cell count is usually elevated with a left shift.
5. Others
a) Urinalysis
(1) Urine specific gravity often low: 1.005–1.012
(2) Proteinuria may occur from secondary glomerulonephropathy.
b) Blood urea nitrogen, creatinine
May reflect prerenal uremia or early renal failure.
c) Electrolyte abnormalities are common from azotemia and vomiting.
d) Metabolic acidosis frequently occurs.

D. Treatment
1. Objectives:
a) Treat shock, correct fluid abnormalities.
b) Start supportive care.
c) Stabilize the animal.
d) Institute treatment for pyometritis.
2. Treat shock.

a) Insert IV catheter
b) Start fluid therapy for shock. (See Table 10-11.)
c) Correct dehydration and other fluid losses.

3. Start supportive care.
   a) Collect diagnostic urine and blood samples.
   b) Correct electrolyte abnormalities.
      Consider supplemental dextrose for hyperkalemia and hypoglycemia.
   c) Correct acid-base derangements
      Consider sodium bicarbonate for metabolic acidosis.
   d) Maintain normal body temperature
      Apply heat if hypothermic.
   e) Begin systemic antibiotics.
   f) Consider 20% mannitol.
      (1) For signs of cerebral edema
      (2) For acute, anuric renal failure
4. Stabilize the animal.

TABLE 10-11. PROTOCOL FOR THE TREATMENT OF PYOMETRA

1. Establish patent airway, O_2.
2. Insert IV catheter.
   a. Multiple electrolyte solutions ± 5% dextrose
      Dog: 50–150 ml/kg over several hours
      Cat: 100–200 ml/aliquot
   b. Treat for shock
3. Collect laboratory sample for CBC, biochemical profile, and blood gases.
4. Start supportive care:
   a. Sodium bicarbonate
   b. Heat
   c. Antibiotics
   d. 20% mannitol
5. Radiograph abdomen.
6. Prepare for ovariohysterectomy.
7. Monitor:
   a. Urine output
   b. PCV, TS
   c. BUN, serum creatinine, electrolytes
   d. Abdominal tenderness
   e. Body temperature

a) Continue fluid therapy.
b) Monitor renal function, body temperature, and other vital signs.
c) Radiograph abdomen.
d) Prepare for surgery.

5. Treat pyometritis.
   a) Ovariohysterectomy
      (1) Treatment of choice for:
         i) All closed pyometras
         ii) Animals that have become toxic from their disease
         iii) Nonbreeding animals
      (2) Caution must be used when anesthetizing ill or uremic patients:
         i) Preanesthetize with atropine or glycopyrrolate.
         ii) Induce with reversible narcotic agent.
         iii) Maintain with light gaseous anesthesia (see Table 10-7).
      (3) At the time of surgery:
         i) Examine uterus closely for evidence of rupture, and if found, lavage abdomen generously with saline and consider installation of antibiotics.
         ii) Consider culture and biopsy of uterus.
         iii) If peritonitis is present, establish drainage of abdomen.
   b) Prostaglandins
      (1) Indicated for open pyometritis in valuable breeding animals or whose owners refuse ovariohysterectomy.
      (2) See works by Burke, Nelson, and Sokolowski in Bibliography for further discussion.

E. Monitor
   1. Packed cell volume, TS q6–12h
   2. Urine output, specific gravity q4–8h

3. BUN, creatinine q24–48h
4. Serum electrolytes q24–48h
5. Abdominal tenderness, effusion
6. Body temperature

V. Dystocia

A. Definition

Dystocia is defined as difficult or abnormal labor. It may occur in both the bitch and the queen, although it is infrequent in the latter.

B. Causes:

1. Maternal
   a) Abnormalities of the pelvis
      i) Old fractures
      ii) Congenital abnormalities
   b) Torsion of uterus
   c) Uterine inertia
   d) Psychological problems
2. Fetal
   a) Malpositioning
   b) Fetal death
   c) Oversized or deformed fetuses
   d) Loss of fetal fluids with inadequate lubrication

C. Clinical signs

1. Are extremely variable
2. Owner excitement and misinterpretation often confuse the situation.
3. It is essential to understand the normal sequence of parturition to determine whether a problem actually exists.

   Note: With normal parturition the mother becomes restless or uneasy and begins nesting 12–48 h prior to the onset of labor. During this time the rectal temperature often drops to 37°C (98°F). A puppy or kitten is usually produced within 4–6 hours after the onset of straining or true labor. The time between delivery of each offspring varies from 10 to 60 min, and the time spent within the pelvic canal should be less than 5 min for each fetus. Total delivery time often depends on the size of the litter and is usually 4–6 h for small litters and 12–18 h for large litters.

4. Signs of dystocia:
    a) Excessive restlessness, panting, abdominal straining, and urinating by the bitch.
    b) Active labor for 4–6 h without production of a fetus.
    c) Intervals between delivery of a fetus greater than 3 h.
    d) Interruption of passage of the fetus through the pelvic canal.
    e) Depression or evidence of toxemia in the bitch.
    f) Failure to deliver all fetuses within 18 h when the number of offspring has previously been determined.
    g) Passage of due date (if known) by 1 week without evidence of impending labor.

D. Diagnosis
1. History
2. Clinical signs
3. Physical examination
    a) Determine cause and urgency of problem.
    b) Palpate abdomen.
    c) Note mammary gland development.
    d) Determine abnormalities of pelvis via rectal examination.
4. Vaginal examination
    a) Detect dilatation of cervix.
    b) Determine presentation of any fetuses.
    c) Detect any fetal movement.
    d) Note torsion of uterus.
5. Abdominal radiography
    a) Define pelvic abnormalities.
    b) Note number, size, presentation of fetuses.
    c) Determine presence of decaying or mummified fetuses.

E. Treatment
1. Depending upon type of dystocia present, four different therapies should be considered:

a) Manual assistance with delivery
b) Stimulation of uterus with drugs
c) Cesarean section
d) Ovariohysterectomy
(See Table 10-12.)

2. Manual assistance
   a) Extract any fetus caught in pelvic canal with gentle traction.
   b) Consider lubrication of canal and the dry fetus.
   c) An episiotomy may be performed to enlarge the vulvar opening.
   d) Use obstetrical instruments cautiously because they may maim the fetus or injure the canal.
   e) If manual extraction fails, consider surgical retrieval via an abdominal approach.
3. Stimulate uterus
   a) Uterine inertia should be suspected in the animal in which the cervix is dilated and normal fetuses are presented to the pelvic canal and yet there are no contractions or only weak contractions occurring.
   b) Attempt to stimulate contractions by digital palpation of vagina (''feathering'').
   c) If no significant contractions occur:
      (1) Administer IV calcium gluconate to prime the uterus.
      (2) Administer oxytocin.
         Note: Do not use in any animal with a closed cervix.
         (See Table 10-12.)
   d) Failure to medically stimulate normal parturition necessitates surgical intervention.
4. Cesarean section
   a) Indicated when:
      (1) Live offspring are desired.
      (2) Cause of dystocia prevents medical delivery.
         Examples:
         i) Narrowed pelvic canal

TABLE 10-12. PROTOCOL FOR THE TREATMENT OF DYSTOCIA

1. Record accurate history.
2. Examine bitch/queen carefully.
   a. Establish approach of labor
      i. Mammary development
      ii. Presence of contractions
      iii. Dilatation of cervix
      iv. Presentation of fetuses—vaginal exam and radiography
   b. Determine anatomy and patency of pelvic canal.
      i. Rectal exam
      ii. Vaginal exam
      iii. Radiography
3. Institute correct therapy.
   a. Manual assistance of offspring caught in pelvic canal
      i. Gentle traction with lubrication
      ii. Episiotomy
      iii. Restrict use of obstetrical instruments.
   b. Stimulate uterus.
      i. Confirm presence of dilated cervix.
      ii. Digital stimulation of vagina
      iii. Ca gluconate
         Dog: 3–15 ml IV slowly
         Cat: 0.5–5 ml IV slowly
            Stop if heart rate increases or nausea occurs.
      iv. Oxytocin
         Dog: 5–15 U IM or IV drip
         Cat: 2.5–5 U IM or IV drop
      v. If no response, repeat Ca gluconate and oxytocin q30min for three doses.
   c. Cesarean section
      i. To save viable offspring
      ii. To allow future pregnancies
      iii. In presence of narrowed pelvic canal, uterine torsion, oversized fetuses, loss of fetal fluids, or depression or toxicity of mother.
   d. Ovariohysterectomy
      i. Offspring are not wanted
      ii. To prevent future pregnancies
      iii. In presence of dead or necrotic fetuses, ruptured uterus, or preexisting genital disease.
4. Supportive care
   a. Dark, quiet cage
   b. Sufficient bedding
   c. Heat
   d. Fluid therapy

ii) Uterine torsion
iii) Loss of fetal fluids
iv) Unresponsive uterine inertia
(3) Mother is to be kept intact for future breeding.
b) Epidural anesthesia is preferred because it causes minimal depression to both the fetuses and the mother.
5. Ovariohysterectomy
Indications:
a) Same as those mentioned for Cesarean section.
b) May be requested by owner if neither offspring are wanted nor future pregnancies are desired.
c) May be preferred if the fetuses are dead and necrotic.
d) Uterus is ruptured and irreparable.
e) Preexisting genital diseases preclude future pregnancies.
F. Postoperative care
1. Until the mother is sufficiently awake and recovered to allow the offspring to nurse, provide the neonates with heat, respiratory stimulation, and oral dextrose.
2. Isolate mother and offspring in a dark, quiet area. Provide adequate warmth and bedding.
3. Consider IV or SQ fluid therapy in debilitated or toxic animals.

BIBLIOGRAPHY

Bovee KC: Medical management of chronic renal failure: control of hyperhosphatemia. p. 1103. In Kirk RW (ed): Current Venterinary Therapy. Vol. 7. WB Saunders, Philadelphia, 1980

Brace JJ, Chew DJ: Urinary System Emergencies. p. 1042. In Kirk RW (ed): Current Veterinary Therapy. Vol. 7. WB Saunders, Philadelphia, 1980

Burk RL, Schaubhut CW: Obstructive urethritis in the female dog. VM/SAC: 896, 1976

Burke TJ: Prostaglandin F_2-alpha in the treatment of pyometritis. Vet Clin N Am 12(1):107, 1982

Cowgill LD: Management of oliguric and anuric renal failure. p. 1087. In Kirk RW (ed): Current Veterinary Therapy. Vol. 7. WB Saunders, Philadelphia, 1980

Crane SW: Evaluation and management of abdominal trauma in the dog and cat. Vet Clin N Am 10(3):655, 1980

Davis LE: Drug therapy in renal disorders. p. 1114. In Kirk RW (ed): Current Veterinary Therapy. Vol. 7. WB Saunders, Philadelphia, 1980

DeHoff WD, Greene RW, Greiner TP: Surgical management of abdominal emergencies. Vet Clin N Am 2(2):301, 1972

DiBartola SP: Acute renal failure: pathophysiology and management. Compend Contin Ed Pract Vet 2(12):952, 1980

DiBartola SP, Chew DJ: Canine urolithiasis. Compend Contin Ed Pract Vet 3(3):266, 1981

Donovan EF: Dystocia. p. 1212. In Kirk RW (ed): Current Veterinary Therapy. Vol. 7. WB Saunders, Philadelphia, 1980

Egger EL, Rigg DL: Treatment of silica urethral obstruction in a dog by retrograde hydropulsion. Compend Contin Ed Pract Vet 5(2):147, 1983

Feeney DA, Barber DL, Johnston GR, Osborne CA: The excretory urogram: part I. Techniques, normal radiographic appearance and misinterpretation. Compend Contin Ed Pract Vet 4(3):233, 1982

Feeney DA, Barber DL, Johnston GR, Osborne CA: The excretory urogram: part II. Interpretation of abnormal findings. Compend Contin Ed Pract Vet 4(4):321, 1982

Finco DR: Nutrition during the uremic crisis. p. 1104. In Kirk RW (ed): Current Veterinary Therapy. Vol. 7. WB Saunders, Philadelphia, 1980

Finco DR, Low DG: Intensive diuresis in polyuric renal failure. p. 1091. In Kirk RW (ed): Current Veterinary Therapy. Vol. 7. WB Saunders, Philadelphia, 1980

Finco DR, Osborne CA, Low DG: Physiology and pathophysiology of renal failure. p. 1453. In Ettinger SJ (ed): Textbook of Veterinary Internal Medicine. Vol. 1. WB Saunders, Philadelphia, 1975

Green RW: Vaginal hyperplasia in the bitch. p. 927. In Kirk RW (ed): Current Veterinary Therapy. Vol. 5. WB Saunders, Philadelphia, 1974

Greiner TP: Genital emergencies. p. 909. In Kirk RW (ed): Current Veterinary Therapy. Vol. 5. WB Saunders, Philadelphia, 1974

Hardy RM, Osborne CA: Canine pyometra: pathophysiology, diagnosis and treatment of uterine and extra-uterine lesions. JAAHA 10:245, 1974

Hardy RM, Senior DF: Canine pyometra. p. 1216. In Kirk RW (ed): Current Veterinary Therapy. Vol. 7. WB Saunders, Philadelphia, 1980

Herran MA, Stein B: Prognosis and management of feline infertility. p. 1231. In Kirk RW (ed): Current Veterinary Therapy. Vol. 7. WB Saunders, Philadelphia, 1980

Hunt CA: Diagnostic peritoneal paracentesis and lavage. Compend Contin Ed Pract Vet 2(6):449, 1980

Jaenike JR: The renal functional defect of post-obstructive nephropathy. J Clin Invest 51:2999, 1972

Klausner JS, Osborne CA: Urinary tract infection and urolithiasis. Vet Clin N Am 9(4):701, 1979

Klausner JS, Osborne CA, Clinton CW, et al: Mineral composition of urinary calculi from miniature schnauzer dogs. J Am Vet Med Assoc 178(10):1082, 1981

Kleine LJ, Thornton GW: Radiographic diagnosis of urinary tract trauma. JAAHA 7(4):318, 1971.

Kleine LJ, Thornton GW: Radiographic diagnosis of urinary tract trauma. Small Anim Vet Med Update Ser 7:2, 1978

Kolata RJ: Abdominal trauma. Compend Contin Ed Pract Vet 1(6):445, 1979

Lees GE, Osborne CA, Stevens JB, Ward GE: Adverse effects caused by polypropylene and polyvinyl urinary catheters. Am J Vet Res 41:1836, 1980

Lees GE, Osborne CA, Stevens JB, Ward GE: Adverse effects of open indwelling urethral catheterization in clinically normal male cats. Am J Vet Res 42:825, 1981

Levinsky NG, Alexander EA: Acute renal failure. p. 806. In Brenner BM, Rector FC (eds): The Kidney. WB Saunders, Philadelphia, 1976

Low DG: Medical management of polyuric renal failure: anabolic agents. p. 1102. In Kirk RW (ed): Current Veterinary Therapy. Vol. 7. WB Saunders, Philadelphia, 1980

Maher TF: Toxic nephropathy. p. 1355. In Brenner BM, Rector FC (eds): The Kidney. WB Saunders, Philadelphia, 1976

Maretta SM, Pask AJ, Greene RW, Si-Kwang L: Urinary calculi associated with portosystemic shunts in six dogs. J Am Vet Med Assoc 178(2):133, 1981

Nelson RW, Feldman EC, Stabenfeldt GH: Treatment of canine pyometra and endometritis with prostaglandin F_2-alpha. J Am Vet Med Assoc 181(9):899, 1982

Oehme FW: Antifreeze poisoning. p. 139. In Kirk RW (ed): Current Veterinary Therapy. Vol. 5. WB Saunders, Philadelphia, 1974

Osborne CA: Urinary tract emergencies. p. 829. In Kirk RW (ed): Current Veterinary Therapy. Vol. 5. WB Saunders, Philadelphia, 1974

Osborne CA: Strategy for nonsurgical removal of canine struvite uroliths. Proc Annu Meet AAHA 49:211, 1982

Osborne CA, Finco DR: Urinary tract emergencies and renal care following trauma. Vet Clin N Am 2(2):259, 1972

Osborne CA, Hammer RF, Klausner JS: Canine silica urolithiasis. J Am Vet Med Assoc 178(8):809, 1981

Osborne CA, Klausner JS, Krawiec DR, Griffith DP: Canine struvite urolithiasis: problems and their dissolution. J Am Vet Med Assoc 179(3):239, 1981

Palminteri A: Clinical appraisal of the narcotic antagonist n-allylnoroxymorphine. J Am Vet Med Assoc 248(11):1396, 1966

Pechman RD: Urinary trauma in dogs and cats: a review. JAAHA 18(1):33, 1982

Penney BE, White RE: Narcotic analgesics in the domestic cat. Vet Clin N Am 8(2):317, 1978

Piermattei DL, Osborne CA: Removal of calculi from the urethra of male dogs by hydropulsion. p. 850. In Kirk RW (ed): Current Veterinary Therapy. Vol. 5. WB Saunders, Philadelphia, 1974

Rich LJ, Sharpnack S: Current concepts and treatment of feline urethral obstruction. p. 837. In Kirk RW (ed): Current Veterinary Therapy. Vol. 5. WB Saunders, Philadelphia, 1974

Rushmer RA: Vaginal hyperplasia and uterine prolapse. p. 1222. In Kirk RW (ed): Current Veterinary Therapy. Vol. 7. WB Saunders, Philadelphia, 1980

Scott RE: Feline urologic diseases. Vet Clin N Am 6(3):479, 1976

Selcer BA: Urinary tract trauma associated with pelvic trauma. JAAHA 18(5):785, 1982

Smith CW, Schiller AG, Smith AR, et al: Effects of indwelling urinary catheters in male cat. JAAHA 17(3):427, 1981

Sokolowski JH: Prostaglandin F_2 alpha-Tham for medical treatment of endometritis, metritis and pyometritis in the bitch. JAAHA 16(1):119, 1980

Stone EA: Surgical management of urolithiasis. Compend Contin Ed Pract Vet 3(7):627, 1981

Thornhill JA: Peritoneal dialysis in the dog and cat: an update. Compend Contin Ed Pract Vet 3(1):20, 1981

Thornhill JA, Cechner PE: Traumatic injuries to the kidney, ureter, bladder and urethra. Vet Clin N Am 11(1):157, 1981

Wildt DE, Seager SWJ: Reproduction control in dogs. Vet Clin N Am 7(4):775, 1977

11

Hematologic Emergencies

ANEMIA

I. Definition

Anemia is a reduction below normal of the number of RBCs, the quantity of hemoglobin, or the volume of packed red cells in the circulating blood. Normal values for these parameters are summarized in Table 11-1.

II. Classification of anemias

A. Acute versus chronic

1. Acute
   a) Condition of short duration or sudden in onset
   b) Clinical signs begin with precipitous drop in PCV to 20% in dogs, 12–15% in cats.
   c) Most commonly associated with blood loss or active blood destruction.
2. Chronic
   a) Insidious or slowly progressive anemia
   b) Animals are presented for emergency evaluation only when they can no longer compensate for their anemic state and become weak or collapsed.
   c) Packed cell volume is often very low:
      (1) Dog ≤ 12–15%
      (2) Cat ≤ 8–10%
   d) Most commonly caused by chronic disease states or bone marrow disorders.
3. Can often be differentiated by history and initial value of PCV.

TABLE 11-1. ERYTHROCYTE PARAMETERS IN THE DOG AND CAT

Parameter	Dog (Normal)	Cat (Normal)
PCV, %	40–55[a]	30–45
Hgb, g/dl	12–18	10–15
Erythrocytes (RBC) × 10^6	5.5–8.5	7.5–10.5
MCV, fl	66–77	39–55
MCHC, g/dl	32–36	32–36
RBC life span, days	120	70
Reticulocytes count, %	0–1.5	0–0.4

[a] Greyhounds and Afghans may normally have PCVs in range of 55–65%.

B. Regenerative versus nonregenerative
  1. Regenerative
    a) A positive bone marrow response is documented, with the appearance of new young RBC (reticulocytes) in the peripheral blood.
    b) Evidence of regeneration:
      (1) Polychromasia, anisocytosis
      (2) Increased number of reticulocytes
      (3) MCV is increased
      (4) MCHC is decreased

      Note: Reticulocytes may not be seen in the peripheral blood for 1–4 days following the stimulation for increased erythropoiesis. This lag phase must be considered when first evaluating acute anemias. Most anemias caused by blood loss or blood destruction are regenerative.
  2. Nonregenerative
    a) There is decreased production of new RBCs.
    b) Evidence of nonregeneration:
      (1) Normal or diminished number of reticulocytes
      (2) Normal or low MCV

(3) Red blood cells usually appear normal on smears.

Note: The presence of nRBC in the peripheral blood may reflect a severe anemia, but does not indicate regeneration unless reticulocytes are also present. Most nonregenerative anemias are associated with chronic disease states or bone marrow disorders.

C. Causes of anemia
 1. Blood loss
  a) Exterior bleeding
   (1) Trauma
   (2) Coagulopathies
   (3) Bloodsucking parasites
  b) Interior bleeding
   (1) Gastrointestinal hemorrhage
    i) Ulcers
    ii) Neoplasms
    iii) Foreign bodies
    iv) Parasites
    v) Viral enteritis
   (2) Trauma
   (3) Coagulopathies
   (4) Bleeding neoplasms
    i) Hemangiosarcoma
    ii) Hemangioma
   (5) Urinary tract lesions
   (6) Iatrogenic following surgery
 2. Blood destruction (hemolysis)
  a) Congenital disorders
   Cause shortened RBC life span
   (1) Pyruvate kinase deficiency
    i) Results in impaired glucose metabolism within the RBC
    ii) Basenji, Beagle
    iii) Young dogs, usually Coombs negative
    iv) Echinospherocytes are common

(2) Hereditary stomatocytosis
- i) Congenital RBC membrane abnormality
- ii) Occurs in chrondrodysplastic Alaskan Malamutes
- iii) Stomatocytes occur in peripheral blood

b) Acquired disorders

(1) Infectious agents
- i) Dogs
  - (*A*) *Babesia canis*
  - (*B*) *Babesia gibsoni*
  - (*C*) *Hemobartonella canis*
    Pathogenic in splenectomized dogs
  - (*D*) *Erlichia canis*
  - (*E*) *Leptospira icterohemorrhagica*
- ii) Cats—*Hemobartonella felis*

(2) Toxic agents (Heinz body anemia)
- i) Dogs
  - (*A*) Raw onions (N-propyl disulfide)
  - (*B*) Methylene blue
  - (*C*) Benzocaine
- ii) Cats
  - (*A*) Methylene blue
  - (*B*) Acetaminophen
  - (*C*) Phenazopyridine
  - (*D*) Benzocaine
  - (*E*) Propylthiouracil

(3) Immune-mediated diseases
- i) Dog—classification of AIHA:
  - (*A*) Class I
    - (*1*) Intravascular agglutination
    - (*2*) Mediated by immunoglobulin G (IgG)

- (*3*) Macroscopic agglutination seen in blood
- (*B*) Class II
  - (*1*) Intravascular hemolysis
  - (*2*) Mediated by immunoglobulin M (IgM) or IgG
  - (*3*) Gross hemolysis seen in blood
- (*C*) Class III
  - (*1*) Extravascular phagocytosis of opsonized RBCs
  - (*2*) Most common form
  - (*3*) Detected only by Coomb's test
- (*D*) Class IV
  - (*1*) Cold hemagglutination
  - (*2*) Mediated by IgM
  - (*3*) Occurs at a temperature below normal body temperature (≤37°C)
  - (*4*) Agglutination seen in blood when cooled to 4°C on a glass slide
- (*E*) Class V
  - (*1*) Cold-acting, nonagglutinating AIHA
  - (*2*) Increased RBC destruction in cold weather
  - (*3*) Diagnosed by Coombs test run at 4°C

ii) Cat—AIHA

Is uncommon and often associated with the FeLV

(4) Miscellaneous causes

- i) Fragmentation of RBC
  - (*A*) Vasculitis
  - (*B*) Splenic torsion
  - (*C*) Dirofiliariasis

(*D*) Hemangiosarcoma and other neoplasms

(*E*) Disseminated intravascular coagulopathy

ii) Hypophosphatemia

iii) Primary and secondary hypersplenism

iv) Liver disease

v) Snake bites

vi) Burns

vii) Heat prostration (DIC)

viii) Fresh water drowning

ix) Neonatal isoimmune erythrolysis

3. Impaired erythropoiesis

a) Nutritional disorders

(1) Iron deficiency

Chronic blood loss

(2) Vitamin B_{12}, folate deficiency

i) Can occur naturally in the dog and cat

ii) Secondary to folate antagonist-type chemotherapy

(b) Chronic disease states

(1) Chronic renal disease

i) Decreased production of erythrocyte-stimulating factor (erythropoietin)

ii) Decreased response of marrow to erythropoietin

iii) Increased demand for RBCs

(2) Chronic infection, inflammation

i) Shortened RBC survival

ii) Impaired marrow response

iii) Impaired transportation of iron

(3) Liver disease

Pathogenesis not well understood

(4) Nonhematogenous neoplasia

i) Impaired iron transport

ii) Reduced RBC lifespan

(5) Miscellaneous endocrine disorders
    i) Hypothyroidism
    ii) Hypoadrenocorticism

c) Bone marrow destruction
  (1) Irradiation
  (2) Chemical agents
    i) Estrogens—exogenous, endogenous
    ii) Chloramphenicol
    iii) Phenylbutazone
    iv) Propylthiouracil
    v) Chemotherapeutic cytotoxic drugs
    vi) Benzene compounds
  (3) Infectious agents
    i) Feline leukemia virus
    ii) *Erlichia canis*
  (4) Immune-mediated RBC aplasia
    Etiology remains to be determined.

d) Myeloproliferative disorders
  (1) Lymphosarcoma
  (2) Granulocytic leukemia
  (3) Plasma cell myeloma
  (4) Erythroleukemia
    i) Reticuloendotheliosis
    ii) Erythemic myelosis
  (5) Myelofibrosis
    The causes of anemia are summarized in Table 11-2.

III. Clinical signs
  A. Pallor
  B. Anorexia, pica
  C. Lethargy
  D. Weakness, exercise intolerance
  E. Syncope, collapse
  F. Dyspnea, polypnea
  G. Tachycardia, pounding pulses
  H. Grade I/II systolic murmur
  I. May also be accompanied by:
    1. Hepatosplenomegaly

TABLE 11-2. CAUSES OF ANEMIA

Blood loss
Exterior bleeding
Interior bleeding
Blood destruction
Congenital hemolytic disorders
Acquired hemolytic disorders
Infectious agents
Toxins
Immune diseases
Impaired erythropoiesis
Nutritional deficiencies
Chronic disease states
Bone marrow destruction
Bone marrow neoplasia

2. Icterus
3. Evidence of bleeding
4. Weight loss, cachexia
5. Hypothermia

IV. Diagnosis

A. Accurate history

1. Onset and duration of signs
2. Note age, sex, breed of animal.
3. Exposure to:
   a) Parasites
   b) Trauma
   c) Toxins
   d) Heat
   e) Other ill animals
4. Medications currently or recently administered
5. Recent illnesses, surgery
6. Incidence of hematologic disorders in littermates, parents, or housemates
7. Current diet and nutritional status
8. Evidence of recent blood loss:
   a) Hematuria
   b) Fresh blood in bowel movements
   c) Melena
   d) Epistaxis
   e) Bleeding from mouth

B. Thorough physical examination
   1. Mucous membrane color
   2. Presence of icterus
   3. Incidence of petechiae, ecchymoses, bruising
   4. General body condition, mental attitude
   5. Presence of murmur, heart rate
   6. Systemic organ abnormalities:
      a) Abnormal lung sounds, pleural effusion
      b) Muffled heart sounds, pericardial effusion
      c) Hepatosplenomegaly
      d) Palpable abdominal mass(es)
      e) Peripheral lymphadenopathy
      f) Renal enlargement, assymetry
      g) Cutaneous, musculoskeletal neoplasms
      h) Ocular masses, inflammation, hemorrhages
   7. Color of feces
   8. Color of urine
   9. Evidence of trauma, ectoparasites, burns, exposure to heat, drowning

C. Hematologic data

Accurate delineation of the cause of anemia and determination of the prognosis is not possible without thorough laboratory evaluation of the patient. Prior to institution of any medical or fluid therapy, laboratory samples should be drawn for analysis. Laboratory tests that are helpful in evaluating anemia are divided below into three groups: those that can be assessed immediately, those that are available within 24–48 h, and those whose results may be delayed. It is necessary for the clinician to closely correlate laboratory results with history and physical examination findings to reach an accurate diagnosis. Figure 11-1 presents a flow chart for use in evaluating anemic patients.

   1. Immediate tests
      a) Examine microhematocrit tube blood sample
         (1) Packed cell volume—denotes severity of anemia
         (2) Icterus, hemolysis—may denote RBC destruction

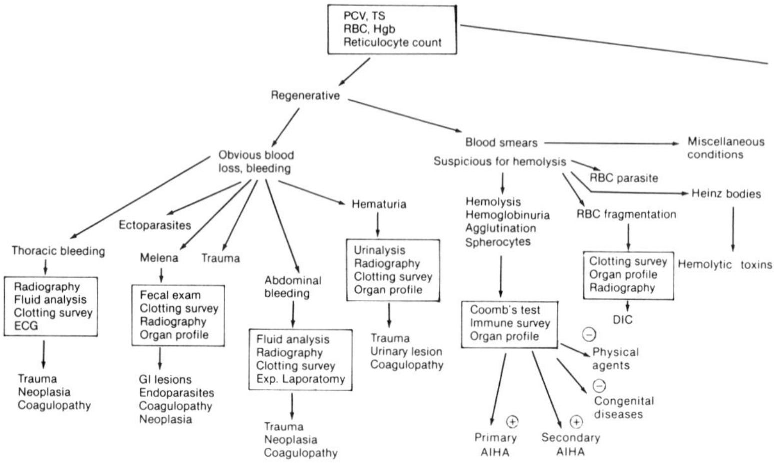

Fig. 11-1. Diagnostic approach to anemia.

(3) Buffycoat
   i) Crude estimate of WBC
   ii) Make buffy coat smears and examine for parasites, inclusion bodies, and erythrophagocytosis.

(4) Reticulocytes—may appear as a light red band or transition zone between the packed red cells and buffy coat.

(5) Total Solids—reflect level of serum proteins and hydration.

b) Examine blood smear (Wright stain)

(1) Red blood cell morphology

On a normal smear there is uniformity of RBC size, shape, and staining color.

   i) Polychromasia
      (*A*) Is a variation in the hemoglobin content of RBC
      (*B*) Is demonstrated by diffuse basophilia
      (*C*) An increase in polychromasia denotes increased RBC pro-

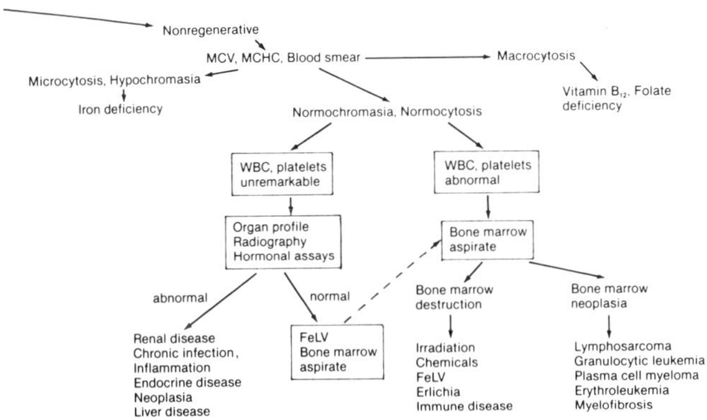

Fig. 11-1. (*Cont.*)

duction or a regenerative response.

(*D*) Greater than three to five polychromatophilic cells per oil immersion field indicates moderate to marked polychromasia.

ii) Anisocytosis

(*A*) Is a variation in RBC size

(*B*) Feline RBCs normally show some anisocytosis.

(*C*) May result from abnormal numbers of either large or small erythrocytes.

(*D*) Closer examination of the RBCs to determine the underlying RBC abnormality should be undertaken.

iii) Hypochromasia

(*A*) Occurs when RBCs retain less stain and appear paler than normal.

(*B*) Hypochromic, microcytic cells are often produced during periods of iron deficiency.

(*C*) Is also reflected by a decrease in MCHC and MCV

iv) Macrocytosis

(*A*) A state of numerous large erythrocytes

(*B*) May occur in responsive anemia due to the presence of reticulocytes that are larger than mature RBCs.

(*C*) Reflected by increase in MCV

(*D*) May also occur in megaloblastoid anemias

v) Spherocytosis

(*A*) Spherocytes are small round, globoid RBCs that have lost their biconcave shape; therefore, no longer have an area of central pallor.

(*B*) Are formed by phagocytes interacting with antibody coated RBCs.

(*C*) Increased number often reflect immune-mediated hemolytic anemia.

(*D*) Are difficult to evaluate in feline blood smears because feline RBCs are normally smaller and denser than canine erythrocytes.

Note: Old RBCs may also become spherocytes, therefore, transfused stored blood may make subsequent blood smears contain spherocytes.

vi) Megaloblastoid RBC

(*A*) Is an enlargement of the RBC

with a disproportionate amount of nuclear material.

(*B*) Occurs with vitamin B_{12} or folate deficiency due to prolongation of the period for Hgb synthesis.

vii) Heinz bodies

(*A*) Appear as pale refractile areas in the RBC under Wright stain.

(*B*) May be large and project from the surface

(*C*) Are areas of denatured Hgb that are visualized as blue bodies at the cell periphery with new methylene blue stains.

(*D*) Are increased in number with hemolytic anemias caused by toxins that oxidize Hgb (Heinz body anemia).

viii) Red blood cell parasites

(*A*) Must be differentiated from particulate debris left behind during the staining process.

(*B*) *Haemobartonella felis* when examined under new methylene blue may appear similar to the staining pattern of punctate reticulocytes.

(*C*) See Bibliography (works by Schalm, Sloss, Soulsby) for a further discussion of their identification.

ix) Rouleaux formation

(*A*) Is stacking or piling of RBCs in a linear fashion or like a role of coins.

(*B*) Is normally seen in feline

blood smears but the significance is unknown.

(*C*) Increased rouleaux formation may occur with severe inflammatory lesions and hyperproteinemia.

(*D*) Must be differentiated from agglutination

x) Acanthocytes

(*A*) Are erythrocytes that have lost their biconcavity and exhibit multiple spicules.

(*B*) Are associated with cholesterol loading of the RBC membrane.

(*C*) May be seen with liver disease and hemangiosarcoma

xi) Red blood cell fragmentation

(*A*) Variety of abnormal erythrocytes and fragments (schistocytes) are seen.

(*B*) Occurs with intravascular hemolysis

(*C*) Is common in DIC, vascular neoplasms, splenic torsion, microangiopathic disorders, and the postcaval syndrome of heartworm disease.

xii) Nucleated red blood cells

(*A*) Appearance of nRBC in the peripheral blood reflects a normal bone marrow response to severe anemia when accompanied by an increase in reticulocytes.

(*B*) May occur in the absence of reticulocytes with lead poisoning, hemangiosarcoma, hyperadrenocorticism, and myeloproliferative diseases.

(2) White blood cell morphology

i) It may be possible on a single blood smear to identify disproportionate numbers of certain white cells or abnormal/malignant white cells.

ii) Inclusions within the WBC should be noted.

Note: During a marked bone marrow response to a severe anemia, the WBC may increase to 20–70,000/mm^3.

(3) Platelets

A crude assessment of the numbers and morphology of platelets should be determined.

c) Determine presence of autoagglutination

(1) Drop small amount of blood onto a glass slide and slowly twirl.

(2) Gross clumping of the RBCs may be due to autoagglutination or rouleaux formation.

(3) Rouleaux formation will disperse when normal saline is added to the slide, but agglutination will persist.

(4) Microscopically, agglutination is seen as irregular clumping or spherical aggregates of erythrocytes.

(5) Autoagglutination often indicates immune-mediated hemolytic anemia.

d) Examine urine via dipstick

(1) Blood—may arise with trauma, coagulopathies, or intrinsic urinary tract disease.

(2) Hemoglobinuria—may indicate intravascular hemolysis.

(3) Urobilinogen—appearance in the urine often denotes RBC destruction.

2. Intermediate tests
   a) Complete blood count
      (1) Assess:
         i) Red blood cell count
         ii) Hemoglobin
         iii) White blood cell count
         iv) Differential
         v) Red blood cell morphology
         vi) Plate numbers
         vii) Presence of nRBC
      (2) Determine RBC indexes:
         i) Mean corpuscular volume (fl)
         $$= \frac{PCV}{\text{RBC} \times 10^{-6}} \times 10$$
         ii) Mean corpuscular hemoglobin concentration (g/dl)
         $$= \frac{\text{Hgb}}{\text{PCV}} \times 100$$
         (See Table 11-1 for normal values.)
         iii) Mean corpuscular volume may be decreased with microcytic anemia and increased with macrocytosis from immature RBCs in responsive anemias.
         iv) Mean corpuscular hemoglobin concentration is usually constant for most species.
   b) Reticulocyte count
      (1) Is determined under new methylene blue stain
      (2) Reticulocytes may be identified as:
         i) Immature versus mature
         ii) Aggregate versus punctate
      (3) The number of aggregate reticulocytes present is the best indicator of bone marrow response.

Note: There is an inherent delay of 1–4 days following the onset of acute anemia before reticulocytes appear.

(4) A responsive or regenerative anemia is defined as:
   i) Absolute reticulocyte count > 60,000/μl
   ii) Observed reticulocyte count (%) >1.5–2.0% in cats and 3–5% in dogs.
   iii) Corrected reticulocyte count (%) >1.0% in cats and 1.5% for dogs (See Table 11-3.)
   iv) Reticulocyte index > 2.0 (see Table 11-3).
   Note: A reticulocyte index > 3.0 is highly suspicious of hemolytic disease. An index < 2.0 indicates hypoproliferation or an RBC maturation defect.

c) Coomb's test

TABLE 11-3. CORRECTIONS FOR RETICULOCYTE COUNTS

I. $$\text{Corrected reticulocyte count (\%)} = \text{Observed reticulocyte count (\%)} \times \frac{\text{Actual PCV}}{\text{Normal PCV}}$$

II. $$\text{Reticulocyte index} = \text{Reticulocyte count (\%)} \times \frac{\text{Actual PCV}}{\text{Normal PCV}} \times \frac{1}{\text{Reticulocyte maturation time (days)}}$$

III. Reticulocyte maturation time for various PCVs

PCV (%)	Maturation time[a] (days)
45	1.0
35	1.5
25	2.0
15	2.5

[a] Insert corresponding maturation time in Equation II.

(1) Direct Coomb's test
Indicates presence of antibodies on the surface of the RBC.

(2) Indirect Coomb's test
   i) Determines presence of antibody against RBCs in serum.
   ii) Is less sensitive than the direct test.

(3) Positive test
   i) May indicate primary autoimmune hemolytic anemia.
   ii) May indicate hemolytic process secondary to some other disease (See Table 11-4).

d) Biochemical organ profile
   i) Note evidence of systemic organ disease.

TABLE 11-4. DISEASES IN THE CAT AND DOG ASSOCIATED WITH COOMB'S-POSITIVE ANEMIA

Infectious
FeLV
Bronchopneumonia
Glomerulonephritis
Parasites
Dirofilaria
Piroplasma
Leishmania
Hemobartonella
Erlichia
Neoplasia
Hemangiosarcoma
Lymphoid neoplasia
Myeloid neoplasia
Metastatic neoplasia of many forms
Immune disease
Systemic lupus erythematosus
Immune-mediated thrombocytopenia
Sjögren's syndrome
Drug interaction

ii) Note bilirubin levels and electrolyte abnormalities.

e) Clotting survey

i) Will help to rule out blood loss secondary to coagulopathies and fragmentation processes such as DIC.

ii) Suggested tests:

(*A*) Platelet count

(*B*) Prothrombin time

(*C*) Partial thromboplastin time

(*D*) Fibrin split products

(*E*) Fibrinogen levels

(*F*) Activated clotting time

(*G*) See section on Bleeding Disorders below.

f) Bone marrow aspirate

(1) Indicated for all nonregenerative anemias

(2) To evaluate presence of:

i) Bone marrow neoplasia

ii) Bone marrow destruction

iii) Red blood cell maturation

g) Other tests

(1) Radiography of chest and abdomen

(2) Aspirate of cutaneous masses, lesions

(3) Aspirate of enlarged spleen, especially in the cat in which myeloproliferative disorders and mast cell tumors may be found. This must be done cautiously because the spleen is often friable.

(4) Urinalysis

(5) Fecal examination

(6) Analysis of fluid retrieved from chest or abdomen

(7) Electrocardiogram—to evaluate intrinsic heart disease or pericardial effusion.

(8) Blood type (for canine patients)

3. Delayed tests

a) Serology

(1) Feline leukemia virus
i) Fluorescent antibody tests
ii) Enzyme-linked immunoadzorbant assay
(2) Leptospira
(3) Erlichia
(4) Parvo virus
b) Clotting factor survey
c) Contrast radiography
(1) Gastrointestinal tract
(2) Urinary tract
d) Immune survey
(1) Antinuclear antibody
(2) Protein electrophoresis
(3) Immune electrophoresis
(4) Platelet factor 3 assay
(5) Rheumatoid factor
e) Hormonal assays
(1) Thyroid hormones
(2) Cortisol assays
f) Exploratory surgery
(1) Abdomen
(2) Thorax

V. Treatment
A. Primary objectives:
1. Combat shock, control hemorrhage.
2. Treat life-threatening emergencies.
3. Determine responsiveness of anemia.
4. Determine cause of anemia.
5. Stabilize animal.
6. Treat or remove cause.
(See Table 11-5.)
B. Combat shock.
1. Ensure patent airway if collapsed.
2. Control any active bleeding.
See Chapters 6 and 7
3. Insert IV catheter
a) Treat shock if present.

TABLE 11-5. PROTOCOL FOR USE IN ANEMIA

1. Ensure patent airway.
2. Insert IV catheter, combat shock.
3. Assess and correct life-threatening emergencies.
4. Draw laboratory samples.
   a. Identify anemia as acute or chronic.
   b. Identify anemia as regenerative or nonregenerative.
5. Consider blood transfusion.
6. Continue diagnostic procedures.
   a. Classify anemia by probable origin.
      i. Blood loss
      ii. Blood destruction
      iii. Inadequate RBC production
   b. Determine cause of anemia.
7. Start supportive care.
   a. Heat
   b. Fluid therapy
   c. Consider blood transfusion
   d. Multiple vitamin supplementation
   e. Isolate animal
8. Treat or remove cause of anemia.
9. Patient monitoring
   a. PCV, TS
   b. Reticulocyte count
   c. Blood smears
   d. CBC
   e. General condition and vital signs

b) Use fluid therapy cautiously—overhydration will dilute concentration of RBC and further decrease O_2 carrying capacity of the blood.

C. Perform thorough physical examination.
   1. Assess any injuries.
   2. Correct any life-threatening injuries.
   3. Note all physical abnormalities.
   4. Try to classify anemia as acute or chronic.

D. Draw laboratory samples.
   1. Packed cell volume, TS
   2. Blood smears
   3. Complete blood count

4. Reticulocyte count
5. Blood type, cross-match (dog)
6. Biochemical organ profile
7. Urinalysis
8. Attempt to classify anemia as regenerative or non-regenerative.

E. Consider blood transfusion.
(See Chapter 1.)
Indications:
1. Rapid blood loss
    a) Packed cell volume ≤ 20% in dog
    b) Packed cell volume ≤ 12–15% in cat

    Note: If blood loss occurs very rapidly, the initial PCV may not reflect the degree of anemia and in fact, may be normal. The decision to administer a transfusion should not be based upon the value of the PCV alone.
2. Collapse of animal from severely low PCV regardless of cause.
3. Blood transfusions should be delayed if at all possible:
    a) If an active hemolytic process is suspected
    b) If blood type or cross-matching has not been performed (dogs)

F. Determine cause of anemia.
1. Classify anemia by probable origin:
    a) Blood loss
    b) Blood destruction
    c) Inadequate red cell production
2. Continue diagnostic tests:
    a) Bone marrow aspirate
    b) Coomb's test
    c) Feline leukemia virus ELIZA
    d) Clotting survey
    e) Radiography
    f) Fluid analysis
    g) Fecal analysis

h) Serology
i) Immune survey
j) Hormonal assays
(See Fig. 11-1.)

G. Start supportive care.
1. Maintain body temperature.
2. Continue fluid therapy.
3. Consider blood transfusion.
4. Multiple vitamin supplementation
5. Consider isolating the patient from other animals.
6. Handle gently, do not stress the animal.

H. Treat or remove the cause.
1. Active blood loss
a) Control hemorrhage.
b) Remove ecto and endoparasites.
c) Administer transfusion.
d) Prepare for exploratory surgery for intrathoracic or intraabdominal bleeding.
2. Active blood destruction
a) Remove hemolytic toxins.
b) Administer antidote to hemolytic toxins (see Chapter 15).
c) Institute tetracycline therapy for blood parasites.
d) Institute corticosteroids for AIHA:
(1) Prednisolone
(2) Hydrocortisone acetate
e) Consider use of immunosuppressive drugs for AIHA:
(1) Cyclophosphamide
(2) Azathioprine
f) Institute therapy for primary systemic diseases and any emergencies caused by physical agents.
3. Inadequate RBC production
a) Supplement diet with iron, vitamin B_{12}, and folate as needed.

b) Remove myelosuppressive agents:
   (1) Stop irradiation.
   (2) Stop chemotherapy.
   (3) Remove sources of estrogen.
   (4) Stop suppressive drugs.
c) Treat chronic disease states.
d) Attempt to stimulate the bone marrow with anabolic drugs such as:
   (1) Methyltestosterone
   (2) Stanazolol
   (3) Oxymetholone
   (4) Nandrolone decanoate
e) Institute chemotherapy for myeloproliferative diseases.

(See Tables 11-6 and 11-7.)

VI. Patient monitoring
   A. Packed cell volume, TS
      q4–6h until > 20% in dog and 15% in cat then q8–24h

TABLE 11-6. DRUG DOSAGES USED IN ANEMIA

Tetracycline HCl (dog)—14 mg/kg PO q8h

Oxytetracycline HCl (cat)—14 mg/kg PO q8h

Prednisolone
   2–4 mg/kg PO, IM q12–24h
   2 mg/kg PO, IM q24h if also administering cyclophosphamide

Hydrocortisone acetate—2–4 mg/kg IM q12–24h

Cyclophosphamide—2 mg/kg PO for 4 consecutive days in each week

Azathioprine—2 mg/kg PO q24–48h

Methyltestosterone—1–2 mg/kg with maximum 25 mg PO q24h

Stanozolol
   Dog: 2–10 mg PO, IM q12h
   Cat: 1–2 mg PO q12h

Oxymetholone—1 mg/kg PO q24h

Nandrolone decanoate—5 mg/kg/week IM with maximum dose of 200 mg

TABLE 11-7. COMMERCIAL PRODUCTS FOR USE IN ANEMIA

Tetracycline HCl—Tetracycline HCl capsules, USP—Purepac Pharmaceutical, Elizabeth, NJ 07207
Oxytetracycline HCl—Medamycin, Med-Teck, Elwood, KS 66024
Prenisolone—Prednisolone tablets, USP—American Pharmaceutical, Passaic, NJ 07055
Hydrocortisone acetate—Hydrocortone acetate, Merck, Sharpe and Dohme, West Point, PA 19486
Cyclophosphamide—Cytoxan, Mead Johnson Pharmaceutical, Evansville, IN 47721
Azathioprine—Imuran, Burroughs Wellcome, Research Triangle Park, NC 27709
Methyltestosterone—Metandren, CIBA Pharmaceutical, Summit, NJ 07901
Stanozolol—Winstrol-V, Winthrop Laboratories, New York, NY 10016
Oxymetholone—Anadrol, Syntex Laboratories, Palo Alto, CA 94304
Nandrolone decanoate—Deca-Durabolin, Organon Pharmaceuticals, West Orange, NJ 07052

B. Reticulocyte count

q48–72h until the anemia is defined as regenerative or nonregenerative

C. Blood smears

Note continued:

1. Agglutination
2. Hemolysis
3. Presence of RBC parasites
4. Red blood cell fragmentation
5. Presence of nRBC

D. Complete blood count

1. Red blood cell count, Hgb
2. White blood cell count, differential
3. Mean corpuscular volume, MCHC
4. Platelet numbers, morphology

E. General condition, vital signs

1. Heart rate, pulse strength
2. Presence of murmur
3. Mucous membrane color

4. Continued icterus
5. Mental alertness
6. Strength
7. Body temperature

BLEEDING DISORDERS

I. Definition

Bleeding disorders arise from abnormalities of the normal hemostatic mechanism. Hemostasis is normally maintained by complex interactions between blood flow, blood vessels, platelets, and circulating coagulation factors. Bleeding disorders may be either inherited or acquired. Patients with clotting disorders that are presented for emergency evaluation most often exhibit persistent bleeding or signs associated with acute anemia.

II. Normal hemostasis
   A. Sequence of events
      1. A blood vessel is damaged and active bleeding begins.
         a) The blood vessel contracts or constricts in an attempt to stem the flow of blood.
         b) Platelets are activated by subendothelial collagen, becoming swollen, and stick to damaged areas.
         c) Platelets begin to release chemical substances such as ADP, epinephrine, and prostaglandins which in turn activate more platelets and promote aggregation.
         d) Platelet aggregation leads to an unstable platelet plug.
      2. The formation of fibrin is needed to stabilize this platelet plug. Fibrin production may be induced via two separate, but closely related pathways:
         a) Intrinsic pathway
            (1) Occurs within the blood vessel. Is a relatively slow process. Is initiated by ex-

posure of factor XII to any nonendothelial substance.

(2) Activation of factor XII leads to a cascade effect whereby factors XI, IX, and VII are activated.

(3) The net result is activation of factor X which is the beginning of the common coagulation pathway. (See Fig. 11-2.)

b) Extrinsic pathway

(1) Requires tissue thromboplastin which resides outside of plasma for its activation

(2) Is a much faster coagulation process

(3) Is initiated when tissue thromboplastin activates factor VII

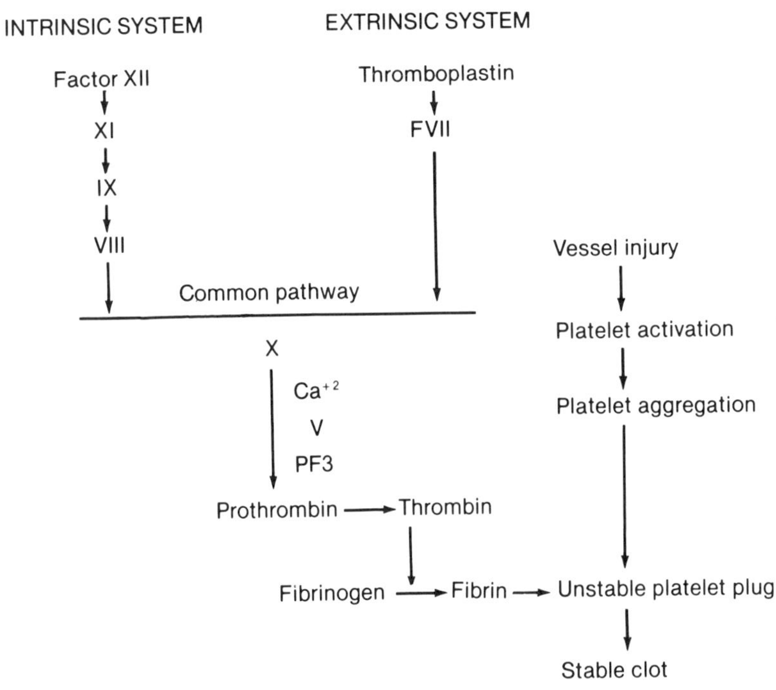

Fig. 11-2. This figure presents the major steps of the normal coagulation process.

(4) Activated factor VII in the presence of calcium ions, activates factor X directly.

c) Common pathway

(1) Activated factor X converts prothrombin (factor II) to thrombin in the presence of calcium ions, platelet factor III, and factor V.

(2) Thrombin in turn converts fibrinogen to fibrin which polymerizes and stabilizes the platelet plug.

(3) The end result is an insoluble clot.

(4) Clot retraction stabilizes the clot even further.

B. Fibrinolysis

Fibrinolysis is the active degradation of the stabilized clot.

1. Activated factor XII promotes release and activation of plasminogen activators.
2. Plasminogen activators may come from vessel walls or from surrounding tissue.
3. They are released following vascular or tissue injury.
4. Plasminogen is then converted to the active fibrinolytic enzyme, plasmin.
5. Plasmin breaks fibrin into fragments, known as fibrin split products.
6. These breakdown products are normally cleared from the circulation by the reticuloendothelial system, especially in the liver.
7. Fibrin split products rise in the circulation when fibrinolysis is increased or the normal clearance mechanisms are impaired.

(See Fig. 11-3.)

III. Causes

A. Inherited defects

1. Blood vessels

a) Primary abnormalities of the blood vessels are rare.

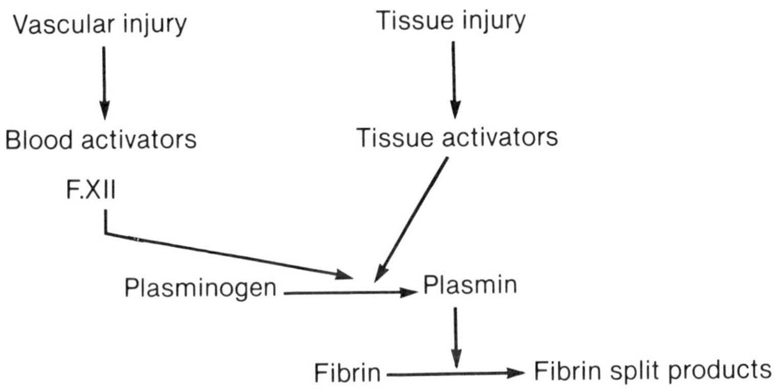

Fig. 11-3. Schematic representation of the fibrinolytic system.

b) A disease similar to Ehlers-Danlos syndrome has been reported in Springer spaniels.

2. Platelets
   a) *Thrombopathies* are inherited defects of platelet function.
      (1) Documented in otter hounds and basset hounds
      (2) Mild to severe spontaneous bleeding episodes may be seen.
   b) *Von Willebrand's disease* is a deficiency of the factor VIII complex.
      (1) *Von Willebrand's factor* (*VWF*) is necessary for normal platelet function, therefore, the clinical disease is usually a manifestation of platelet dysfunction.
      (2) VWF occurs with varying degrees of severity in a large number of breeds of dogs:
         i) Doberman pinscher
         ii) German shepherd
         iii) Golden retriever
         iv) Miniature schnauzer
         v) Scottish terrier, and so forth.

3. Coagulation factors
   a) Factor XII deficiency (Hageman trait)
      (1) Does not usually cause a bleeding tendency
      (2) Documented in cats as a laboratory finding, but not as a clinical disease
   b) Factor XI deficiency
      (1) Reported in:
         i) Springer spaniels
         ii) Great Pyrenees
         iii) Kerry blue terriers
         iv) Cats
      (2) Minor spontaneous bleeding problems are common.
      (3) Surgery may induce protracted hemorrhage that begins within 24 h of the procedure.
   c) Factor X (Stuart factor) deficiency
      (1) Reported in cocker spaniels
      (2) Clinical severity varies
      (3) Young animals tend to show more severe, often lethal hemorrhaging.
      (4) Is probably lethal in the homozygous state
   d) Factor IX deficiency (Christmas disease)
      (1) Also called Hemophilia B
      (2) Documented in:
         i) Cairn terrier
         ii) Black and Tan coonhound
         iii) Scottish terrier
         iv) Malamute
         v) St. Bernard
         vi) Cocker spaniel
      (3) Sex-linked recessive, therefore males are usually affected, with females being carriers.
      (4) Clinically similar in appearance to Hemophilia A.
   e) Factor VIII deficiency (Hemophilia A)

(1) Also known as classic Hemophilia
(2) Sex-linked recessive trait:
  i) Females are carriers
  ii) Males are affected
(3) Many breeds have been reported to have this disease:
  i) Mixed-breed dogs
  ii) Irish setters
  iii) German shepherd
  iv) Labrador retrievers
  v) Golden retrievers
  vi) Weimaraners
  vii) Samoyeds
  viii) English bulldogs
  ix) Miniature and standard poodles
  x) Cats
  xi) and many others
(4) The disease varies from mild to severe.
(5) Bleeding episodes are first noted soon after weaning.
(6) Subcutaneous hematomas, melena, epistaxis, and hemarthroses are common.
(7) Surgical procedures routinely induce bleeding.

f) Factor VII deficiency
(1) Reported in:
  i) Alaskan malamutes
  ii) Beagles
(2) Exhibit mild bleeding tendencies and an increased susceptibility to demodecosis.

g) Factor II (prothrombin) deficiency
(1) Reported in boxers, cocker spaniels
(2) May produce mild to severe bleeding

h) Factor I deficiency
(1) Hypofibrinogemia
  i) St. Bernard
  ii) Sporadic cases have been seen in mixed-breed dogs.
  iii) Severe or lethal hemorrhaging

(2) Dysfibrinogemia
- i) Russian wolfhound
- ii) Mild bleeding that is often worse after trauma or surgery

B. Acquired disorders
1. Blood vessels
   - a) Aging changes
   - b) Vasculitis
   - c) Immune-mediated disorders of blood vessels
   - d) Hyperadrenocorticism
   - e) Drug therapy
2. Platelet disorders
   - a) Thrombocytopenia
     - (1) Decreased production
       - i) Irradiation
       - ii) Drug induced:
         - (*A*) Estrogen
         - (*B*) Phenylbutazone
         - (*C*) Dapsone
         - (*D*) Cytotoxic drugs
       - iii) Chronic infections
       - iv) Myeloproliferative diseases
       - v) Infectious agents
         - (*A*) Feline leukemia virus
         - (*B*) *Erlichia canis*
       - vi) Cyclic hematopoiesis
       - vii) Idiopathic causes
     - (2) Increased destruction
       - i) Immune-mediated disease
       - ii) Infectious diseases
         - (*A*) *Erlichia canis*
         - (*B*) *Rickettsia rickettsia*
         - (*C*) Viruses
       - iii) Postvaccination with modified-live virus vaccine
       - iv) Endotoxemia/septicemia
       - v) Neoplasia
       - vi) Drug-induced:

- (*A*) Cytotoxic drugs
- (*B*) Quinidine
- (*C*) Digitoxin
- (*D*) Gold salts
- (*E*) Phenylbutazone
- (*F*) Dapsone, and so forth

(3) Platelet sequestratoin
- i) Splenomegaly
- ii) Hypersplenism
- iii) Hepatomegaly
- iv) Hypothermia

(4) Increased utilization
- i) Protracted/severe hemorrhage
- ii) Vasculitis
- iii) Microangiopathy
- iv) Disseminated intravascular coagulation
- v) Septicemia

b) Thrombocytopathia

Is a qualitative or functional defect in platelet function.

(1) Drug induced
- i) Aspirin
- ii) Corticosteroids
- iii) Phenylbutazone
- iv) Aminophylline
- v) Furosemide
- vi) Levamisole
- vii) Cephalosporins, nitrofurantoin
- viii) Carbenicillin
- ix) Phenothiazine tranquilizers
- x) Dextrans
- xi) Antihistamines, and so forth

(2) Systemic illnesses
- i) Uremia
- ii) Myeloproliferative diseases
- iii) Hepatic cirrhosis
- iv) Systemic lupus erythematosis

3. Coagulation factors
   a) Vitamin K deficiency
      (1) Vitamin K is necessary for the production of factors II, VII, IX, X.
      (2) Causes of vitamin K deficiency:
         i) Inadequate dietary intake
         ii) Decreased production in the gut
            (*A*) Antibiotics
            (*B*) Diffuse small bowel disease
            (*C*) Pancreatic exocrine insufficiency
         iii) Malabsorption
         iv) Warfarin toxicity (see Chapter 15)
   b) Liver disease

      Many clotting factors are synthesized in the liver, therefore severe, diffuse liver disease or hepatic cirrhosis may result in deficiencies of clotting factors.
   c) Circulating anticoagulants
      (1) Exogenous agents:
         i) Heparin
         ii) Coumadin
      (2) Endogenous agents:
         i) Heparin released from mast cell tumors
         ii) Monoclonal immunoglobulins
         iii) Antibodies to clotting factor proteins
         iv) Lupus anticoagulants
   d) Disseminated intravascular coagulopathy
      (1) Simultaneous activation of the clotting and fibrinolytic systems leads to widespread microvascular thrombosis, consumption of clotting factors, depletion of platelets and, therefore, a significant tendency to bleed.
      (2) Disseminated intravascular coagulopa-

thy may develop with any stimulus that activates the coagulation system.

(3) It may arise with the following conditions:

i) Infectious diseases
- (*A*) Canine hepatitis
- (*B*) Feline panleukopenia
- (*C*) Leptospirosis
- (*D*) Dirofilariasis
- (*E*) Feline infectious peritonitis

ii) Neoplasia
- (*A*) Hemangiosarcoma
- (*B*) Myeloproliferative diseases

iii) Miscellaneous
- (*A*) Liver disease
- (*B*) Acute pancreatitis
- (*C*) Acute gastric dilatation-volvulus
- (*D*) Heatstroke
- (*E*) Hemolytic diseases
- (*F*) Amyloidosis
- (*G*) Massive trauma

The causes of clotting disorders are summarized in Table 11-8.

IV. Clinical signs

A. Epistaxis
B. Petechia of mucous membranes
C. Ecchymoses, cutaneous bruises
D. Subcutaneous hematomas
E. Hemarthrosis
F. Hyphemá, retinal, or vitreal hemorrhages
G. Melena, hematuria
H. Bleeding into body cavities
I. Gingival bleeding
J. Protracted bleeding following surgery, trauma, estrus, or parturition
K. Weakness, collapse

TABLE 11-8. CAUSES OF BLEEDING DISORDERS

Abnormalities of blood vessels
- Inherited—Ehler-Danlos syndrome
- Acquired
  - Infection, inflammation, aging
  - Drug therapy, hyperadrenocorticism

Platelet disorders
- Inherited
  - Thrombopathia
  - Von Willebrand's disease
- Acquired
  - Thrombocytopenia
  - Thrombopathia

Abnormalities in clotting factors
- Inherited—deficiencies of factors I, II, VII, VIII, IX, X, XI
- Acquired
  - Vitamin K deficiency
  - Liver disease
  - Circulating anticoagulants
  - DIC

L. Anemia

M. Hypovolemic shock

N. Central nervous system signs may occur with cerebral vascular accidents.

V. Diagnosis

A. History

1. Age, sex, breed of patient
2. Description of previous and current bleeding episodes:
   a) Age of onset
   b) Location
   c) Precipitating cause
   d) Severity
   e) Duration
   f) Frequency
   g) Type
   h) Previous therapy
3. Medical history of parents and siblings
4. Evidence of toxin ingestion or exposure to chemicals, drugs, physical agents, trauma

5. List of drugs currently administered to patient
6. Previous or recent surgical procedures
7. Previous illnesses or clinical signs associated with other organ diseases
8. Previous therapy administered for bleeding problems

B. Physical examination
1. Characterize the hemorrhage.
   a) Platelet abnormalities often cause petechiae, ecchymoses, epistaxis, hematuria, and melena.
   b) Clotting factor deficiencies may also cause deep hemorrhaging into joints, subcutaneous spaces, and body cavities.
2. Examine for evidence of trauma and recent surgeries.
3. Determine extent of hemorrhages and number of organs involved.
   Examine: eyes, mouth, skin, joints, feces, and urine.
4. Note other systemic signs:
   a) Icterus, hemolysis
   b) Lymphadenopathy
   c) Hepatosplenomegaly
   d) Abdominal masses
   e) Heart murmurs
   f) Dyspnea
   g) Abdominal pain
   h) Body temperature

C. Laboratory analysis of coagulation
1. Platelet tests
   a) Platelet count
      (1) Direct method (unopette method)
         i) Must be performed on fresh, unrefrigerated blood in EDTA
         ii) Normal = 150–300,000/mm^3
         iii) Bleeding is usually noted with counts $<50,000/mm^3$.

(2) Indirect method
   i) Assess the number of platelets per oil immersion field on a blood smear.
   ii) Normal = three to four per field
   Normal = 1 platelet to 20 RBC
   (See Table 11-9.)

b) Platelet function tests
   (1) Whole blood clot-retraction tests
   A whole blood clot will retract from the sides of glass containers with a normal quality and quantity of platelets.

TABLE 11-9. NORMAL COAGULATION PARAMETERS

Test	Normal Values
Platelet count	150–300,000/mm^3
Clot retraction	1–2 h at 37°C
Skin bleeding time	1–5 min
Cutical bleeding	1–5 min
PTT	
Dog:	14–25 sec
Cat:	14–28 sec
Man:	25–40 sec
ACT	
Dog:	60–90 sec
Cat:	mean = 70 sec
PT	
Dog:	7–10 sec
Cat:	5–9 sec
RVVT	
Dog and cat:	8–14 sec
TT	
Dog and cat:	6–9 sec
Fibrinogen	
Dog and cat:	150–200 mg/dl
FSP	
Dog and cat:	<2 μg/ml

(2) Platelet aggregation and adhesiveness tests
   i) Evaluate platelet function in the presence of certain reagents
   ii) Require specialized coagulation laboratories
(3) Skin bleeding time
   i) A lancet is used to create a small wound on the planum nasale of dogs or the ear pinnae of cats.
   ii) Although crude, may be used to evaluate both platelet and vascular clotting ability.
(4) Cutical bleeding time
   i) Cut one of the nails short enough to expose the artery.
   ii) Measure the time that lapses until the bleeding stops.

c) Platelet morphology
   (1) Significance of morphologic changes:
      i) Large—are usually younger active platelets
      ii) Giant—rapid platelet turnover
      iii) Fragmented—microangiopathy
      iv) Abnormal shapes—neoplasia
   (2) Note inclusions and parasites.

d) Bone marrow examination
   (1) Useful to evaluate presence and number of megakaryocytes in animals with thrombocytopenia.
   (2) Normal = one to two megakaryocytes/bone marrow spicule

e) Immune tests
   (1) To diagnose immune disease as source of thrombocytopenia
   (2) Example:
      i) Coomb's test
      ii) Platelet factor 3

iii) Rheumatoid factor
iv) Antinuclear antibody assay

2. Intrinsic system tests

   Will detect deficiencies in factors XII, XI, X, IX, VIII, V, prothrombin, and fibrinogen.

   a) Partial thromboplastin time
      (1) May be performed with (APTT) or without (PTT) a surface activator
      (2) Utilizes citrated plasma
      (3) Controls should be run with plasma from normal animals of the same species.
      (4) When used with human plasma the normal values are considerably longer.
      (5) Any result >7 sec longer than the control should be considered abnormal.
      (6) Becomes prolonged with a reduction of 30% or more of affected clotting factor
   b) Activated clotting time (ACT)
      (See Table 11-10.)

TABLE 11-10. COMMERCIAL PRODUCTS FOR USE IN BLEEDING DISORDERS

Activated coagulation time—Vacutainer 3Z06XF534, Berton, Dickenson, Rutherford, NJ 07070

FSP latex agglutination test—Thrombo-Wellcotest, Burroughs-Wellcome, Research Triangle Park, NC 27709

RVVT—Stypven test, Burroughs-Wellcome, Research Triangle Park, NC 27709

Prednisone—Prednisone tablets, USP, American Pharmaceuticals, Passaic, NJ 07055

Hydrocortisone acetate—Hydrocortone acetate, Merck, Sharpe and Dohme, West Point, PA 19486

Vincristine—Oncovin, Eli Lilly, Indianapolis, IN 46285

Cyclophosphamide—Cytoxan, Mead Johnson Pharmaceutical, Evansville, IN 47721

Azathioprine—Imuran, Burroughs Wellcome, Research Triangle Park, NC 27709

Vitamin K_1—Aquamephyton, Merck, Sharpe and Dohme, West Point, PA 19486

Heparin—Heparin sodium, USP, Eli Lilly, Indianapolis, IN 46285

(1) Allows the use of whole blood instead of plasma
(2) The contact activator in the test also improves the precision of the procedure.
(3) The clotting time may also become prolonged with severe thrombocytopenia ($<10{,}000/mm^3$).

3. Extrinsic system tests
   a) Abnormalities include deficiencies of factors II, VII, X, V, and fibrinogen.
   b) These tests often reflect liver function and presence of warfarin toxicity because they test the vitamin K-dependent clotting factors.

   Actual tests
   a) One-stage prothrombin time (PT)
      (1) Utilizes citrated plasma
      (2) Is not very accurate in detecting mild deficiencies
      (3) The sample is abnormal if results are >5 sec longer than the control.
   b) Russell's viper venon time test (RVVT)
      (1) Is used to differentiate factor VII deficiency from other extrinsic abnormalities
      (2) Also assesses platelet function
      (3) Measures factors I, II, V, X, and platelets
      (4) Does not measure factor VII
      (5) A patient with a normal RVVT and prolonged PT has a factor VII deficiency.
      (6) Utilizes citrated plasma
4. Individual tests
   a) Thrombin time (TT)
      (1) Utilizes citrated plasma
      (2) Measures the reactivity of fibrinogen to thrombin
      (3) Is independent of intrinsic and extrinsic factors
      (4) Is prolonged by abnormalities of fibrinogen

b) Fibrinogen assay
   (1) Is the only coagulation factor present in high enough quantities to be routinely measured.
   (2) Decreased levels are seen in:
      i) Liver disease
      ii) Disseminated intravascular coagulopathy
      iii) Hereditary hypofibrinogenemia
c) Fibrin split products (FSP)
   (See Table 11-10.)
   (1) Increased levels (>10 μg/ml) of FSP usually reflect increased fibrinolysis.
   (2) The half-life of FSP is approximately 9–12 h.
   (3) Increased levels of FSP are suggestive, although not specific for DIC.
d) Individual factor survey
   (1) Certain coagulation laboratories* are capable of assaying for individual clotting factors.
   (2) It is often necessary to take advantage of this service in diagnosing specific inherited factor deficiencies.
   (3) One of the most common factors assayed is factor VIII.
   (4) Factor VIII has three distinct components:
      i) Immunologically active portion = factor VIII:related antigen (FVIII:RA)
      ii) Biologically active portion = factor VIII:coagulant (FVIII:C)
      iii) Platelet function—related portion = factor VIII:von Willebrand's factor (FVIII:VWF)

* W. Jean Dodds, DVM, Division of Laboratories and Research, New York State Department of Health, Albany, New York, 12201.

In Hemophilia A, FVIII:RA is normal or increased and FVIII:C is decreased; in Von Willebrand's disease both FVIII:RA and FVIII:C are decreased and FVIII:VWF is decreased or absent.

Figure 11-4 provides a diagnostic approach to bleeding disorders.

D. Other laboratory tests
   1. Complete blood count, reticulocyte count
   2. Blood smear
      Evaluate for RBC and platelet morphology.
   3. Biochemical profile
   4. Urinalysis
   5. Bone marrow aspirate
   6. Blood type
   7. Immunologic survey

VI. Treatment
   A. Primary objectives:
      1. Combat shock
      2. Control hemorrhage
      3. Classify type of clotting disorder
      4. Institute specific therapy for coagulopathy.
         Remove cause.
      5. Start supportive care.
         (See Table 11-11.)
   B. Combat shock.
      1. Ensure patent airway if collapsed
      2. Insert large-gauge IV catheter
         a) Institute fluid therapy.
         b) Consider glucocorticoid administration.
   C. Control hemorrhage.
      1. Direct pressure, pressure bandages.
      2. Arterial ligation
      3. Topical epinephrine, hemostatics
      4. Consider whole blood transfusion:
         a) For rapid decline in PCV ≤20% in the dog and ≤12–15% in the cat
         b) For active, persistent bleeding
      5. Draw diagnostic blood samples first.

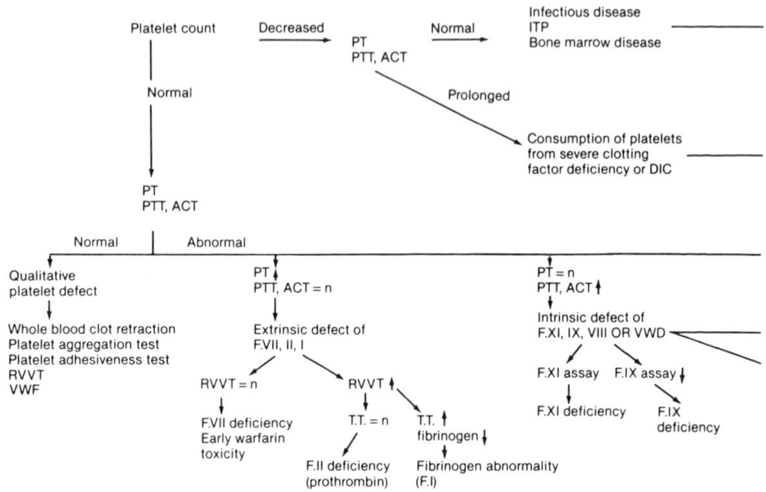

Fig. 11-4. Diagnostic approach to clotting disorders. ↑ = prolonged or increased; n = normal; ↓ = decreased.

D. Perform thorough physical examination.
   1. Determine extent of multiple organ involvement.
   2. Characterize type of hemorrhage.
   3. Note other contributing illnesses.

E. Classify type of clotting disorder.
   1. Draw laboratory samples
   2. Clotting survey:
      a) Platelet count
      b) Prothrombin time
      c) Fibrin split products
      d) Partial thromboplastin time or ACT
      e) Fibrinogen
   3. Blood type
   4. Complete blood count, retriculocyte count
   5. Subdivide disorder into likely origin:
      a) Disorder of blood vessels
      b) Platelet abnormality
      c) Abnormality of clotting factors

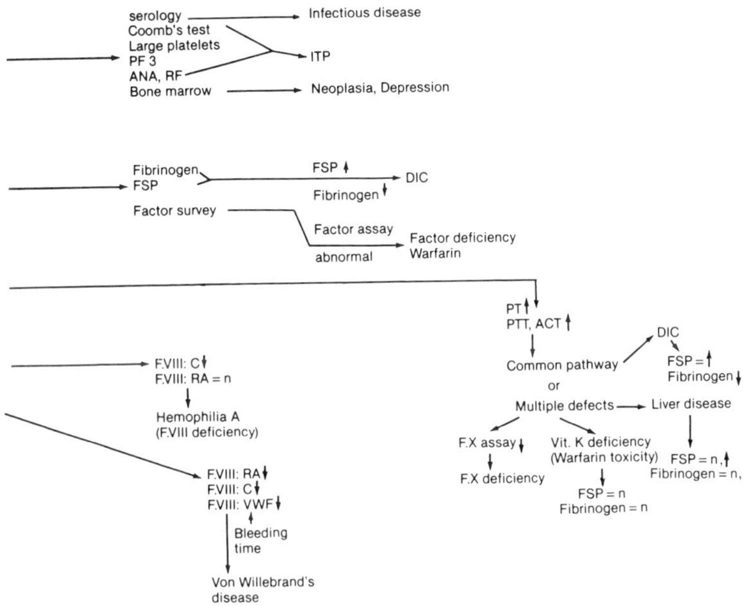

Fig. 11-4. (*Cont.*)

   d) Disseminated intravascular coagulopathy
   e) Inherited versus acquired
   (See Fig. 11-4.)
6. Perform secondary diagnostic tests.
   a) Examine blood smear for RBC and platelet morphology
   b) Biochemical organ profile
   c) Immune survey
   d) Clotting factor assay
   e) Platelet function tests
   f) Russell's viper venom time, TT
   g) Bone marrow aspirate
   h) Serology
7. From interpretation of laboratory data, determine cause of clotting disorder.

F. Institute specific therapy.
   1. Remove all anticoagulants.

TABLE 11-11. PROTOCOL FOR BLEEDING DISORDERS

1. Ensure patent airway.
2. Insert IV catheter, treat shock.
3. Control hemorrhage.
4. Perform thorough physical examination.
5. Draw initial laboratory samples.
   a. Clotting survey
      Platelet count
      PT, PTT, or ACT
      FSP
      Fibrinogen
   b. CBC, reticulocyte count
   c. Blood type
6. Classify clotting disorder by probable origin.
   a. Blood vessel abnormality
   b. Platelet disorder
   c. Clotting factor abnormality
   d. DIC
7. Stabilize the animal.
   a. Consider blood transfusion.
   b. Continue diagnostic tests.
   c. Remove inciting causes or contributing factors.
   d. Start supportive care.
8. Institute specific therapy.
   a. Replacement therapy
      i. Whole blood
      ii. Fresh or frozen plasma
      iii. Plasma cryoprecipitates
   b. Immune therapy
   c. Vitamin K_1 supplementation
   d. Coagulation inhibitors for DIC
9. Patient monitoring
   a. PCV, TS
   b. Clotting survey
   c. Signs of continued bleeding
   d. Vital signs

2. Terminate all antiplatelet drugs.
3. Stop all bone marrow depressants.
4. Platelet disorders
   a) Replacement therapy
      (1) Fresh whole blood
         i) Blood should be <8 h old.

- ii) Collect blood in plastic bags.
- iii) Do not refrigerate.
- iv) Give without a filter.
- v) Twelve to 20 ml/kg IV
- vi) Two hundred and fifty milliliters of blood supplies approximately 50 million platelets.

(2) Platelet-rich plasma

- i) Centrifuge fresh acid citrate dextrose blood at 1,500 rpm for 3–5 min.
- ii) Draw off plasma.
- iii) Six to 10 ml/kg IV BID is preferred if other components of whole blood are not needed.

b) Immune therapy

(1) Corticosteroids

- i) Prednisone
- ii) Hydrocortisone acetate

(2) Vincristine

(3) For refractory cases consider:

- i) Azathioprine
- ii) Cyclophosphamide
  - (*A*) Must be used cautiously
  - (*B*) Chemical-induced cystitis may induce hematuria.
- iii) Splenectomy

(See Tables 11-10 and 11-12.)

5. Clotting factor abnormalities

a) Replacement therapy

(1) Whole blood

- i) Indicated for bleeding severe enough to cause anemia
- ii) Indicated for factor XI deficiency
- iii) Twelve to 20 ml/kg IV

(2) Plasma

- i) Fresh or frozen
- ii) Indicated for:

TABLE 11-12. COMMON DRUG DOSAGES USED IN BLEEDING DISORDERS

Prednisone, 2–4 mg/kg PO, IM q12–24h

Hydrocortisone acetate, 2–4 mg/kg IM q12–24h

Vincristine, 0.01–0.025 mg/kg IV q24h × 1–3 days

Cyclophosphamide, 2 mg/kg PO, IV q24h × 1–4 days
 (Use in clotting disorders only if other drugs are ineffective)

Azathioprine, 2 mg/kg PO q24h × 1–3 days

Vitamin K_1
 Dog—10–15 mg PO, IM q8–12h × 6–21 days
 Cat—2.5–5 mg PO, IM q8–12h × 6–21 days

Heparin—10 U/kg IV q6–12h

Fresh frozen plasma
 Factor I deficiency—12–20 ml/kg IV q24h × 3–5 days
 Factor VII deficiency—12–20 ml/kg IV q4h as needed
 Factor VIII deficiency—6–10 ml/kg IV q8–12h × 3–5 days
 Factor IX deficiency—6–10 ml/kg IV q12–h × 3–5 days
 Factor X deficiency—6–10 ml/kg IV q24h combined with vitamin K_1
 Von Willebrand's disease—6–10 ml/kg IV q12h × 3–5 days

Plasma cryoprecipitates
 Factor I deficiency—6–10 ml/kg IV q24h × 1–5 days
 Factor VIII deficiency—6–10 ml/kg IV q12h × 3–5 days
 Von Willebrand's disease—6–10 ml/kg IV q12h × 1–3 days

(*A*) Nonanemic patients

(*B*) Deficiencies of factors I, VII, VIII, IX, X, and VWD. (See Table 11-12.)

(3) Plasma cryoprecipitates

i) Concentrated plasma rich in fibrinogen and factor VIII.

ii) Cryoprecipitate is formed by freezing fresh plasma and then thawing it in a refrigerator; the cryoprecipitate forms at the plasma surface and can be siphoned off.

iii) Indicated for deficiencies of factors I, VIII, and VWD

b) Vitamin K_1 Therapy
   (1) Indicated for:
      i) Vitamin K deficiencies
      ii) Warfarin toxicity
      iii) Liver disease
      iv) Overdosage of anticoagulants
      v) Deficiency of factor X
   (2) Vitamin K_1 is preferred over vitamin K_3 because K_3 must be converted to K_2 in animals and is poorly stored in the liver.

6. Disseminated intravascular coagulopathy
   a) Removal of the inciting cause
      Is the most important therapy.
   b) Fluid therapy
      (1) Correct hypovolemia.
      (2) Prevent venous stasis.
      (3) Helps to dilute anticoagulants
   c) Coagulation inhibitors
      Although controversial, the following agents are proposed:
      (1) Heparin—10 U/kg IV q6–12h
      (2) Aspirin—10–25 mg/kg PO q24h
   d) Replacement therapy
      (1) Whole blood
      (2) Fresh plasma
         i) If RBCs not required
         ii) Incubate plasma with 5–10 U/kg heparin for 30 min.
         iii) Give 10 ml/kg IV q3–6h.
      (3) Plasma cryoprecipitate
         Ten to 20 ml IV q3h

G. Start supportive care.
   1. Continued fluid therapy
   2. Antibiotics
   3. Maintain normal body temperature.
      (See Chapters 4, 10, and 12 for specific therapy of bleeding into each of the major organs.)

VII. Patient monitoring
    A. Packed cell volume, TS q4–12h
    B. Platelet count q48–72h
    C. Prothrombin time, PTT, or ACT q48–72h
    D. Fibrinogen, FSP q48–72h
    E. Signs of continued hemorrhaging
        1. Petechiation
        2. Hematuria
        3. Melena
        4. Hematoma formation at venapuncture and injection sites
    F. Mucous membrane color
    G. Body temperature

BIBLIOGRAPHY

Badylak SF: Hemolytic anemia in the dog. Compend Contin Ed Pract Vet 2(9):685, 1980

Badylak SF: A pathophysiologic approach to the diagnosis of hemolytic anemia in the dog. Compend Contin Ed Pract Vet 3(9):827, 1981

Campbell KL, Greene CE: Factor IX deficiency (hemophilia B) in a Scottish terrier. J Am Vet Med Assoc 182(2):170, 1983

Cotter SM, Brenner RM, Dodds WJ: Hemophilia A in three unrelated cats. J Am Vet Med Assoc 172(2):166, 1978

Cramer DV, Lewis RM: Reticulocyte response in the cat. J Am Vet Med Assoc 160(1):61, 1972

Davenport DJ, Breitschwerdt EB, Carakostas MC: Platelet disorders in the dog and cat. Part I: Physiology and pathogenesis. Compend Contin Ed Pract Vet 4(9):762, 1982

Davenport DJ, Breitschwerdt EB, Carakostas MC: Platelet disorders in the dog and cat. Part II: Diagnosis and management. Compend Contin Ed Pract Vet 4(10):788, 1982

Dodds WJ: Bleeding disorders. p. 1679. In Ettinger SJ (ed): Textbook of Veterinary Internal Medicine. Vol. 2. WB Saunders, Philadelphia, 1975

Dodds WJ: Inherited hemorrhagic defects. p. 438. In Kirk RW (ed): Current Veterinary Therapy. Vol. 6. WB Saunders, Philadelphia, 1977

Dorland's Illustrated Medical Dictionary. 24th Ed. WB Saunders, Philadelphia, 1965

Drazner FH: Clinical implication of disseminated intravascular coagulation. Compend Contin Ed Pract Vet 4(12):974, 1982

Duncan JR, Prasse KW: Clinical examination of bone marrow. Vet Clin N Am 6(4):597, 1976

Feldman BF: Coagulopathies of small animals. J Am Vet Med Assoc 179(6):559, 1981

Feldman BF: Disseminated intravascular coagulation. Compend Contin Ed Pract Vet 3(1):46, 1981

Feldman BF: Anemias associated with blood loss and hemolysis. Vet Clin N Am 11(2):265, 1981

Feldman BF: Hypoproliferative anemias and anemias caused by ineffective erythropoiesis: depression or nonresponsive anemias. Vet Clin N Am 11(2):277, 1981

Feldman BF, Madewell BR, O'Neill S: Disseminated intravascular coagulation: antithrombin, plasminogen, and coagulation abnormalities in 41 dogs. J Am Vet Med Assoc 179(2):151, 1981

Feldman BF, Soares J, Kitchell BE, et al: Hemorrhage in a cat caused by inhibition of factor XI (plasma thromboplastin antecedent) J Am Vet Med Assoc 182(6):589, 1983

Green RA: Hemostasis and disorders of coagulation. Vet Clin N Am 11(2):289, 1981

Guyton AC (ed): Textbook of Medical Physiology. 6th Ed. WB Saunders, Philadelphia, 1981

Hardy WD: Feline leukemia virus: its related diseases and control. Vet Clin N Am 7(1):93, 1977

Hardy WD: Feline leukemia virus non-neoplastic diseases. JAAHA 17(6):941, 1981

Hill BL, Zenoble RD, Dodds WJ: Prothrombin deficiency in a Cocker spaniel. J Am Vet Med Assoc 181(3):262, 1982

Johnstone IB: Current concepts of hemostasis. Compend Contin Ed Pract Vet 3(12):1071, 1981

Johnstone IB: Inherited defects of hemostasis. Compend Contin Ed Pract Vet 4(6):483, 1982

Kier AB, Bresnahan JF, White FJ, et al: Factor XII deficiency in domestic cats. Can J Comp Med 44:309, 1980

Kociba GJ: The diagnosis of hemostatic disorders. Vet Clin N Am 6(4):609, 1976

MacEwen EG, Patnaik AK, Wilkins RJ: Diagnosis and treatment of canine hematopoietic neoplasms. Vet Clin N Am 7(1):105, 1977

Maggio L: Anemia in the cat. Compend Contin Ed Pract Vet 1(2):474, 1979

Morgan RV: Blood dyscrasias associated with testicular tumors in the dog. JAAHA 18(6):970, 1982

Mount ME, Feldman BF, Buffington T: Vitamin K and its therapeutic importance. J Am Vet Med Assoc 180(11):1354, 1982

Rebar AH, Boon GD: An approach to the diagnosis of bleeding disorders in the dog. JAAHA 17(2):227, 1981

Ruehl W, Mills C, Feldman BF: Rational therapy in disseminated intravascular coagulation. JAVMA 181(1):76, 1982

Schalm OW, Jain NC, Carroll EJ: Veterinary Hematology. 3rd Ed. Lea & Febiger, Philadelphia, 1975

Searcy GP: The differential diagnosis of anemia. Vet Clin N Am 6(4):567, 1976

Sloss MW (ed): Veterinary Clinical Parasitology. 4th Ed. Iowa State University Press, Ames, 1970

Soulsby EJL: Helminths, Arthropods and Protozoa of Domestic Animals. 6th Ed. Williams and Wilkins, Baltimore, 1968

Weiser MG: Correlative approach to anemia in dogs and cats. JAAHA 17(2):286, 1981

Werner LL: Coombs' positive anemias in the dog and cat. Compend Contin Ed Pract Vet 2(2):96, 1980

12

Respiratory Emergencies

UPPER AIRWAY OBSTRUCTION

I. Definition

Occlusion or narrowing of any part of the airway may result in impaired respiration. The major sequela of this impairment is decreased oxygenation of the blood with inadequate delivery of O_2 to the tissues. When *airway obstruction* severely diminishes the air exchange process, a life-threatening emergency exists.

II. Causes

A. Trauma may produce an obstruction via:

1. Facial fractures
2. Mandibular fractures
3. Epistaxis
4. Lacerations of larynx and trachea
5. Fractures of larynx and trachea
6. Soft tissue swelling

B. Infections

May compromise the nasal passage, pharynx, and larynx

C. Foreign material

Examples:

1. Bones
2. Wood
3. Food
4. Toys
5. Vomitus
6. Mucus

7. Water
8. Plant material

D. Angioneurotic edema
   Produces laryngeal edema uncommonly in animals
E. Tumors
   1. Primary tumors of the airway
   2. Tumors of surrounding soft tissues
   3. Metastatic tumors
F. Neuromuscular disorders
   1. Myasthenia gravis
   2. Esophageal paralysis
   Predispose to aspiration of ingesta
G. Iatrogenic manipulation
   Intubation often causes laryngeal spasms in cats.
F. Anatomic conformations
   1. Often predispose certain breeds of dogs to airway collapse
   2. May be the most common cause of airway obstruction in the dog
   3. Clinical features of these disorders are summarized in Table 12-1.

III. Clinical signs
   A. Noisy, stridulous, or stertorous breathing
   B. Choking and retching of white froth
   C. Dyspnea, polypnea
   D. Cyanosis
   E. Pawing or clawing at face and throat
   F. Coughing
   G. Exercise intolerance, collapse
   H. Intolerance to heat, with predisposition to heat stroke
   I. Anxiety, pacing, hysteria
   J. ± Pyrexia

IV. Diagnosis
   A. History
      1. Previous episodes with similar clinical signs
      2. Recent trauma
      3. History of chewing or playing with foreign objects
      4. Recent allergic reaction
      5. Breed, age, sex of animal

TABLE 12-1. ANATOMIC CAUSES OF AIRWAY OCCLUSION

Anatomic Conformation	Pathophysiology	Breeds
Stenotic nares	Occlusion of nares develops from collapse of the lateral alar cartilage and overlying rhinarium.	Brachycephalic breeds
Elongation of soft palate	Soft palate often overlies the epiglottis. Palate is often thickened and obstructs the glottis.	Brachycephalic breeds, beagle, cocker spaniel
Eversion of lateral ventricles of larynx	Develops over time from excessive negative pressure in the larynx/pharynx during inspiration in dogs with narrowed airways.	Brachycephalic breeds, especially English bulldog
Laryngeal paralysis	Congenital	Bouvier, English bulldog, Siberian husky
	Acquired Idiopathic, bilateral	Giant-breed dogs, especially St. Bernard
	Unilateral Traumatic Lymphosarcoma	 Any breed of dog or cat Cats
Hypoplasia of trachea	Congenital defect where there is inadequate growth of the tracheal rings. Often accompanied by elongation of soft palate and/or eversion of laryngeal saccules.	English Bulldog
Tracheal collapse	Proposed causes: Hereditary predisposition Dietary factors Obesity Demineralization of tracheal cartilages Inflammation Small airway disease Dorsoventral collapse is the most common.	Yorkshire terrier, Chihuahua, Pomeranian, toy and miniature poodle, other nonbrachycephalic toy breeds

B. Physical examination
   1. Extreme care must be used in examining all animals with airway obstruction because they are susceptible to collapse and respiratory arrest when stressed.
   2. Examine head and neck for:
      a) Obvious facial injuries
      b) Epistaxis
      c) Wounds
      d) Stenotic nares
      e) Oral foreign bodies or tumors
      f) Soft tissue swellings
   3. Palpate head and neck for swelling, crepitance, deformity, and pain.
   4. Auscultate upper airway and thorax.
   5. Characterize and localize abnormal respiratory sounds.
   6. Perform thorough general examination to determine other underlying systemic disorders.

C. Radiography
   1. Plain radiography
      Skull, larynx, neck, thorax—examine for:
      a) Radiopaque foreign bodies
      b) Soft tissue swelling, masses
      c) Fractures, dislocations of facial bones, mandible, hypoid apparatus
      d) Tracheal collapse
      e) Subcutaneous emphysema
      f) Pulmonary and cardiac abnormalities
   2. Fluoroscopy
      a) Often necessary to delineate tracheal collapse
      b) Watch for dorsoventral occlusion of trachea:
         (1) Cervical collapse occurs with inspiration.
         (2) Intrathoracic collapse usually develops upon expiration.
   3. Contrast radiography
      Will help to confirm paralysis of the esophagus

D. Direct examination of pharynx and larynx
   1. Perform under light anesthesia.
   2. Consider if foreign bodies, tumors, or anatomic defects are suspected.
   3. Abnormal anatomic findings include:
      a) An elongated soft palate usually overlies the epiglottis and is often thickened, redundant, and inflamed.
      b) Everting saccules are seen as thin, pink membranous tissue which prolapses into the laryngeal inlet, especially during inspiration.
      c) In laryngeal paralysis, vocal folds fail to abduct upon inspiration, retain a midline position, and obviously narrow the laryngeal opening. Assymetrical abduction may occur with laryngeal hemiplegia.

E. Other tests
   1. Electromyography
      Confirms denervation of laryngeal muscles and esophagus.
   2. Bronchoscopy
      May be necessary to confirm presence of lower airway obstruction from:
      a) Tumors
      b) Tracheal whiplash
      c) Foreign material
   3. Laboratory workup
      a) Complete blood count
      b) Biochemical organ profile
      c) Arterial blood gases

V. Treatment
   A. Primary objectives:
      1. Establish a patent airway.
      2. Institute and assist ventilation.
      3. Start supportive care.
      4. Determine cause.
      5. Remove or correct cause.
   B. Establish a patent airway.

1. Separate the animal from its owner.
2. Take the animal to a central treatment area or intensive care ward.
3. Intubate if unconscious.
4. Begin O_2 therapy.
5. Suction all blood and foreign material from the mouth.
6. If the obstruction appears partial and if the patient is not collapsed, sedate and place the animal in an O_2 cage.
7. Keep excitement and handling to a minimum.
   (See Table 12-2.)

C. Determine site of obstruction.
   1. Perform preliminary examination of pharynx and larynx during intubation of any collapsed animal.
   2. Most upper airway obstructions produce stridulous sounds which are loudest at the larynx and pharynx.
   3. The point of maximum airway obstruction is usually the site where respiratory noise is noted as the loudest.
   4. Tracheal collapse usually causes a low-pitched honking sound which may be accompanied by coughing.
   5. Consider radiography if lower airway obstruction is suspected. This must be undertaken with the utmost care.
   6. Consider emergency bronchoscopy for distal tracheal tumors or injuries.
   7. If respiratory distress occurs from an upper airway obstruction and relief is not provided by sedation, O_2 therapy and supportive care, consider a tracheostomy.

D. Technique for tracheostomy

   Note: If the animal is unconscious and the obstruction prohibits intubation, tracheostomy should be performed immediately, with little time taken for sterile preparation of the site.

TABLE 12-2. PROTOCOL FOR THE TREATMENT OF AIRWAY OBSTRUCTION

1. Separate animal from owner; move it to the intensive care unit.
2. Establish patent airway.
   a. Intubate if collapsed or unconscious.
   b. Remove oral foreign material and blood.
   c. Perform tracheostomy.
3. Institute O_2 therapy.
4. Start supportive care.
   a. IV fluid therapy
   b. Sedation
   c. Antibiotics
   d. Corticosteroids
   e. Bronchodilators
   f. Maintain normal body temperature.
5. Further diagnostic procedures
   a. Radiography—survey films, fluoroscopy
   b. Laryngoscopy
   c. Bronchoscopy
   d. Electromyography
6. Assess and treat coexisting problems.
7. Prepare for surgery.
   a. Removal of foreign bodies or tumors
   b. Repair of fractures and wounds
   c. Incision and drainage of abscesses
   d. Correct anatomic defects.
      i. Stenotic nares—resection of lateral alar cartilage
      ii. Elongated soft palate—surgical resection
      iii. Everted laryngeal ventricles—remove saccules
      iv. Laryngeal paralysis—unilateral laryngectomy with removal of vocal cord, arytenoid cartilage, and aryepiglottic fold
      v. Cervical tracheal collapse—C-ring prostheses, tracheal plication
8. Continue postoperative care of tracheostomy tube
   a. Suction q2–4h using aseptic technique.
   b. Nebulization with saline or acetylcysteine diluted with saline or installation of 1 ml saline into tracheal tube to liquefy secretions q2-8h
   c. Maintain normal hydration with SQ or IV fluids.
   d. Antibiotics
   e. Monitor body temperature.
   f. Periodically radiograph chest for signs of pneumonia.

1. Carefully induce anesthesia and intubate.
2. Place animal in dorsal recumbency.
3. Shave hair and sterilely prepare the skin from the point of the jaw to the thoracic inlet.
4. Make an incision over the trachea immediately caudal to the larynx or caudal to the obstruction.
5. Separate bluntly the two sternohyoid muscles (Figure 12-1A).
6. Incise the trachea between the cartilagenous rings. See Figure 12-1A, B. For high obstructions, make the incision between rings 2, 3, and 4.
7. Enlarge the incision with a Trousseau dilator or sharp scalpel blade. Care must be taken not to lacerate the endotracheal tube. See Figure 12-1B.
8. Withdraw the endotracheal tube and insert a tracheostomy tube. See Table 12-3 and Figure 12-1C.
9. If the tracheostomy tube is supplied with an obturator, remove it.
10. Tie the tracheostomy tube in place with umbilical tape and/or suture it to the skin of the neck.
11. Sterile endotracheal tubes may be used in giant-

TABLE 12-3. COMMERCIAL PRODUCTS USED IN TREATING AIRWAY OBSTRUCTIONS

Tracheostomy tube—Portex, Portex, Wilmington, MA 01887

Acetylcysteine—Mucomyst, Mead Johnson Pharmaceutical, Evansville, IN 47721

Morphine—Morphine sulfate Carpuject, Winthrop Laboratories, New York, NY 10016

Meperidine HCl—Demerol HCl, Winthrop Laboratories, New York, NY 10016

Fentanyl-droperidol—Innovar-Vet, Pitman-Moore, Washington Crossing, NJ 08560

Oxymorphone—Numorphan, Endo Laboratories, Garden City, NY 11530

Dexmethasone
Azium, Schering, Kenilworth, NJ 07033
Dexate-SP, Burns Biotec Laboratories, Omaha, NB 68103

Prednisolone—Prednisolone, Purepac Pharmaceutical, Elizabeth, NJ 07207

Aminophylline—Aminophyllin, Searle Laboratories, Chicago, IL 60680

Theophylline—Theophyl, Knoll Pharmaceutical, Whippany, NJ 07981

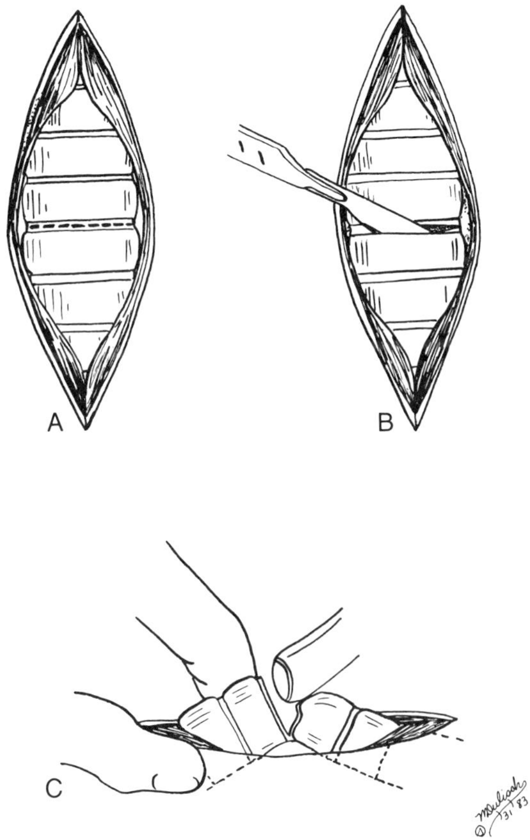

Fig. 12-1. Technique for insertion of a tracheostomy tube. The sternohyoid muscles are bluntly separated and trachea is exposed (A). The trachea is incised between the cartilagenous rings and the incision is enlarged with a scalpel blade (A, B). The trachea is gently lifted upward and the tracheostomy tube is inserted (C).

breed or thick-necked dogs in which ordinary tracheostomy tubes cannot be adequately secured.

12. Suction the airway and ensure patency of the tube.
13. Anesthesia may be maintained through the tracheostomy tube if further surgical procedures are to be performed at the same time.

E. Start supportive care.
   1. Treat shock with IV fluid therapy and corticosteroids.
   2. Rapidly cool any hyperthermic animal. See protocol in section on Heat Prostration, Chapter 9.
   3. Consider antibiotics.
   4. Consider corticosteroids for angioneurotic edema.
   5. Patients with mild to moderate cases of tracheal collapse may often be managed medically with:
      a) Bronchodilators
         (1) Aminophylline
         (2) Theophylline
      b) Sedation
         (1) Morphine SO_4
         (2) Meperidine HCl
         (3) Fentanyl-droperidol
      c) Oxygen therapy
      d) Nebulization with normal saline

   See Table 12-4

F. Determine cause of obstruction.
   1. May already be obvious from site of occlusion or found during initial examination.
   2. Radiography may be attempted when the animal is stable.
   3. Perform further diagnostic tests:
      a) Laryngoscopy
      b) Fluoroscopy
      c) Bronchoscopy
      d) Electromyography
   4. Determine presence of multiple airway abnormalities.
   5. Diet all brachycephalic and toy breeds with anatomic abnormalities in anticipation of corrective surgery.
   6. Draw all laboratory samples.

G. Assess and treat other problems.
   1. Stop external and internal hemorrhaging.
   2. Correct hyperthermia.

TABLE 12-4. DRUG DOSAGES FOR USE IN AIRWAY OBSTRUCTION

Drug	Dosage
Morphine	Dog: 0.1–0.4 mg/kg SQ q8–12h Cat: 0.05 mg/kg SQ q12h
Meperidine HCl	0.25–2.0 mg/kg SQ q8–12h
Fentanyl-droperidol	0.1–0.3 ml/25 kg IM
Oxymorphone	Dog: 0.1 mg/kg IV Cat: 0.02 mg/kg IV
Dexamethasone	0.02–0.2 mg/kg IV, SQ q8h
Prednisolone	0.01–0.25 mg/kg IM, PO q8h
Aminophylline	Dog: 6–11 mg/kg IV, IM, PO q6–8h Cat: 4 mg/kg IM, PO q12h
Theophylline	Dog: 6–11 mg/kg IV, IM, PO q6–8h

3. Combat pulmonary edema.
4. Monitor fluid therapy carefully in cardiac patients.
5. Assess neurologic status in patients with head trauma.
6. Assess extent of any allergic reaction.
7. Determine presence of multiple anatomic deformities.

H. Remove or correct the cause.
   1. Trauma
      a) Keep nostrils and mouth free of blood.
      b) Stabilize animal over 24–72 h, then repair facial and mandibular fractures, wounds, and lacerations.
      c) Use cold compresses in first 24 h for soft tissue swelling.
   2. Infections
      a) Continue systemic antibiotics.
      b) Use hot compresses on areas of diffuse cellulitis.
      c) Incise and drain abscesses.
   3. Foreign material
      Remove under sedation or anesthesia.

4. Angioneurotic edema
   a) Continue corticosteroids.
   b) Remove source of allergen.
5. Tumors
   a) Perform surgical excision.
   b) Anastomosis of trachea may be required for primary neoplasms.
   c) Euthanasia should be considered for widespread metastasis.
6. Neuromuscular disorders
   a) Institute specific therapy and specialized feeding procedures.
   b) Continue antibiotics and nebulization for pneumonia.
7. Anatomic abnormalities
   a) Stenotic nares
      Resect lateral alar cartilage.
   b) Elongation of soft palate
      Surgically shorten palate.
   c) Everted laryngeal ventricles
      Remove saccules.
   d) Laryngeal paralysis
      (1) Unilateral laryngectomy with removal of vocal cord, arytenoid cartilage, and aryepiglottic fold
      (2) Unilateral or bilateral arytenoid cartilage lateralization
   e) Cervical tracheal collapse
      (1) Attempt stabilization with sedation and slowly discontinue O_2.
      (2) If animal cannot be stabilized medically, consider reconstruction of trachea with C-ring protheses and tracheal plication.
   f) Intrathoracic tracheal collapse is very difficult to treat.
      (1) Continue medical therapy with O_2, sedation, bronchodilators.

(2) Treat coexisting cardiac or small airway disease.

VI. Postoperative care and monitoring
  A. Tracheostomy tube care
    1. Tracheostomy tubes require continuous nursing care.
    2. Thick mucus accumulates because the tube itself is irritating and the normal warming and humidifying mechanisms of the nasal passages are bypassed.
    3. These secretions may adhere to the free end of the tube and compromise its patency.
    4. The steps taken for maintenance of the tracheostomy tube are summarized in Table 12-2.
    5. If the tube becomes prematurely plugged, it may be replaced.
    6. Following removal of the tube, the site is left open to heal by second intention. Suturing of the skin may cause subcutaneous and mediastinal emphysema. Cleanse the site daily until healing is complete.
  B. Monitor vital signs
    1. Mucous membrane color
    2. Capillary refill time
    3. Respirations
      a) Frequency and effort
      b) Continued abnormal airway and lung sounds
    4. Heart rate and pulse strength
    5. Body temperature
    6. Mental alertness
    7. Strength, tolerance to handling and examination
  C. Monitor specific abnormalities
    1. Watch animal with epistaxis and facial injuries for renewed bleeding or continued soft tissue swelling.
    2. Watch for recurrence of soft tissue swelling accompanying infections, trauma, and allergic reactions.

3. Watch postoperative patients for:
   a) Coughing, gagging
   b) Aspiration of secretions
   c) Inhalation of food
   d) Onset of bronchopneumonia
   e) Onset of inflammation or infection at surgical site
   f) Continued abnormal respiratory sounds or cyanosis
   g) Development of secondary laryngeal paralysis following surgery of the trachea
   h) Dehiscence at surgical sites of tumor excision or tracheal anastomoses
   i) Development of strictures at surgical site

PARENCHYMAL/EXCHANGE DISEASES

I. Definition

Oxygen and carbon dioxide pass through several layers of respiratory membrane as they are exchanged in the lungs. These are (1) the alveolar surfactant and fluid layer, (2) the alveolar epithelium with basement membrane, (3) the thin interstitial space, and (4) the capillary basement membrane and endothelium. Any process that alters the thickness or the surface area and the pressure difference across these membranes, and affects the regional perfusion alters the overall rate of gaseous exchange. When ventilation-perfusion abnormalities result in severe impairment of oxygenation, a respiratory emergency arises. The discussion in this section will be confined to four such disease processes: (1) pneumonia, (2) pulmonary contusion, (3) pulmonary edema, and (4) feline asthma.

II. Pneumonia

A. The most common life-threatening types are:
   1. Acute fulminating bronchopneumonia
   2. Smoke inhalation

3. Aspiration pneumonia
   a) Ingesta or food
   b) Water (near-drowning)
      Fresh or salt water

B. Pathophysiology
   1. Inflammatory exudate and/or foreign material occlude the aveoli.
   2. The total surface area for air exchange is decreased.
   3. Diminished surfactant activity leads to atelectasis.
   4. Ventilation-perfusion abnormalities occur as blood is shunted by nonventilated alveoli.
   5. Aspiration of salt water causes movement of interstitial fluid into the alveoli, compromising ventilation even further.
   6. Exposure to carbon monoxide dramatically changes gas pressure across the pulmonary membrane, resulting in binding of Hgb and impediment of O_2 unloading in the peripheral tissues.
   7. Direct damage to the airways may also result from contact with acidic ingesta, soot particles, or other noxious gases. This impairs ciliary action and predisposes to mucosal edema, as well as decreasing surfactant activity.
   8. Failure to alleviate these events will result in the development of widespread pulmonary edema, a decrease in compliance, and alterations in circulating blood volume, serum electrolytes, tissue perfusion, and oxygenation.

C. Clinical signs
   1. Polypnea, dyspnea
   2. Cyanosis
   3. Productive coughing
   4. Weakness, fatigue
   5. Depression, lethargy, anorexia
   6. Shock
   7. Orthopnea
   8. ± Pyrexia

9. ± Purulent nasal and ocular discharge.
10. Smoke inhalation victims may exhibit:
    a) Loss of consciousness
    b) Burns on face, lips, mouth
    c) Singed whiskers and hair
    d) Hoarseness, stridor
    e) Cherry-red mucous membranes from extreme heat or carbon monoxide poisoning
    f) Laryngeal edema
11. Patients who have nearly drowned may show:
    a) Loss of consciousness
    b) Fluid from mouth and nose
    c) Hypothermia
    d) Shallow, slow respirations
    e) Slow, weak pulses
    f) Respiratory and/or cardiac arrest

D. Diagnosis
1. History
    a) Recent upper airway infection
    b) Recent exposure to infectious respiratory disease
    c) Exposure to fire, heat, noxious gases
    d) Previous episodes of regurgitation or vomiting
    e) Previously diagnosed esophageal paralysis
    f) Known incidence of near-drowning
2. Physical examination
    a) Auscultate for:
        (1) Moist rales and rhonchi
        (2) Wheezing, other abnormal respiratory sounds
        (3) Muffled lung and heart sounds may occur in areas of severe atelectasis and consolidation.
    b) Examine:
        (1) Consistency of ocular and nasal discharge and sputum
        (2) Color of mucous membranes
        (3) Evidence of exposure to fire or heat

(4) Evidence of near-drowning
(5) Symptoms of other systemic disorders
(6) Body temperature
(7) Mental attitude and strength

3. Radiography of chest
   a) Determine pattern and distribution of pathologic changes. (See Table 12-5.)

TABLE 12-5. RADIOGRAPHIC CHANGES WITH PARENCHYMAL DISEASES

Disease	Radiographic Signs
Pneumonia	
Bronchopneumonia	Alveolar or mixed alveolar-bronchial pattern; air bronchograms present; changes present in multiple lobes and throughout the lobes
Aspiration	Most commonly affect ventral portions of middle lobes; may be uni- or bilateral; mixed alveolar-interstitial pattern; air bronchograms present unless consolidated
Inhalation	Early changes confined to interstitial pattern with peribronchial infiltrates; late changes show mixed alveolar-interstitial pattern with air bronchograms present; early changes are widespread and diffuse; later changes may affect dependent portions of lungs, mimicking aspiration
Pulmonary contusion	Irregular, patchy areas of mixed alveolar-interstitial patterns or consolidation; often contain air bronchograms; may be associated with rib fractures, pneumothorax, or atelectasis
Pulmonary edema	
Cardiogenic	
Dog	Hilar, mixed alvelar-interstitial densities
Cat	Diffuse, peripheral alveolar or mixed pattern
Electric shock, snakebite, inhalation	Generalized, severe mixed pattern; often most pronounced in diaphragmatic lobes; bilateral, symmetrical; air bronchograms present
Hypoproteinemia	Mixed pattern with air bronchograms late; often accompanied by hydrothorax
Feline asthma	Increased interstitial densities and peribronchial markings; increased thoracic size; straightening of diaphragm; hyperlucency of lungs; ± aerophagia; emphysematous bullae with chronic asthma

b) Examine for evidence of concurrent airway and cardiac disease.
c) Contrast radiography may be indicated if esophageal paralysis is suspected.

4. Laboratory tests
   a) Complete blood count
   b) Transtracheal aspirate
      (1) Fluid analysis, cytology
      (2) Culture and sensitivity
   c) Arterial blood gas determinations
   d) Measurement of carboxyhemoglobin levels in venous or arterial blood
   e) Bronchoscopy for direct visualization and biopsy of the airways may be indicated in smoke inhalation or aspiration of solid foreign material.
   f) Microscopic examination of sputum
   g) Electrocardiography for detection of coexisting arrhythmias and heart disease.

E. Treatment
   1. Primary objectives:
      a) Remove animal from source of injury.
      b) Maintain patency and function of airways.
      c) Treat infection.
      d) Enhance removal of secretions.
      e) Start supportive care.
   2. Remove animal from source of injury.
      a) Remove animal from site of fire.
      b) Remove animal from water.
      c) Begin cardiopumonary resuscitation if comatose from respiratory or cardiac arrest.
      d) See section on Cardiac Arrest, Chapter 2
   3. Ensure a patent airway.
      a) Suction all secretions and foreign material from mouth and airway.
      b) Intubate if collapsed, comatose.
      c) Administer O_2:

(1) Mask, cage, endotracheal tube
(2) Forty percent for most types of pneumonia
(3) One hundred percent for carbon monoxide poisoning

d) Consider performing a tracheotomy if the airway is compromised from laryngeal edema, laryngeal spasm, or accumulation of secretions.

e) Consider positive pressure ventilation
(1) Indicated in patients with severe inhalation pneumonia and drowning victims
(2) May be accomplished via an endotracheal or tracheostomy tube

(See Table 12-6.)

4. Combat shock.
   a) Insert an IV catheter.
   b) Begin fluid therapy.
   c) Consider short-acting corticosteroids.
5. Begin diagnostic tests.
   a) Radiography of thorax
   b) Complete blood count, TTA
   c) Arterial blood gas analysis
   d) Measurement of venous carboxyhemoglobin levels
   e) Bronchoscopy
   f) Electrocardiogram
6. Institute specific therapy.
   a) Enhance removal of secretions
      (1) Nebulization with normal saline
      (2) Maintain normal body hydration with SQ or IV fluids.
      (3) Institute physiotherapy.
         i) Deep breathing
         ii) Positive pressure ventilation
         iii) Chest percussion (coupage)
         iv) Forced turning or exercise

TABLE 12-6. PROTOCOL FOR THE TREATMENT OF PNEUMONIA

1. Ensure patent airway.
   a. Suction foreign material, secretions.
   b. Intubate if necessary.
   c. Consider tracheotomy for airway obstruction.
2. O_2 therapy
   a. 100% for carbon monoxide poisoning
   b. 40% for pneumonia
   c. Consider assisted ventilation.
3. Perform diagnostic workup.
   a. Radiography of chest
   b. Transtracheal aspiration
   c. CBC
   d. Blood gas determination
   e. Bronchoscopy
4. Start therapy.
   a. Nebulization with normal saline
   b. Physiotherapy
      i. Positive pressure ventilation
      ii. Deep breathing
      iii. Chest percussion (coupage)
   c. Fluid therapy
   d. Bronchodilators
   e. Antibiotics
   f. Analgesics
   g. Consider corticosteroids for inhalation injury.
5. Patient monitoring
   a. Mucous membrane color
   b. CRT
   c. Respiratory rate and effort
   d. Type of lung sounds
   e. Body temperature
   f. Blood gas determination
   g. Periodic radiography of chest
   h. ECG

b) Treat infections.
   (1) Bacterial bronchopneumonias and aspiration pneumonia from ingesta or vomitus usually require immediate institution of antibiotics.
   (2) In the case of smoke inhalation and near-drowning, prophylactic use of antibiotics should be avoided.

(3) Choose the antibiotic based on culture results.

c) Bronchodilators

Helpful in reversing bronchial spasm and constriction

d) Sodium bicarbonate

(1) Often indicated following prolonged cyanosis, atelectasis, or respiratory arrest

(2) Evaluate need by blood gas determinations.

e) Analgesics, sedatives

(1) May be used in selected patients exhibiting extreme pain from burns or other injuries

(2) Are contraindicated in fulminating bacterial pneumonia and near-drowning

f) Corticosteroids

(1) May be indicated in the early treatment (first 12–24 h) of inhalation injuries

(2) Are contraindicated in fulminating bacterial pneumonia and near-drowning

(See Tables 12-7 and 12-8.)

7. Start supportive care.
   a) Assess and stabilize other injuries.
   b) Maintain body temperature if hypothermic.
   c) Institute local treatment for ocular and cutaneous burns.
   d) Consider mannitol and dexamethasone for cerebral edema following prolonged hypoxia (especially after near-drowning).
   e) See also the protocol in the section on Pulmonary Edema below.

F. Patient monitoring

1. Vital signs
   a) Mucous membrane color
   b) Capillary refill time
   c) Respiratory rate, effort
   d) Body temperature

TABLE 12-7. COMMON DRUG DOSAGES FOR PARENCHYMAL DISEASES

Drug	Dosage
Bronchodilators	
Aminophylline	Dog: 6–11 mg/kg IV, IM, PO q6–8h Cat: 4 mg/kg IM, PO q12h
Theophylline	Dog: 6–11 mg/kg IV, IM, PO q6–8h
Analgesics, sedatives	
Morphine	0.1–0.4 mg/kg SQ q8–12h
Diazepam	Dog: 5–15 mg IV Cat: 2.5–5.0 mg IV
Hydrocodone bitartrate	0.2–0.5 mg/kg PO q8h
Diuretics	
Furosemide	2–4 mg/kg IV, IM q4–12h
Ethacrynate sodium	0.2–0.4 mg/kg IV, IM q4–12h
Corticosteroids	
Dexamethasone	0.1–0.2 mg/kg IV, SQ q8h
Prednisolone	0.1–0.25 mg/kg IM, PO q8h
Hydrocortisone sodium succinate	8–20 mg/kg IV once
Prednisolone sodium succinate	11–25 mg/kg IV once
Others	
Digoxin	Dog: 0.007 mg/kg PO, IM q12h Cat: 0.003–0.005 mg/kg PO, IM q12h
Ouabain	0.01 mg/kg IV q30–120 min
2% nitroglycerin ointment	$\frac{1}{8}$–$\frac{1}{2}$ in. topically q6h
Hydralazine	Dog: 0.55 mg/kg PO q12h

e) Heart rate
   (1) Monitor closely for arrhythmias.
   (2) See section on Arrhythmias, Chapter 2.
f) Neurologic status

2. Type and distribution of lung sounds
3. Amount and consistency of airway secretions
4. Monitor thoracic radiographs q24–48h.
5. Monitor blood gases q4–24h.
6. Monitor CBC q24–48h.
7. Monitor ECG.
8. Watch closely for onset of acute respiratory distress syndrome: hyperventilation and respiratory alkalosis unresponsive to oxygen therapy. (See Chapter 1.)

TABLE 12-8. COMMERCIAL PRODUCTS FOR USE IN PARENCHYMAL-EXCHANGE DISEASES

Aminophylline—Aminophyllin, Searle Laboratories, Chicago, IL 60680

Theophylline—Theophyl, Knoll Pharmaceuticals, Whippany, NJ 07981

Morphine—Morphine sulfate Carpujet, Winthrop Laboratories, New York, NY 10016

Diazepam—Valium, Roche Laboratories, Nutley, NJ 07110

Hydrocodone bitartrate—Hycodan, Endo Laboratories, Garden City, NY 11530

Furosemide—Lasix, American Hoechst, Somerville, NJ 08876

Ethacrynate sodium—Sodium Edecrin, Merck, Sharpe and Dohme, West Point, PA 19486

Dexamethasone
Azium, Schering, Kenilworth, NJ 07033
Dexate-SP, Burns Biotec Laboratories, Omaha, NB 68103

Prednisolone—Prednisolone, Purepac Pharmaceutical, Elizabeth, NJ 07207

Hydrocortisone sodium succinate—Solu-Cortef, Upjohn, Kalamazoo, MI 49001

Prednisolone sodium succinate—Solu-Delta-Cortef, Upjohn, Kalamazoo, MI 49001

Digoxin—Lanoxin, Wellcome Animal Health Division, Kansas City, MO 64108

Ouabain–Ouabain, Eli Lilly, Indianapolis, IN 46285

2% Nitroglycerine ointment–Nitro-Bid ointment, Marion Laboratories, Kansas City, MO 64137

Hydralazine—Apresoline HCl, CIBA Pharmaceutical, Summit, NJ 07901

Isoproterenol—Isuprel, Breon Laboratories, New York, NY 10016

Epinephrine—Adrenalin, Parke-Davis, Morris Plains, NJ 07950

III. Pulmonary contusion

A. Definition and cause

Pulmonary contusion is bruising or hemorrhage into lung parenchyma and is most often caused by blunt thoracic trauma. Pulmonary contusion may be associated with fractures of the ribs, pneumo- or hemothorax, and herniation of the diaphragm. Resiliency of the rib cage allows pulmonary contusions to also occur alone. Air exchange is reduced in the same manner as in pneumonia.

B. Clinical signs

1. Mild contusions

- a) Tachypnea
- b) ± Apprehension

2. Severe contusions
    - a) Cyanosis
    - b) Dyspnea, orthopnea
    - c) Shock
    - d) Weakness, collapse
    - e) Hemoptysis
        - (1) Is infrequent
        - (2) Warrants a guarded prognosis
3. Other signs of trauma
    - a) Limb fractures
    - b) Rib fractures
    - c) Lacerations
    - d) Blunt abdominal trauma
    - e) Cardiac arrhythmias
    - f) Shock

C. Diagnosis

1. History of trauma
2. Physical findings
    - a) Evidence of trauma
    - b) Clinical signs referable to respiratory system
3. Radiography of chest
    - a) See Table 12-5.
    - b) Radiographic changes may not be apparent immediately, but develop over the first 4 h.
    - c) Radiographic lesions may continue to worsen for the first 24 h following the injury.

D. Treatment

1. Objectives:
    - a) Combat shock.
    - b) Maintain adequate oxygenation.
    - c) Provide supportive care during period of resolution.

      See Table 12-9
2. Combat shock.
    - a) Insert IV catheter.
    - b) Begin fluid therapy.

TABLE 12-9. PROTOCOL FOR THE TREATMENT OF PULMONARY CONTUSION

1. Ensure patent airway.
2. Treat for shock, control hemorrhage, and correct life-threatening injuries.
3. Institute oxygen therapy.
4. Start medical therapy.
   a. Corticosteroids
   b. Bronchodilators
   c. Consider diuretics.
   d. Consider antibiotics.
   e. Consider nebulization with ethanol.
5. Consider further diagnostic workup.
   a. Thoracic radiographs
   b. Blood gas determination
6. Monitor
   a. Respiratory rate and effort
   b. Mucous membrane color, CRT
   c. Lung sounds
   d. Repeat radiographs in 24–48 h

---

c) Consider corticosteroids and sodium bicarbonate.

d) Assess and treat other life-threatening emergencies.

3. Ensure a patent airway.
   a) Intubate if collapsed.
   b) Suction secretions from airway.
   c) Administer O_2 via mask, endotracheal tube, or cage.
   d) Consider positive pressure ventilation if intubated.
4. Institute medical therapy.
   a) Indicated early in course:
      (1) Corticosteroids
      (2) Diuretics
   b) Indicated throughout course:
      (1) Bronchodilators
      (2) Oxygen
   c) Antibiotics should be considered if evidence of infection is found.

d) Nebulization with ethanol-saline in a 1:2 dilution may be attempted for severe contusions to facilitate removal of blood and fluid.

E. Patient monitoring

Note: Severe pulmonary contusions are associated with high mortality rates because it is not possible to mechanically remove the blood and secretions from the terminal airways and alveoli. Careful monitoring and continued therapy are required until resolution of the contusion is documented.

1. Vital signs
2. Radiographs of chest q24–48h until resolution occurs (usually within 3–7 days).
3. Arterial blood gases q24–48h

IV. Pulmonary edema

A. Definition

Pulmonary edema is the accumulation of excessive amounts of fluid within the lung. Edema begins as an increase in water in the interstitium and progresses to fluid within the alveoli. An emergency arises when this fluid accumulation diminishes oxygenation of the blood to a level that is life-threatening.

B. Pathophysiology

1. There are four mechanisms by which pulmonary edema occurs:
   a) Increased pulmonary capillary hydrostatic pressure
   b) Decreased plasma oncotic pressure
   c) Altered pulmonary capillary permeability
   d) Pulmonary lymphatic insufficiency
2. Abnormalities of both pulmonary capillary hydrostatic and oncotic pressures favor movement of fluid out of the capillaries and into the interstitial and alveolar spaces.
3. Capillary permeability may be increased from direct insult to endothelial cells or disruption of their biochemical functions.
4. Impaired lymphatic drainage leads to retention of interstitial fluid.

5. Inhibition or inactivation of surfactant further contributes to the development of edema.
6. In some instances the pathogenesis of the edema is not well understood.

C. Classification of causes of pulmonary edema
   1. Increased pulmonary capillary pressure
      a) Cardiac disease, especially left heart failure
      b) Excessive parenteral fluid administration
   2. Decreased capillary oncotic pressure (hypoproteinemia)
      a) Liver disease
      b) Malnutrition, malabsorption
      c) Protein-losing enteropathy
      d) Protein-losing nephropathy
      e) Chronic hemorrhaging
   3. Altered capillary permeability
      a) Smoke inhalation
      b) Near-drowning
      c) Acute respiratory distress syndrome (shock lung)
      d) Endotoxins
         (1) Uremia
         (2) Vasoactive substances
      e) Exotoxins
         (1) Snake venom
         (2) Alpha-naphthyl thiourea (ANTU) poisoning
      f) Disseminated intravascular coagulopapthy
   4. Lymphatic insufficiency
      Infiltrative neoplasms
   5. Cause unknown
      a) Electrical shock
      b) Head injuries
      c) Seizures
      d) Drug induced

D. Clinical signs
   1. Moist, productive cough
   2. Cyanosis
   3. Orthopnea, dyspnea

4. Hemorrhagic froth from the nose and mouth
5. Apprehension
6. Moist rales upon auscultation

E. Diagnosis
1. History
   a) Previously diagnosed heart disease
   b) Exposure to:
      (1) Smoke
      (2) Near-drowning
      (3) ANTU poison
      (4) Venomous snakes
      (5) Electrical cords
      (6) Drugs
   c) Intolerance to exercise or stress
   d) Classic clinical signs
   e) Currently administered fluid therapy: type and quantity
2. Physical examination
   a) Check for oral and facial burns.
   b) Discern evidence of trauma.
   c) Note neurologic status.
   d) Determine presence of:
      (1) Heart murmurs
      (2) Arrhythmias
      (3) Peripheral venous distention
      (4) Ascites
   e) Observe overall state of nutrition.
   f) Examine for snakebites, exposure to toxins.
   g) Ascertain evidence of hypoproteinemia:
      (1) Ventral-dependent edema
      (2) Hydrothorax
      (3) Ascites
   h) Note evidence of other systemic illnesses.
   i) Observe age, sex and breed of animal.
3. Radiography of thorax
   See Table 12-5.
4. Laboratory tests
   a) Complete blood count

b) Biochemical organ profile
c) Urinalysis
d) Blood gas determination
e) Clotting survey
f) Sulfobromophthalein retention
g) Intestinal absorption studies

5. Other tests
    a) Electrocardiogram
    b) Measurement of CVP
    c) Echocardiography
    d) Nonselective angiography
    e) Percutaneous biopsy of liver, kidney, thoracic masses

F. Treatment
1. Objectives:
    a) Improve oxygenation of blood.
    b) Combat the edema.
    c) Determine and remove the cause.
2. Ensure a patent airway.
    a) Remove the animal from the owner and take it to a central treatment area or intensive care ward.
    b) Intubate and begin positive pressure breathing if collapsed.
    c) Administer O_2 via mask or cage.
    d) Handle gently. Minimize stress.
3. Consider insertion of IV catheter.
    a) To provide access to a vein for IV administration of medications
    b) Fluid therapy is contraindicated.
    c) Draw all blood samples for laboratory analysis.
4. Start medical therapy.
    a) Diuretics
        (1) Furosemide
        (2) Ethacrynate sodium
            (See Tables 12-7 and 12-8.)
    b) Bronchodilators

(1) Aminophylline
(2) Theophylline

c) Nebulization
(1) Ethanol-saline in a 1:2 dilution
(2) Reduces surface tension and foaming in the larger airways
(3) Facilitates removal of the edema fluid

d) Consider sedation.
(1) Helpful during cardiogenic pulmonary edema to decrease anxiety and stress
(2) Drug of choice is morphine sulfate.
(3) Contraindicated in patients with head injuries, seizures, and other forms of neurogenic pulmonary edema because it may increase intracranial pressure.

5. Determine cause.

a) Electrocardiography
(1) May be performed with animal standing if it is too stressed to lie down.
(2) Note evidence of heart disease.

b) Radiography of thorax
Attempt radiography when the animal is stable enough to leave the O_2 cage.

c) Complete blood count, organ profile, UA
(1) Note any hypoproteinemia.
(2) Determine presence of liver or renal disease.
(3) Watch for evidence of multiple organ dysfunction.

d) Blood gas determination

e) Catagorize probable origin of edema:
(1) Cardiac disease
(2) Liver disease
(3) Intestinal disorder
(4) Protein-losing nephropathy
(5) Toxin or drug induced
(6) Secondary to physical agents
(7) Neurogenic disorder

(8) Neoplasia
(9) Disseminated intravascular coagulopathy
(10) Overhydration

6. Institute specific therapy.
   a) Decrease workload of heart
      (1) Cage rest
      (2) Digitalization
      (3) Vasodilator therapy
         i) Is useful in both cardiac and neurogenic forms of pulmonary edema because vasodilators decrease resistance to cardiac outflow.
         ii) Must be used cautiously because they are hypotensive
      (4) Specific medications for feline cardiomyopathy
   b) Corticosteroids
      (1) Consider their use in:
         i) Electrical shock
         ii) Anaphylaxis
         iii) Smoke inhalation
         iv) Snakebites
   c) Plasma transfusion
      For hypoproteinemia
   d) Remove or treat cause.
      (1) Terminate fluid therapy, offending drug therapy.
      (2) Consider mannitol for head injuries.
      (3) Institute therapy for underlying systemic disorders.
7. Phlebotomy
   a) Should be considered in all cardiac patients that fail to stabilize with conventional therapy
   b) May also be beneficial in other forms of pulmonary edema
      (See Table 12-10.)
8. Start supportive care.

TABLE 12-10. PROTOCOL FOR THE TREATMENT OF PULMONARY EDEMA

1. Ensure patent airway; institute O_2 therapy.
   a. Mask
   b. O_2 cage
   c. Intubation, positive pressure ventilation
2. Consider insertion of IV catheter.
3. Start medical therapy.
   a. Decrease workload of heart
      i. Cage rest
      ii. Sedation
      iii. Digitalization
   b. Improve ventilation.
      i. Bronchodilators
      ii. Endotracheal suctioning
      iii. Nebulization with ethanol: saline
   c. Eliminate excessive fluid.
      i. Diuretics
      ii. Vasodilators
      iii. Phlebotomy
         Dog: remove 8 ml/kg, may be repeated in 2 h
         Cat: remove 6–10 ml/kg
   d. Stabilize membranes.
      Corticosteroids
   e. Supportive care
      i. Antibiotics
      ii. Sodium bicarbonate
4. Begin diagnostic workup when stable.
   a. Radiography
   b. Electrocardiography
   c. CBC, organ profile, urinalysis
   d. Blood gas determinations
5. Monitor:
   a. Respiratory rate and effort
   b. Pulse and heart rate
   c. Blood pressure
   d. CVP
   e. PCV, TS, BUN
   f. Urine output
   g. Body weight

a) Antibiotics
b) Sodium bicarbonate
c) Maintain body temperature.
d) Maintain patency of IV line.
e) See also protocol for CHF, Chapter 2.

G. Patient monitoring
  1. Respiratory rate and effort
     Note:
     a) Open-mouthed breathing
     b) Orthopnea
     c) Cyanosis
     d) Capillary refill time
     e) Presence of oral or nasal froth
     Auscultate thorax for rales.
  2. Heart and pulse rate
     Note arrhythmias and pulse deficits.
  3. Central venous pressure
     See Chapters 1 and 2, especially section on CHF.
  4. Blood pressure
     Particularly useful to monitor effects of vasodilating drugs
  5. Packed cell volume, TS, BUN
     a) Monitor for onset of dehydration and prerenal azotemia.
     b) Assess level of hypoproteinemia and response to therapy.
  6. Urine output
     a) Especially during therapy with diuretics
     b) Monitor urine specific gravity and protein.
     c) Consider quantification of any protein loss.
  7. Body weight
     a) Should be expected to drop, as medical therapy increases the elimination of edema fluid.
     b) Readjust medication dosages as the body weight changes.
  8. Electrocardiogram

V. Feline asthma
  A. Definition
     Feline asthma is an allergic condition characterized by reversible bronchospasm and bronchiolar obstruction. Acute asthma might be more accurately classified with diseases that cause airway obstruction. Because obstruction occurs in the terminal small airway, feline

asthma has been included in this section under exchange diseases.

B. Cause

Although specific allergens are not often defined, the following have been incriminated as causative factors:

1. Dust from cat litter
2. Smoke
3. Household dust particles
4. Kapok
5. Talc

C. Clinical signs

1. Sudden onset of dyspnea
2. Forceful, prolonged expiration
3. Open-mouthed breathing
4. Cyanosis
5. Orthopnea
6. Anxiety
7. Drooling
8. Increased bronchovesicular lung sounds
9. Expiratory wheezing, coughing
10. Abdominal distention with aerophagia
11. Clawing at the face

D. Diagnosis

1. History
    a) Intermittent episodes of wheezing, gagging, and/or coughing.
    b) Episodes may be worse after eating, handling, exercise, or going outside.
    c) Seasonal incidence may be noted.
    d) Anorexia and depression may also occur.
2. Physical examination
    a) Presence of suspicious clinical signs and physical findings
    b) Note productivity of coughing and sensitivity of trachea.
    c) Auscultate closely for crackling expiratory sounds, expiratory wheezing, and a diffuse increase in bronchovesicular sounds.

  - d) Note duration and any prolongation of inspiratory and expiratory phases of respiration.
  - e) Discern any increased expiratory effort.
3. Radiography of thorax
   - a) See Table 12-5.
   - b) Bullous emphysematous lesions may be seen in chronic cases.
   - c) Atelectasis is rarely seen following severe, recurrent episodes.
4. Laboratory data
   - a) Complete blood count

     Eosinophilia is noted in some cats.
   - b) Transtracheal aspirate or bronchoscopy

     Demonstration of increased numbers of eosinophils and occasional mast cells.
   - c) Skin-testing

     Although not routinely successful in cats, it may help to determine specific allergens involved.

E. Treatment
1. Objectives:
   - a) Relieve bronchospasm.
   - b) Eliminate airway obstruction.
   - c) Avoid contact with allergen.
2. Institute O_2 therapy.
   - a) It is preferable to place animal in O_2 cage because most cats do not tolerate O_2 masks.
   - b) Minimize handling and stress.
   - c) Draw blood for CBC.
3. Arrest the allergic reaction.
   - a) Institute corticosteroid therapy
   - b) The ultra-short-acting steroids may be administered in life-threatening situations, or asthma complicated by shock.
   - c) Most patients will respond to oral or injectable prednisolone or dexamethasone.
4. Start bronchodilators.

   Two classes of agents are available:

a) Xanthine derivatives
   Are often used in combination with corticosteroids during episodes of moderate respiratory distress.
b) Sympathomimetics
   (1) Are usually reserved for severe or life-threatening episodes
   (2) Are used in combination with xanthine derivatives and corticosteroids

(See Tables 12-8 and 12-11.)

5. Complete diagnostic workup.
   a) Radiography of thorax
   b) If stable, perform TTA or bronchoscopy.
6. Decrease exposure to allergens.
   a) Replace clay kitty litter with shredded newspaper, wood shavings, or damp sand.
   b) Stop application of all flea powders.
   c) Discourage owners from smoking.
   d) Replace dirty furnace or air filters.
   e) Consider skin-testing.

TABLE 12-11. PROTOCOL FOR THE TREATMENT OF FELINE ASTHMA

1. Institute O_2 therapy.
2. Start medical therapy—choose from the following:
   a. Corticosteroids
      i. Prednisolone sodium succinate—1–3 mg/kg IV
      ii. Hydrocortisone sodium succinate—1–3 mg/kg IV
      iii. Dexamethasone—0.05–0.1 mg/kg IM, SQ q6–8h
      iv. Prednisolone—0.5 mg/kg IM, PO q8–12h
   b. Xanthine derivatives
      i. Aminophylline—2 mg/kg IV in 100 ml 5% D/W IV q8–12h; or 50 mg PO q8h
      ii. Theophylline—0.1 mg/kg IV, IM q8h
   c. Sympathomimetics
      i. Isoproterenol—dilute 0.2 mg in 10 ml normal saline; give 0.2–0.3 ml of dilution IM q30 min; or 0.2 mg in 100 ml 5% D/W IV q8h to effect
      ii. Epinephrine—0.1 mg SQ q4–6h; or 0.2 mg in 100 ml 5% D/W IV q8–12h to effect
3. Draw blood for CBC.
4. Radiograph thorax.
5. If stable, perform TTA, bronchoscopy.

F. Patient monitoring
   1. Respiratory rate and effort
   2. Mucous membrane color
   3. Lung sounds, continued coughing
   4. Radiographic changes
      Repeat radiographs in 2–14 days.

PLEURAL CAVITY DISEASE

I. Definition

Pleural cavity disease includes the problems that decrease functional capacity of the lungs by assuming space in the pleural cavity and injuries that disrupt the respiratory bellows by damaging the integrity of the thoracic wall. These diseases must be differentiated from systemic problems that compromise respiration by causing pressure upon or restricting excursions of the diaphragm, namely, ascites, gastric dilatation, intraabdominal neoplasms or hemorrhage, pregnancy, and abdominal pain. Table 12-12 summarizes the causes of pleural cavity disease.

II. Classification
   A. Pneumothorax
      1. Pathophysiology
         a) Is the accumulation of free air in the pleural cavity
         b) As air escapes into the pleural cavity, nega-

TABLE 12-12. CLASSIFICATION OF PLEURAL CAVITY DISEASE

Pneumothorax
Pleural effusion
Chylothorax
Pyothorax
Hydrothorax
Hemothorax
Neoplastic effusion
Infectious, inflammatory effusion
Diaphragmatic hernia
Flail chest

tive pleural pressure is lost, and the lungs undergo elastic recoil and collapse.

c) Tension pneumothorax is a condition in which a tear in the pleura forms a one-way valve so that air accumulates in the pleural space during inspiration and is not expelled during expiration.

d) Tension pneumothorax causes rapid clinical deterioration because severe pulmonary atelectasis and decreased venous return to the heart occur within a short time.

2. Causes
   a) Trauma
      (1) Is the most common cause
      (2) ± Rib fractures
      (3) Blunt, nonpenetrating blows produce:
         i) Pleural lacerations
         ii) Parenchymal lacerations
         iii) Tracheobronchial ruptures
      (4) Penetrating injuries allow leakage of atmospheric air into the chest.
   b) Spontaneous forms
      (1) Rupture of bullous emphysematous lung lesions
      (2) Rupture of granulomatous lung lesions
   c) Iatrogenic causes
      (1) Intrathoracic surgical procedures
      (2) Resuscitative efforts
      (3) Overzealous positive pressure ventilation
      (4) Surgical procedures near the diaphragm or ribs
   d) Following pneumomediastimum from trauma to the trachea or esophagus

B. Pleural effusion
   1. Pathophysiology
      a) Pleural effusion is abnormal fluid accumulation in the pleural cavity.

b) Normally there are several milliliters of fluid in the pleural cavity to diminish friction between the lungs, heart, and parietal pleura.
c) This normal fluid is formed by transudation from the parietal pleura and is removed by absorption into capillaries and lymphatics of both the visceral and parietal pleura.

2. Classification
   a) Hemothorax
      (1) Is blood in the pleural cavity
      (2) Causes:
         i) Trauma to lung parenchyma
         ii) Rupture of cardiac or intrathoracic blood vessels
         iii) Clotting disorders
         iv) Bleeding neoplasms, especially hemangiosarcoma
         v) Lung lobe torsion
   b) Chylothorax
      (1) Indicates the presence of intestinal lymph or chyle within the pleural space
      (2) Occurs with rupture of the thoracic duct from:
         i) Trauma
         ii) Herniation of diaphragm
         iii) Thromboembolization of the cranial vena cava
         iv) Thoracic surgical procedures
         v) Undetermined causes
   c) Hydrothorax
      (1) Is the presence of transudate in the pleural cavity
      (2) Pure transudate is usually caused by hypoproteinemia.
      (3) Modified transudate develops with any long standing condition such as heart failure and cardiomyopathy.
   d) Pyothorax

(1) Is pus or septic effusion in the pleural space
(2) Causes:
i) Penetrating thoracic wounds
ii) Penetrating esophageal wounds
iii) Extension of infection from the lungs, mediastinum, or abdomen
iv) Complication of hematogenous infections
v) Migration of foreign bodies
vi) Iatrogenic contamination of a preexisting pleural effusion

e) Neoplastic effusion
(1) Causes:
i) Anterior mediastinal lymphoma
ii) Mesothelioma
iii) Metastatic carcinomas and adenocarcinomas
iv) Hemangiosarcoma
(2) This effusion may be distinguishable from inflammatory effusion by the presence of neoplastic cells.

f) Inflammatory, aseptic effusion
Most commonly arises from:
(1) Lung lobe torsion (dogs)
(2) Feline infectious peritonitis (cats)

C. Diaphragmatic hernia
1. Pathophysiology
a) A blunt blow exerts increased pressure to the peritoneal side of the diaphragm.
b) If the glottis is open, there is no equalizing pressure on the thoracic side of the diaphragm and the diaphragm ruptures.
c) Displacement of the lungs by abdominal viscera and disruption of the respiratory bellows leads to inadequate air exchange.
2. Causes
a) Blunt trauma

   b) Falling from heights
   c) Congenital malformations
   d) See also section on Hernias, Chapter 7.
D. Flail chest
  1. Pathophysiology
   a) Flail chest occurs with fractures of both the proximal and distal portions of consecutive ribs.
   b) The chest wall is unstable and moves paradoxically, being drawn inward with inspiration and forced outward with expiration.
   c) May occur with consecutive fractures of the proximal ribs in young animals when the costal cartilages are still very pliable.
   d) Often accompanied by pulmonary contusion
  2. Causes
   a) Automobile accidents
   b) Attacks by a larger animal

III. Clinical signs
 A. General symptoms
  1. Mild resting polypnea to severe dyspnea
  2. Cyanosis
  3. Abduction of the forelimbs
  4. Reluctance to lie down
  5. Coughing
  6. Increased abdominal respiratory efforts
  7. Pain, apprehension
  8. Increased susceptibility to stress
  9. Shock, pallor
  10. ± Pyrexia
 B. Specific signs
  1. Pneumothorax
   a) Diminished lung sounds dorsally
   b) Hyperresonance with chest percussion, especially dorsally
   c) Rib fractures
   d) Thoracic wounds
   e) Subcutaneous emphysema

2. Pleural effusion
    a) Diminished lung sounds ventrally
    b) Muffled heart sounds
    c) Displacement of the apex beat of the heart
    d) Pleural friction rubs upon auscultation
    e) Dullness ventrally with chest percussion
    f) Decreased compressibility of the anterior thorax may be noted with some neoplasms
    g) Subcutaneous limb edema and ascites may occur with hydrothorax of any cause.
    h) Cardiac disease may be accompanied by murmurs or arrhythmias.
3. Diaphragmatic hernia
    a) Unilateral or ventral muffling of heart and lung sounds and dullness with percussion
    b) Auscultation of gut sounds within the chest
    c) Conspicuous absence of abdominal organs with abdominal palpation
    d) External evidence of trauma
    e) Dysphagia, vomiting, and retching may occur with chronic or congenital hernias.
    f) Rarely, gastric dilatation may occur within the chest, resulting in tympany with percussion.
4. Flail chest

    Obvious deformity of the chest which moves paradoxically with breathing

IV. Diagnosis

A. History

1. Determine onset of respiratory distress.
2. Documented traumatic incident:
    a) Automobile accident
    b) High-rise fall
    c) Attack by another animal
    d) Penetrating wounds from projectiles
3. Previously diagnosed systemic illnesses:
    a) Liver or cardiac disease
    b) Hypoproteinemia
    c) Bleeding disorders

   d) Primary lung parenchymal disease
   e) Foreign bodies of trachea or esophagus
   f) Incidence of recent surgical procedures
   g) Evidence of any other concurrent illnesses

B. Physical examination
  1. Auscultation
     a) Determine type and presence of lung sounds.
     b) Note areas where lung sounds are diminished or absent.
     c) Discern any muffling of heart sounds and abnormal heart sounds or murmurs.
     d) Listen for pleural friction rubs, airway noise, and intrathoracic gut sounds.
  2. Percussion

     Note areas of dullness, hyperresonance, or tympany.
  3. Palpation
     a) Attempt to locate any bite wounds, lacerations, or fractures of the thoracic cage.
     b) Determine whether abdominal organs are in their normal positions.
  4. Examine other body systems

     Detect evidence of chronic systemic diseases:
     a) Weight loss
     b) Pyrexia
     c) Weakness
     d) Dehydration
     e) Heart murmurs, arrhythmias
     f) Hepatomegaly
     g) Subcutaneous edema
     h) Ascites
     i) Peripheral venous distention
     j) Note any signs of external trauma.
     k) Discern any bleeding at other sites.

C. Radiography of thorax
  1. Plain radiographs
     a) Delineate:
        (1) Rib fractures
        (2) Pulmonary parenchymal injuries

(3) Pneumothorax
(4) Presence of pleural effusion

b) May allow definitive diagnosis of diaphragmatic hernia if abdominal viscera are visualized within the chest.

c) If thoracic detail is obscured by fluid within the chest, remove as much fluid as possible via thoracentesis and repeat the radiographs.

2. Contrast radiography

a) May be necessary to confirm the presence of a diaphragmatic hernia

b) Pneumoperitoneography with 20–30 ml of carbon dioxide will help define small tears. A horizontal, upright beam radiograph is taken with the animal in a ventrodorsal position. The intact diaphragm is well outlined by air.

c) Barium administered PO outlines displacement of the gastrointestinal tract.

D. Thoracentesis

1. Techniques

a) Thoracentesis should be attempted in animals with severe pneumothorax and pleural effusion that are severely compromised, before the stress of radiography.

b) Shave hair and sterilely prepare the skin.

c) Air is best aspirated dorsally at the seventh to ninth intercostal spaces.

d) Fluid is best aspirated ventrally at the seventh or eighth intercostal space. Care must be taken to avoid the apex beat of the heart.

e) A 20- or 22-gauge 1.5-in. needle, three-way stopcock, and 20-ml syringe are used.

f) Tranquilization may be needed in some patients.

g) Tension pneumothorax should be suspected if the syringe plunger is forcibly pushed back by positive pleural pressure or with removal of large quantities of air.

h) As much fluid as possible is removed and a small quantity is saved for laboratory analysis and culture.

2. Fluid analysis
   a) Note:
      (1) Physical appearance
      (2) Specific gravity
      (3) Total protein
      (4) White blood cell count
      (5) Red blood cell count
      (6) Cytology
      (7) Presence of chyle, microorganisms
   b) Blood aspirated accidentally from the intercostal or thoracic arteries will clot and platelets will be seen in smears made from the fluid.
   c) Bloody effusion does not clot.
   d) True chylous fluid will clear from a milky white to a translucent straw color after being alkalinized and mixed with ether.
   e) Transudate generally has a specific gravity <1.013 and a total protein <1.0 g/dl.
   f) Table 12-13 provides data to be used in the differential diagnosis of pleural effusions.

E. Other diagnostic tests
   a) Complete blood count
   b) Urinalysis
   c) Biochemical organ profile
   d) Clotting survey
   e) Arterial blood gases
   f) Measurement of CVP
   g) Electrocardiography
   h) Echocardiography
   i) Contrast lymphangiography
   j) Feline leukemia virus ELIZA
   j) Feline infectious peritonitis titer, serum electrophoresis
   k) Nonselective angiography

TABLE 12-13. CHARACTERISTICS OF PLEURAL EFFUSION

Type of Effusion	Color	Specific Gravity	Total Protein (g/dl)	Clots	Cytology
Pure transudate	Clear to pure yellow	<1.018	1.0–3.0	No	<300 cells/mm^3 Cells seen are mostly mononuclear
Modified transudate	Pale yellow to blood-tinged	1.018–1.030	1.0–5.0	Does not usually	Cellularity is greater than transudate. RBC ≥ 25,000/mm^3 Lymphocytes are increased. Reactive mesothelial cells are seen and may be mistaken for neoplastic cells.
Hemorrhagic effusion	Blood red	1.030–1.045	3.0–7.5	Does not clot if long-standing	Blood elements resemble peripheral blood. PCV—10–40% Neoplastic cells may be seen with hemangiosarcoma. Platelets are not seen in smears
Chyle	Milky white	—	—	No	Contains large numbers of lymphocytes and small number of RBC Chylomicrons stain bright orange with Sudan III. Will clear when alkalinized and mixed with equal parts of ether
Septic effusion (pyothorax)	Cloudy, purulent	1.021–1.033	3.0–5.5	No	Malodorous Toxicity and degeneration (karolysis, karyorrhexis, and pyknosis) of neutrophils are seen. Free or phagocytized bacteria or fungal elements are seen.
Aseptic, inflammatory effusion (FIP)	Straw-yellow	1.027–1.045	4.1–8.5	Yes	Thick, viscious, stringy consistency Only moderate numbers of RBCs and WBCs seen. Neutrophils predominate and are not toxic. No microorganisms are seen.
Neoplastic effusion	Clear yellow to serosanguinous	1.015–1.045	1.5–7.5	May clot	± Malignant cells seen and must be differentiated from reactive mesothelial cells.

V. Treatment
  A. Objectives:
    1. Evacuate all air and fluid from the pleural cavity.
    2. Correct any defects in the thoracic wall and diaphragm.
    3. Treat or remove the cause.
  B. Establish patent airway.
    1. Intubate if collapsed.
    2. Administer O_2.
  C. Treat shock.
    1. Insert IV catheter.
    2. Begin fluid therapy.
    3. Consider corticosteroids.
  D. Perform preliminary examination of chest.
    1. Apply airtight bandage over penetrating "sucking" wounds and flail segments.
    2. Examine for abnormalities in percussion and auscultation.
       (See Table 12-14.)
  E. Assess status of animal.
    1. Perform systemic examination.
      a) Examine for other life-threatening injuries.
      b) Control any external hemorrhaging.
    2. For severe respiratory distress:
      a) Perform immediate thoracentesis with a needle and syringe.
      b) Minimize handling and stress.
      c) Administer O_2.
      d) Consider insertion of indwelling chest tube.
    3. For mild to moderate distress:
      a) Radiograph thorax.
      b) Perform thoracentesis.
        (1) Evacuate air and/or fluid.
        (2) Determine type of effusion.
        (3) Attempt to determine source of effusion.
      c) Reradiograph thorax
      d) Consider insertion of chest tube for:
        (1) Severe pneumothorax

TABLE 12-14. PROTOCOL FOR THE TREATMENT OF PLEURAL CAVITY DISEASE

1. Establish patent airway; institute O_2 therapy.
2. Treat for shock.
3. Perform thoracic examination.
   a. Auscultation
   b. Percussion
   c. Bandage penetrating wounds, flail segments.
4. Assess status of animal.
   a. Severe distress
      i. Perform immediate thoracentesis.
      ii. Consider insertion of chest tube.
      iii. O_2 therapy
   b. Mild to moderate distress
      i. Radiograph thorax—survey and contrast films.
      ii. Perform thoracentesis.
      iii. Consider insertion of chest tube.
      iv. O_2 therapy
   c. No distress
      i. Radiograph thorax.
      ii. Cage rest
      iii. Observation
5. Perform diagnostic workup.
   a. Thoracic fluid analysis
   b. CBC, biochemical profile
   c. Clotting survey
   d. ECG, CVP
6. Start supportive care.
   a. Fluid therapy
   b. Antibiotics
   c. $\pm$Sodium bicarbonate
7. Monitor
   a. Respiratory rate and effort; if rate >60 breaths/min, consider inserting a chest tube or increasing frequency of chest tube evacuation.
   b. Mucous membrane color; CRT
   c. Patency of one-way valve
   d. Serial thoracic radiographs
8. Prepare for surgery.
   a. Herniorrhaphy
   b. Repair wounds and rib fractures.
   c. Exploratory thoracotomy
   d. Ligate thoracic duct.
   e. Lobectomy
9. Remove any medical causes of pleural cavity disease by appropriate therapy.

(2) Tension pneumothorax
(3) Large quantities of pleural effusion
(4) Pleural effusion that is likely to recur

4. Technique for insertion of chest tube:
   a) The hair is shaved and the skin is sterilely prepared.
   b) If time allows, the skin and musculature are infiltrated with a local anesthetic one to two ribs caudal to the thoracic insertion site.
   c) The tube is inserted in the dorsal aspect of the seventh to eight intercostal space for prolonged evacuation of air.
   d) The tube is inserted ventrally in the same intercostal space for continued drainage of fluid.
   e) One or more tubes uni- or bilaterally may be inserted.
   f) A stab incision is made through the skin.
   g) The chest tube with trochar is advanced cranially to the desired site, and with a quick, forceful movement is advanced through the intercostal muscles and into the thorax. (See Fig. 12-2.)
   h) The trochar is removed, the tube is cross-clamped, and the free end of the tube is attached to a three-way stopcock, one-way valve, or continuous evacuation pump.
   i) See Table 12-15.
   j) The clamp is released and patency of the tube is ensured.
   k) A pursestring suture is placed in the skin where the tube exits.
   l) The tube is fixed to the chest by placing stay sutures through a tape butterfly surrounding the free end of the tube.
   m) A light chest wrap is applied to protect the tube from dislodgement.

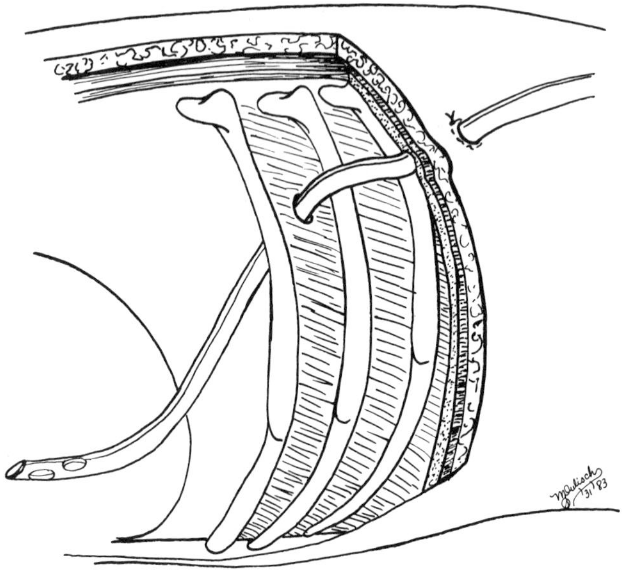

Fig. 12-2. Technique for insertion of an indwelling chest tube. A stab incision is made one or two rib spaces caudal to the site of insertion into the chest. A pursestring suture placed in the skin where the tube exits helps to maintain an airtight seal and prevents slippage of the tube.

TABLE 12-15. COMMERCIAL PRODUCTS FOR USE IN PLEURAL CAVITY DISEASE AND RESPIRATORY ARREST

Indwelling chest tube—Argyle trochar catheter with Sentinel Eye and Sentinel line, Argyle Division of Sherwood Medical, St. Louis, MO 63103

One-way air valve—Heimlich Chest Drain Valve, Bard-Parker, Rutherford, NJ 07070

Continuous evacuation pump—PLEUR-EVAC, Deknatel, Division of Howmedica, Queens Village, NY 11429

Naloxone HCl—Narcan injection, Endo Laboratories, Garden City, NY 11530

Levallorphan tartrate—Lorfan, Roche Laboratories, Nutley, NJ 07110

Doxapram—Dopram injectable, A.H. Robins, Richmond, VA 23220

5. No respiratory distress is present:
    a) Radiograph thorax.
    b) Perform thoracentesis.
        (1) A single aspiration of air may be sufficient to relieve mild cases of pneumothorax.
        (2) Remove as much pleural fluid as possible.
    c) Cage rest and observation may be all that is required for mild cases of pneumothorax with minimal polypnea ($<$60 respirations/min) and mild cases of traumatic hemothorax.

F. Start supportive care.
    a) Oxygen therapy
    b) Antibiotics
    c) $\pm$ Sodium bicarbonate
    d) Continued fluid therapy

G. Stabilize animal and prepare for surgery.
1. Indication for exploratory thoracotomy:
    a) Persistent arterial or neoplastic intrathoracic bleeding
    b) Unresponsive spontaneous or tension pneumothorax
    c) Recurrent pneumothorax
    d) Penetrating wounds
    e) Neoplasms unresponsive to other therapy
    f) Suspected pericardial disease
    g) Unresponsive pyothorax
2. Repair wounds and rib fractures.
3. Repair diaphragmatic hernias.
    See Chapter 7.
4. Lobectomy is indicated in:
    a) Lung lobe torsions
    b) Pneumothorax from emphysematous or granulomatous lung lesions
    c) Irreversible atelectasis of a lung lobe
5. Ligation of thoracic duct

Is the treatment of choice for persistent chylothorax

- H. Start specific medical therapy.
  1. Correct or reverse hypoproteinemia.
  2. Institute appropriate therapy for
     a) Cardiac disease
     b) Clotting disorders
     c) Chylothorax
     d) Pyothorax
  3. Begin chemotherapy for neoplasms.
  4. Palliative measures are currently the only therapy available for certain neoplasms and FIP.

VI. Patient monitoring

- A. Respiratory rate and effort
  1. Resting respiratory rate should be <60 breaths/min.
  2. With rates >60 breaths/min:
     a) Consider insertion of chest tube.
     b) Examine any tube already inserted for patency.
- B. Capillary refill time, mucous membrane color
- C. Heart rate and rhythm
- D. Maintain patency of chest tube.
  1. Fluid or blood aspirated through a one-way valve may cause the rubber leaflets to stick together.
  2. Replace one-way valve as often as needed.
  3. Tubes used to drain fluid should be aspirated every 2–6 h or any time the respiratory rate increases.
- E. Arterial blood gases q24–48h
- F. Central venous pressure
- G. Electrocardiogram
- H. Body temperature
- I. Complete blood count, serum electrolytes
- J. Serial radiographs of thorax q24–48h
  1. Radiographs are useful to check the position of chest tubes after their insertion.
  2. Serial radiographs will allow evaluation of resolution of both pneumothorax and pleural effusion.

RESPIRATORY ARREST

I. Definition

Respiratory arrest is the cessation of breathing. It is imperative for the clinician to know that respiratory arrest demands immediate correction and should take precedence over all other emergency care. Approximately 3–5 min can lapse between respiratory arrest and the development of cardiac failure and arrest.

II. Cause

- A. May result from any of the respiratory emergencies discussed in this chapter
- B. May follow states of respiratory insufficiency from:
  1. Chronic heart disease
  2. Thromboembolism following treatment of heartworm disease
  3. Chronic pulmonary parenchymal disease of any type
- C. Depression of respiratory centers
  1. Brain injuries
  2. Increased intracranial pressure
  3. Hypoxia
  4. Infection
  5. Overdosage of depressant drugs, such as:
     - a) Narcotics
     - b) Tranquilizers
     - c) Barbiturates
     - d) Gaseous anesthetics
- D. Paralysis of respiratory muscles
  - a) Fractures of cervical spinal cord with involvement of the phrenic nerve
  - b) Myasthenia gravis
  - c) Organophosphate poisoning
  - d) Overdosage of paralytic agents, such as succinylcholine
- E. Severe spasms of respiratory muscles, such as those seen in terminal tetanus, may contribute to respiratory arrest.

F. Because respiratory arrest usually precedes or accompanies cardiac arrest, the causes of cardiac arrest should be reviewed. See Chapter 2.

III. Clinical signs
- A. Slow, irregular respirations
- B. Labored respirations
- C. Absence of chest movements
- D. Cessation of airflow
- E. Cyanosis
- F. Signs of hypoxia that precede respiratory arrest include:
  - a) Restlessness, anxiety
  - b) Tachycardia, arrhythmias
  - c) Nausea, vomiting
  - d) Dilatation of pupils
  - e) Involuntary muscle twitching

IV. Diagnosis
- A. Physical examination
  1. The state of respiratory arrest should be obvious.
  2. Rapid evaluation of the cardiovascular system should be undertaken.
  3. A thorough physical examination is indicated to determine a probable cause.
- B. Ancillary tests
  1. Used primarily to determine the etiology and assess the extent of damage caused by respiratory arrest.
  2. Include:
     - a) Complete blood count
     - b) Biochemical organ profile
     - c) Urinalysis
     - d) Electrocardiogram
     - e) Arterial blood gases
     - f) Radiography of chest and abdomen
     - g) Measurement of CVP

V. Treatment
- A. Objectives:
  1. Establish a patent airway.
  2. Begin artificial respiration and O_2 therapy.
  3. Reestablish normal, spontaneous respiration.

4. Avoid cardiac arrest.
5. Remove the cause.

B. Establish a patent airway.
1. Intubate.
2. Remove any foreign debris or obstructive material.
3. Institute 100% O_2 therapy with intermittent positive pressure ventilation.
4. See Table 12-16.
5. If circumstances do not allow intubation, begin mouth-to-nostril breathing.
   a) Dog: 10–12 breaths/min
   b) Cat: 12–15 breaths/min
6. In the absence of a source of O_2, begin positive pressure ventilation with room air via an AMBU bag.
7. Perform a tracheotomy if upper airway obstruction prevents intubation.

C. Start fluid therapy.
1. Insert an IV catheter.
2. Begin administration of a multiple electrolyte solution or 5% D/W.

D. Record ECG.
1. Note any cardiac abnormalities.
2. Institute therapy as indicated. See Chapter 2.

E. Eliminate respiratory depressants.
1. Terminate anesthesia and flush gaseous anesthetics from O_2 lines.
2. Use antagonistic drugs to reverse the effects of narcotics:
   a) Naloxone HCl
   b) Levallorphan tartrate
      (See Tables 12-15 and 12-16.)
   c) Consider the use of respiratory stimulants, such as doxapram.

F. Cardiac arrest
If this crisis develops follow the protocol outlined in Chapter 2.

G. Remove cause.

TABLE 12-16. PROTOCOL FOR THE TREATMENT OF RESPIRATORY ARREST

1. Establish patent airway.
   a. Remove obstructions, foreign material.
   b. Intubate.
   c. Consider tracheostomy.
2. Artificial respiration
   a. Intubation with O_2
      i. Positive pressure–end-inspiratory pressure of 15–20 cm H_2O
      ii. High O_2 flows—15 ml/kg/min with minimum of 1 liter
      iii. Rate
         Dog: 10–12 breaths/min
         Cat: 12–15 breaths/min
   b. Intubation with room air delivered via AMBU bag
      i. Positive pressure—watch for wide excursions of chest
      ii. Rates—same as above (2.a.iii)
   c. Mouth-to-nostril breathing
      i. Attempt positive pressure.
      ii. Rates—same as above
3. Call for help.
4. Insert IV catheter—5% D/W or multiple electrolyte solution.
5. Record ECG.
6. Eliminate depressant agents.
   a. Stop anesthesia.
   b. Narcotic antagonists
      i. Naloxone HCl
         Dog: 0.02–0.04 mg/kg IV
         Cat: 0.02–0.03 mg/kg IV
      ii. Levallorphan tartrate
         Dog: 0.02–0.2 mg/kg IV
         Cat: 0.22–0.45 mg/kg IV
   c. Respiratory stimulants
      i. Doxapram—1–4 mg/kg IV
7. See protocol for cardiac arrest, Chapter 2.
8. Monitor
   a. Mucous membrane color and CRT
   b. Respiratory rate and ventilation
   c. Pulse, heart rate and rhythm
   d. Pupils
   e. CVP, blood gases
   f. ECG
9. Investigate and remove cause of respiratory failure.

Once a diagnosis of the cause is determined, begin specific therapy for that disorder.

VI. Patient monitoring
   A. Discontinue assisted respiration once spontaneous respirations are noted.
   B. Continuously monitor:
      1. Capillary refill time
      2. Mucous membrane color
      3. Electrocardiogram
      4. Pupils
         As hypoxia is reversed the pupils change from dilated to midsized and become responsive to light.
      5. Level of consciousness, response to stimuli
         Improvement also closely parallels the reversal of hypoxia.
      6. Pulse strength and rate
         Compare it to heart rate.
   C. Arterial blood gases
      Help to evaluate adequacy of therapy
   D. Central venous pressure
      1. Used to assess response to fluid therapy
      2. May help to determine underlying cause
   E. When stable:
      1. Leave the animal in O_2 cage for 4–24 h.
      2. Watch closely for signs of recurrence for at least 24 h.
      3. Minimize handling and stress.
      4. Institute long-term management of any predisposing systemic diseases.

BIBLIOGRAPHY

Berg J: Chylothorax in the dog and cat. Compend Contin Ed Pract Vet 4(12):986, 1982

Bonagura JD: Pulmonary edema. p. 243. In Kirk RW (ed): Current Veterinary Therapy. Vol. 7. WB Saunders, Philadelphia, 1980

Bryan RD, Frome RW: Tracheal leiomyoma in a dog. J Am Vet Med Assoc 178(10):1069, 1981

Carpenter JL: Bronchial asthma in cats. p. 208. In Kirk RW (ed): Current Veterinary Therapy. Vol. 5. WB Saunders, Philadelphia, 1974

Creighton SR, Wilkins RJ: Pleural effusions. p. 253. In Kirk RW (ed): Current Veterinary Therapy. Vol. 7. WB Saunders, Philadelphia, 1980

Crow SE: Neoplasms of the respiratory tract. p. 249. In Kirk RW (ed): Current Veterinary Therapy. Vol. 7. WB Saunders, Philadelphia, 1980

Crowe DT: Traumatic pulmonary contusions, hematomas, pseudocysts, and acute respiratory distress syndrome: an update—Part I. Compend Contin Ed Pract Vet 5(5):396, 1983

Ettinger SJ, Ticer JW: Diseases of the trachea. p. 604. In Ettinger SJ (ed): Textbook of Veterinary Internal Medicine. Vol. 1. WB Saunders, Philadelphia, 1975

Farrow CW: Near-drowning. p. 182. In Kirk RW (ed): Current Veterinary Therapy. Vol. 7. WB Saunders, Philadelphia, 1980

Farrow CW: Inhalation injury. p. 186. In Kirk RW (ed): Current Veterinary Therapy. Vol. 7. WB Saunders, Philadelphia, 1980

Guyton AC: Textbook of Medical Physiology. 6th Ed. WB Saunders, Philadelphia, 1981

Hardie EM, Kolata RJ, Stone EA, Steiss JE: Laryngeal paralysis in three cats. J Am Vet Med Assoc 179(9):879, 1981

Harpster NK: Pulmonary edema. p. 219. In Kirk RW (ed): Current Veterinary Therapy. Vol. 5. WB Saunders, Philadelphia, 1974

Harvey CE: Upper airway obstruction surgery: overview of results. JAAHA 18(4):535, 1982

Harvey CE, O'Brien JA: Management of respiratory emergencies in small animals. Vet Clin N Am 2(2):243, 1972

Harvey HJ, Sykes G: Tracheal mast cell tumor in a dog. J Am Vet Med Assoc 180(9):1097, 1982

Haskins SC: Cardiopulmonary resuscitation. Compend Contin Ed Pract Vet 4(2):170, 1982

Hedlund CS, Taugner CH: Tracheal surgery in the dog—Part II. Compend Contin Ed Pract Vet 5(9):738, 1983

Hunt CA: Chest trauma-specific injuries. Compend Contin Ed Pract Vet 1(8):624, 1978

Kagan KG: Thoracic trauma. Vet Clin N Am 10(3):641, 1980

Kleine LJ: Radiologic aspects of thoracic trauma in the dog and cat (Part I). Compend Contin Ed Pract Vet 1(3):199, 1979

Kleine LJ: Radiologic aspects of thoracic trauma in the dog and cat (Part II). Compend Contin Ed Pract Vet 1(4):287, 1979

Kolata RJ: Management of thoracic trauma. Vet Clin N Am 11(1):103, 1981

Kolata RJ, Burrows CF: The clinical features of injury by chewing electrical cords in dogs and cats. JAAHA 17(2):219, 1981

Krahwinkel DJ: Thoracic trauma. p. 268. In Kirk RW (ed): Current Veterinary Therapy. Vol. 7. WB Saunders, Philadelphia, 1980

McKiernan B: Diseases of the canine and feline tracheobronchial tree. p. 229. In Kirk RW (ed): Current Veterinary Therapy. Vol. 7. WB Saunders, Philadelphia, 1980

McKiernan B: Canine and feline pneumonia. p. 235. In Kirk RW (ed): Current Veterinary Therapy. Vol. 7. WB Saunders, Philadelphia, 1980

Moise NS, Spaulding GL: Feline bronchial asthma: pathogenesis, pathophysiology, diagnostics, and therapeutic considerations. Compend Contin Ed Pract Vet 3(12):1091, 1981

O'Brien JA, Harvey CE: Diseases of the upper airway. p. 565. In Ettinger SJ (ed): Textbook of Veterinary Internal Medicine. Vol. 1. WB Saunders, Philadelphia, 1975

Orsher AN, Kolata RJ: Acute respiratory distress syndrome: case report and literature review. JAAHA 18(1):41, 1982

Osborne CA, Perman V: Pleural effusion. p. 234. In Kirk RW (ed): Current Veterinary Therapy. Vol. 5. WB Saunders, Philadelphia, 1974

Rodkey WG: Initial assessment, resuscitation and management of the critically traumatized small animal patient. Vet Clin N Am 10(3):561, 1980

Schaer M, Zaki FA, Harvey HJ, O'Reilly WH: Laryngeal hemiplegia due to neoplasia of the vagus nerve in a cat. J Am Vet Med Assoc 174(5):513, 1979

Short CE: Therapy of respiratory emergencies. p. 277. In Kirk RW (ed): Current Veterinary Therapy, Vol. 7. WB Saunders, Philadelphia, 1980

Suter PF, Head JR: Mediastinal, pleural, and extrapleural diseases. p. 767. In Ettinger SJ (ed): Textbook of Veterinary Internal Medicine. Vol. 1. WB Saunders, Philadelphia, 1975

Tams TR, Scherding RG: Smoke inhalation injury. Compend Contin Ed Pract Vet 3(11):986, 1981

Taugner CH, Hedlund CS: Tracheal surgery in the dog—Part I. Compend Contin Ed Pract Vet 5(8):599, 1983

Ticer JW, Brown SG: Thoracic trauma. p. 629. In Ettinger SJ: (ed): Textbook of Veterinary Internal Medicine. Vol. 1. WB Saunders, Philadelphia, 1975

Venker-van Haagen AJ: Laryngeal paralysis in young Bouviers. p. 290.

In Kirk RW (ed): Current Veterinary Therapy. Vol. 7. WB Saunders, Philadelphia, 1980

Venker-van Haagen AJ, Bouw J, Hartman W: Hereditary transmission of laryngeal paralysis in Bouviers. JAAHA 17(1):75, 1981

Venker-van Haagen AJ, Hartman W, Goedegebuure SA: Spontaneous laryngeal paralysis in young Bouviers. JAAHA 14(6):714, 1978

Walshaw R, Ford RB: Canine upper respiratory diseases. p. 214. In Kirk RW (ed): Current Veterinary Therapy. Vol. 7. WB Saunders, Philadelphia, 1980

White RJ: Acute respiratory failure. p. 190. In Kirk RW (ed): Current Veterinary Therapy. Vol. 5. WB Saunders, Philadelphia, 1974

Wykes PM: Canine laryngeal diseases. Part I. Anatomy and disease syndromes. Compend Contin Ed Pract Vet 5(1):8, 1983

Wykes PM: Canine laryngeal diseases. Part II. Diagnosis and treatment. Compend Contin Ed Pract Vet 5(2):105, 1983

Yoshioka MM: Management of spontaneous pneumothorax in twelve dogs. JAAHA 18(1):57, 1982

13

Bites and Stings of Venomous Animals and Toad Poisoning

Carol S. O'Neill Foil
Don R. Waldron

VENOMOUS ARTHROPODS

I. Definition

This section will deal with envenomations produced by the bites or stings of spiders, scorpions, and ticks. The clinical signs produced by arthropod envenomations vary greatly depending on the species involved. The emergency clinician should be aware that, just as is the case in snakebite, every exposure to a poisonous animal does not result in significant envenomation. Furthermore, because of protection afforded by their haircoats and, in some cases because of inherent resistance to the toxins, envenomation by arthropods is probably much less common among small animals than among humans. Nevertheless, because of widespread knowledge among pet owners of the appearance and nature of venomous arthropods, the veterinary clinician may be called upon to provide information and reassurance more frequently than to provide real emergency therapy. For this reason, some comparative medicine information is provided herein concerning venomous arthropods.

II. Spiders

A. *Latrodectus spp.*—black widow spider, Australian red-back spider, katipo

1. Biology

a) Distribution and habitat
   (1) There are five Latrodectus species with a worldwide distribution for the genus.
   (2) The *black widow spider* occurs throughout the United States and Canada.
   (3) The *red-back spider* occurs throughout Australia.
   (4) The *katipo* occurs in coastal areas of New Zealand south to Dunedin on South Island.
   (5) The red-back and black widow spiders have similar habitats, being found in quiet dark areas under houses, among garden rubbish, and in infrequently disturbed outbuildings.

b) Description
   (1) Members of the genus are small ($<$3 cm) and unaggressive.
      i) Only the females are considered dangerous. They may be extremely aggressive when protecting egg masses.
      ii) The females have globose, shiny black abdomens with distinctive red to orange hourglass markings (black widow) or stripes (red-back).

2. Pathophysiology of envenomation
   a) *Latrodectus spp*. produce a *neurotoxin* which acts at presynaptic nerve processes by increasing Ca^{2+} permeability of the nerve cell membrane.
   b) Ca^{2+} influx causes release of and depletion of neurotransmitters at affected synapses.
   c) Resultant clinical signs derive from a patchy derangement of skeletal and autonomic motor pathways.

3. Clinical signs
   a) Signs are highly variable. They are listed gen-

erally according to chronological events and degree of severity.

(1) No clinical signs
(2) Local pain, redness, swelling
(3) Rapid regional swelling, tenderness in regional lymph nodes
(4) Generalized pain—especially abdominal cramping
(5) Nausea, vomiting, salivation
(6) Ataxia, convulsions, flaccid paralysis
(7) Coma and respiratory failure (RARE)!

b) Differential diagnosis
 (1) Acute abdomen syndrome (see Chapter 7)
 (2) Other neuromuscular toxins

c) Dogs have been reported to be relatively resistant to the toxin of *Latrodectus spp.* (See Editorial, Lancet, 1980, in Bibliography). Clinical envenomation of dogs or cats has rarely been reported. No recent deaths have been reported.

4. Treatment

Note: therapy is based upon the clinical severity. (See Table 13-1.)

Assess severity:

a) Local signs and pain only
 (1) Cold compresses (avoid hypothermia)
 (2) Short-acting corticosteroids
  i) Hydrocortisone sodium succinate
  ii) Prednisolone sodium succinate
 (3) Mild analgesics
  i) Aspirin
  ii) Other nonsteroidal antiinflammatory agents
 (4) Exercise may relieve pain.
 (5) *No* restrictive bandages or tourniquets are indicated.

b) Systemic signs (See Table 13-1.)

TABLE 13-1. PROTOCOL FOR USE WITH EXPOSURE TO THE BLACK WIDOW OR RED-BACK SPIDER (*Latrodectus spp.*)

1. Obtain definitive history, identification of spider.
2. Assess severity of injury. *Do not apply tourniquets*!
3. If no systemic signs:
   a. Cold compress (avoid hypothermia)
   b. Short-acting corticosteroids
      i. Hydrocortisolone sodium succinate, 8–20 mg/kg IV
      ii. Prednisolone sodium succinate, 11–25 mg/kg IV
      iii. Dexamethasone, 1–6 mg/kg IV, SQ
   c. Mild analgesics
      i. Aspirin, 10 mg/kg q12h (dogs)
      ii. Other nonsteroidal antinflammatory drugs
      iii. Pentazocine lactate, 0.3–0.7 mg/kg IM (dogs)
4. If systemic signs are seen, begin:
   a. 10% calcium gluconate, 5–10 ml IV slowly
      Observe for relief of symptoms.
   b. If no relief occurs, give methocarbamol, 44.4–222.2 mg/kg IV.
   c. If signs persist, consider:
      i. Morphine SO_4
         Dog: 1 mg/kg IM
         Cat: 0.1 mg/kg IM
      ii. Meperidine HCl
         Dog: 10 mg/kg IM PRN
         Cat: 3 mg/kg IM PRN
   d. As a last resort, consider use of antivenom.
      Dose: one vial IM
      Must be used with caution!
5. Monitor for 24 h
   For return of clinical signs, antivenom dose may be repeated.

(1) 10% Ca gluconate
   i) Observe for relief of symptoms.
   ii) If no relief occurs, see step 2.

(2) Methocarbamol
   i) Observe for relief of symptoms.
   ii) If no relief occurs, see step 3.

(3) Narcotic analgesics
   i) Observe for relief of symptoms.
   ii) If no relief occurs, see step 4.

(4) Antivenom (See Table 13-13 for source)
   i) One vial IM is sufficient.

ii) May be repeated if no relief occurs.
iii) Observe for adverse reaction (anaphylaxis).
iv) Because of the possibility of anaphylaxis and/or serum sickness, the use of antivenom may cause more morbidity than any possible envenomation.

B. Atrax (funnel-web spiders)
1. Biology
a) Distribution and habitat
(1) The only dangerous species is restricted to an area in New South Wales within a 160-km radius of Sydney.
(2) Funnel-web spiders roam freely and commonly in suburban environments. Webs which are tubular or tunnel shaped are constructed in burrows or crevices in rocks or around house foundations. Colonies with hundreds of individuals may be formed.
b) Description
(1) The Sydney funnel-web spider is large (up to 6–7 cm) and robust.
(2) The male spider is the more dangerous, and it is an aggressive spider.
2. Pathophysiology of envenomation
a) Atraxotoxin is a complex of *neurotoxins* which act directly on nerve fibers.
b) The toxin causes widespread release of neurotransmitters affecting both autonomic and motor nerves.
c) Fortunately, the actions of the toxin, while being rapid in onset, are short-lived.
3. Clinical signs
a) Dogs and cats are reportedly resistant to the effects of atraxotoxin (see Sutherland, 1978, Bibliography). Experimentally, only minor

transient cardiovascular signs have been observed. Therefore, the emergency clinician is likely to receive inquiries only when an exposure has actually been observed by a client who is aware of the toxic potential of the spider.

b) Signs reported in people and experimental monkeys are given for comparative purposes. These develop within minutes of envenomation.
   (1) Local pain
   (2) Piloerection and fasciculation of skeletal muscles
   (3) Tachycardia, hypertension, coma
   (4) Gross muscle contraction, salivation, lacrimation. Death from asphyxiation at this stage.
   (5) Spontaneous remission of signs in survivors
   (6) A second phase may ensue with progressive, potentially fatal hypotension and apnea.

4. Treatment
   a) No therapy other than the treatment of local pain and swelling is likely to be necessary for the dog or cat.
   b) Management of human cases involves the following procedures:
      (1) Immediate application of an arterial tourniquet
      (2) Immobilization of affected limb and immediate transport to hospital
      (3) Release of tourniquet only after all necessary preparations for therapy have been completed.
      (4) Observation for development of systemic signs.
      (5) Treatment of signs
         i) IV diazepam—maximum dose

ii) Atropine to effect
iii) Short-term barbiturate anesthesia
iv) Maintenance of airway
v) Monitoring of blood pressure for 24 h
vi) Specific rabbit antivenom has recently been developed. (See Table 13-13.)

C. *Loxosceles spp.* brown spiders, fiddleback spiders
1. Biology
a) Distribution and habitat
(1) *Loxosceles spp.* are most widespread in the Americas. They have only recently been reported in Australia where they are not considered of great medical importance.
(2) *Loxosceles reclusa* (brown recluse spider) is the most important species in the United States. It is most prevalent in the southern half of the Missouri-Ohio-Mississippi River basin.
(3) The spider is found outdoors under stationary objects or indoors in undisturbed storage areas.
b) Description
This is a relatively small, nonaggressive, nocturnal, active spider. It is brown with a darker brown fiddle-shaped mark on the dorsal carapace.
2. Pathophysiology of envenomation
a) The mode of action of the complex venom is poorly understood. It is a complex of *necrotizing* enzymes and other proteins.
b) The brown recluse bite often eventuates in an enlarging necrotic ulcer involving the site of the bite and migrating outward and downward. Without treatment the ulceration may continue

actively for months and become grossly disfiguring.

3. Clinical signs
   a) There is little local pain or any immediate adverse reaction. Therefore, the veterinary emergency clinician is unlikely to be called unless a bite of a brown recluse is observed by an informed client.
   b) The development of clinical signs is gradual:
      i) Within 2–6 h, slight pain and erythema are seen.
      ii) Later a blister may develop which is surrounded by firm swelling.
      iii) Within a variable period of time, necrosis is observed with the formation of a black eschar; ulceration follows.
      iv) The ulcer continues to enlarge for a variable period of time, then becomes indolent.
   c) In humans, various systemic signs, including fever, rash, joint pain, and intravascular hemolysis have been reported to occur. These presumably have an immunologic basis.
4. Treatment
   a) There is no specific therapy.
   b) Some have advocated immediate excision of observed bites. However, every bite does not cause an ulcer, so that delay of surgery until necrosis has begun would be more conservative. The development of a blister at the site of a known brown recluse bite is an indication for surgical excision of the bite wound.
   c) Surgical excision should include the entire affected area.
   d) There is no evidence that corticosteroids, local or systemic, affect the outcome of a brown recluse spider bite.

III. Scorpions
   A. Definition
      1. There are many groups of scorpions distributed throughout the world. The majority, including all those found in Australia, are of minor medical importance.
      2. The scorpion of major importance which is found in the United States and Mexico is *Centuroides sculpturatus*.
   B. *Centuroides sculpturatus*
      1. Biology
         a) This scorpion occurs within the United States only in the state of Arizona.
         b) It is frequently found near human dwellings clinging to the undersurface of debris or under the bark of trees.
         c) It may be recognized by its yellowish cephalothorax which lacks any stripe.
      2. Pathophysiology of envenomation
         a) Centuroides produces a *neurotoxin* which affects both skeletal and autonomic motor neurons.
         b) Although experimental evidence is lacking, dogs and cats must be either relatively resistent to the toxin or rarely envenomated, because there are few reports of envenomation in these species.
      3. Clinical signs
         a) Local pain. Most species of scorpion produce only this sign. In the United States, only *Centuroides sculpturatus* produces a serious envenomation.
         b) Systemic signs reported in people envenomated by *Centuroides sculpturatus*:
            (1) May be no local pain
            (2) Difficulty swallowing
            (3) Nervousness, behavioral abnormalities
            (4) Respiratory distress

(5) Opisthotonic spasms
(6) Salivation, gastric distension
(7) Mydriasis, nystagmus, blindness
(8) Micturition, defecation, penile erection
(9) Respiratory arrest
(10) Hypertension
(11) Cardiac arrest

4. Treatment (See Table 13-2.)
   a) Control local pain.
      (1) Cold packs (avoid hypothermia)
      (2) Short-acting corticosteroids
         i) Hydrocortisone sodium succinate
         ii) Prednisolone sodium succinate
      (3) Analgesics *Note*: narcotic analgesics have been reported to be contraindicated in Centuroides envenomation (See Stahnke, 1978, Bibliography).
         i) Aspirin

TABLE 13-2. PROTOCOL FOR STING OF *Centuroides sculpturatus*

1. Obtain definitive history, identification of scorpion.
2. Control local pain.
   a. Apply cold packs (avoid hypothermia).
   b. Administer short-acting corticosteroids.
      i. Hydrocortisone Na succinate, 8–20 mg/kg IV
      ii. Prednisolone Na succinate, 5–25 mg/kg IV
      iii. Dexamethasone, 1–6 mg/kg IV, SQ
   c. Analgesics
      i. Aspirin, 10 mg/kg PO (dogs)
      ii. Other nonsteroidal antiinflammatory agents
         Note: Narcotic analgesics are contraindicated.
3. If systemic signs occur:
   a. Induce barbiturate anesthesia.
      i. Pentobarbital Na, Up to 30 mg/kg IV to effect (dogs)
      ii. Sodium thiopental, 3–15 mg/kg IV to effect
      iii. Thiamylal sodium, 8–20 mg/kg IV then to effect
   b. Maintain patent airway.
   c. Assist respiration.
   d. Administer specific antivenom (See Table 13-13) according to package insert.

ii) Other nonsteroidal antiinflammatory agents

b) If systemic signs occur:
(1) Barbiturate anesthesia
(2) Maintain airway and respiration.
(3) Specific antivenom (See Table 13-13.)

IV. Tick paralysis

A. Definition

1. Tick paralysis is a neuromuscular disorder caused by a poorly defined toxin which is injected by some ticks into their hosts. In most cases, the host is exposed to the toxin several days after attachment and engorgement of an adult female tick.
2. Tick paralysis has been reported in dogs and cats in association with infestation by a number of species of hard (Ixodid) ticks. The species of ticks most commonly implicated are *Dermacentor andersoni* in the western United States, *Dermacentor variabilis* in the southeastern United States, and *Ixodes holocyclus* in eastern coastal Australia. Because the latter tick is associated with a more severe paralysis syndrome necessitating more vigorous emergency protocols, it will be discussed under a separate heading.

B. Tick paralysis in North America

1. Biology
a) *Dermacentor andersoni* (Rocky Mountain spotted fever tick) and *Dermacentor variabilis* (American dog tick) have been most often associated with cases of tick paralysis. However, *Rhipicephalus spp.* and other species of hard ticks have been occasionally reported to cause tick paralysis.
b) These are three-host ticks. The engorged female tick (in place for 5–9 days) is responsible for toxin production.
c) *Dermacentor species* are wood ticks which have ornate scuta. They are most abundant in

the late spring and summer. The dog is the preferred host for *Dermacentor variabilis*, while horses and cattle are preferred by adult *D. andersoni*.

2. Pathophysiology of envenomation
   a) Some adult female ticks, after engorgement for several days, secrete a large polypeptide in the saliva which acts as a *neurotoxin*.
   b) Factors which contribute to the production of the toxin are not understood. Some local tick populations have a very high percentage of potentially toxic females. In some geographic localities, intoxication is unknown despite the presence of ticks.
   c) The tick paralysis factor causes a progressive block in conduction of terminal nerve fibers. This results in failure to release neurotransmitter at end plates.
   d) Experimental evidence demonstrates that nerve fibers are affected most at the nodes of Ranvier. For this reason, longer nerve fibers are affected more severely than shorter fibers. Also smaller (slower) fibers are more severely affected. This explains why terminal motor neurons and more posteriorly located motor functions are preferentially affected (See Murnaghan and O'Rourke, 1978, Bibliography).
3. Clinical signs and diagnosis
   a) Tick paralysis is a symmetrical paresis or paralysis of dogs that begins on the rear limbs and ascends to involve the forelimbs. In North America, cats are not affected.
   b) The paresis is characterized by motor weakness, hypotonicity, ataxia, and hyporeflexia.
   c) Within 1–4 days, if left untreated, the disease may progress to cause respiratory paralysis and death.

d) Cranial nerves, sensory function, and consciousness are not usually affected until secondary complications have ensued. Occasionally facial palsy may be observed and the voice may change.

e) The differential diagnosis includes botulism (type C) and polyradiculoneuritis (or coonhound paralysis).

   (1) In cases of botulism there may be a history of carrion ingestion. The disease is usually rapidly progressive and does not usually have an ascending course. Cranial nerve involvement may be severe.

   (2) Polyradiculoneuritis may follow exposure to a raccoon. There are more often sensory abnormalities present (hyperesthesia). Muscle wasting may develop rapidly. There is no response to dipping for ticks. Electromyography may be used to differentiate this from tick paralysis.

f) Tick paralysis is diagnosed by history of tick exposure and by finding one or more adult engorged female ticks on the patient. All patients with lower motor neuron paresis and intact cranial nerve and sensory functions should be carefully searched for ticks; ear canals and even nasal passages should be inspected. Regression of signs should occur following an effective insecticidal dip. In North America, signs of tick paralysis will abate within 24 h of removing the tick.

4. Treatment

   a) The dog should be thoroughly treated with an effective insecticidal dip. (Commercial dips labeled for use against ticks.)

   b) Failure to remove the offending tick can result in death within 1–4 days.

C. Tick paralysis in Australia

1. Biology

a) Tick paralysis in Australia is caused by *Ixodes holocyclus*. Common names are scrub tick, dog tick, and bottle tick. Other species of Ixodes are occasionally associated with paralysis.

b) The tick and the disease are found in the scrub or bush country along the eastern coastline from Queensland to Victoria.

c) The natural hosts for *Ixodes holocyclus* are marsupials. Tick populations have become very large in areas where predator eradication has allowed host populations to build up.

2. Pathophysiology of intoxication

a) The pathomechanisms of the action of the *neurotoxin*, holocyclotoxin, are similar to that for tick paralysis in other geographic areas. The intoxication is, however, more severe and more persistent.

b) In addition to the inhibition of release of neurotransmittors from terminal motor processes, there are central and autonomic effects. Central respiratory depression and elevated systemic blood pressure are observed. The latter is apparently a result of central sympathetic stimulation (See Ilkiw, 1983, Bibliography).

c) The paralyzing polypeptide secreted by female *Ixodes holocyclus* is relatively resistant to the actions of host proteases (See Stone, 1979, Bibliography). This accounts for the progression of signs after removal of all ticks.

d) Unlike paralyzing ticks in North America, repeated exposure to *Ixodes holocyclus* may induce immunity to the toxin in host species (See Wright et al., 1983, Bibliography).

3. Clinical signs and diagnosis

a) Unlike North American tick paralysis, both dogs and cats are affected in Australia. This is a common and severe endemic disease of dogs in some parts of of Australia.

b) Signs are seen 6–7 days after attachment of a female tick.

c) Early signs include altered voice, cough, and dysphagia. This is followed by slight incoordination in the rear legs.

d) The paralysis ascends rapidly and will progress even if ticks are removed. Paralysis may be accompanied by violent retching and by mydriasis.

e) Most severely affected dogs become completely paralyzed but have consciousness and sensory function intact. Respiratory rate may be depressed and a grunting and convulsive respiratory effort is characteristic.

f) Systemic blood pressure is elevated. Various cardiac arrythmias (either tachyarrhythmias or bradyarrythmias) may be seen.

g) In dogs not supported by intensive veterinary care, the mortality rate is very high.

h) The differential diagnosis includes type C botulism. In cases presented in an advanced state, snake bite may have to be considered.

i) Diagnosis is made by finding the offending tick or ticks or a recent history of tick bite and by the lack of any of the other clinical signs of snake envenomation.

4. Treatment (See Table 13-3.)

a) Ticks should be sought and carefully removed. Engorged ticks must not be severed or squeezed while still attached to the patient. An effective insecticidal dip should be applied.

b) Early therapy is of paramount importance. If clinical signs are present, the patient should receive hyperimmune serum. (See Table 13-13.)

c) Respiration should be supported. In advanced cases, tracheostomy and intermittent positive

TABLE 13-3. PROTOCOL FOR TICK PARALYSIS IN AUSTRALIA

1. Perform thorough inspection for ticks. Remove all ticks carefully. Apply effective insecticidal dip.
2. If any clinical signs are present, give hyperimmune serum.
   a. Give 0.5 ml/kg IM to start.
   b. Repeat as needed.
3. Supportive care
   a. Support respiratory function.
      i. Tracheostomy if needed
      ii. Intermittent positive pressure ventilation if needed
   b. Avoid stress. Tranquilize if necessary.
      Acepromazine 0.05–0.1 mg/kg slowly IV or IM
   c. Avoid dehydration.
      i. Balanced electrolyte solution IV
      ii. Use cautiously to avoid exacerbating hypertension
   d. Treat systemic hypertension.
      1. Phenoxybenzamine 1 mg/kg diluted in 20 ml saline, slowly IV. Repeat q 12–24 h.
      2. Or acepromazine 0.05–0.1 mg/kg slowly IV to maximum dose of 6 mg
   e. Avoid aspiration of food or vomitus.
      i. Keep patient NPO if gag reflex is diminished.
      ii. Tracheostomy
4. Monitor
   a. For progression of signs
      Administer more hyperimmune serum.
   b. Respiration
      i. For respiratory paralysis
      ii. For passive congestion (turn patient frequently)
   c. Blood pressure, if possible (See Chapter 1)

pressure ventilatory (IPPV) assistance may be required. Care must be taken to avoid patient aspiration of vomitus.

d) Avoidance of stress is desirable. Tranquilization may be necessary.

e) Fluids may be administered if dehydration is suspected, but do so cautiously to avoid exacerbating systemic hypertension and passive pulmonary congestion.

f) Recently workers have advocated the use of α-adrenergic blocking agents to treat the systemic hypertension (See Ilkiw, 1983).

(1) Phenoxybenzamine HCL (See Ilkiw, 1983).
(2) An alternative is the use of acepromazine as an α-blocker and tranquilizer.

SNAKE ENVENOMATION

I. Definition
   A. Snake venoms are complex, potentially lethal animal toxins containing enzymes and nonenzymatic proteins. The severity of snake bite is dependent on many factors, including the snake species, size of the snake, volume of venom injected, and the size of the patient.
   B. Early administration of antivenom and supportive therapy are the basis for successful treatment of snake envenomation. Because of the high cost of antivenom and the possibility of serious adverse reactions to it, every effort should be made to confirm severity of envenomation before administration of antivenom.
   C. Extreme caution is advised in the use of first aid or in hospital surgical procedures in snakebite. Morbidity may be increased by the incautious use of incision/excision techniques.

II. Venomous snakes
   A. North American pit vipers (*Crotalidae*)
      1. Biology
         a) Medically important pit vipers are represented by three genera in the United States.
            (1) Genus Crotalus or large rattlesnakes includes the eastern and western diamondback rattlesnakes.
            (2) Genus Agkistrodon, or moccasins, includes the cottonmouth water moccasin and copperhead.
            (3) Genus Sistrurus or groundrattlers includes the northern massasauga and the southern pygmy rattlesnake.

2. Pathophysiology of envenomation

   Pit viper venoms are in general hemotoxic, vasculotoxic, and necrogenic.

   a) *Venom hemorrhagins* are agents that have a direct lytic effect on endothelial cells or endothelial cell junctions of capillaries allowing red blood cells, serum, and proteins to reach the interstitial space. Platelet aggregation is inhibited by these venom constituents.
   b) *Venom myotoxins* are polypeptides that act on the sarcoplasmic reticulum and sarcolemma of skeletal muscle allowing increased sodium (Na^+) and water influx into muscle cells. Cellular swelling and death follow this influx. Muscle necrosis is a delayed phenomenon following envenomation.
   c) *Enzymes* are found in all snake venoms and are involved in many of the pathologic processes of pit viper envenomation.
      (1) Defibrination of blood is caused by "thrombin-like" enzymes.
      (2) Phospholipase A causes lysis of erythrocytes and induces prostaglandin synthesis, causing vasodilation and reduced arterial pressure.
   d) *Mojave rattlesnake venom* is unique among North American pit vipers in that it is primarily a presynaptic neurotoxin and is capable of causing severe neurologic signs including respiratory arrest and death.

3. Clinical signs and diagnosis
   a) The clinical signs of pit viper envenomation include local and systemic signs. The severity of envenomation should be estimated by careful serial physical examinations.
      (1) Local signs
         i) One, two, or several fang puncture wounds that ooze serum or blood.

- ii) Pain and swelling are characteristic early signs of pit viper envenomation.
- iii) Ecchymotic hemorrhage locally is common.
- iv) Swelling and sensitivity of regional lymph nodes may be seen.
- v) Skin and muscle necrosis are delayed consequences of envenomation.

(2) Systemic signs
- i) Hypovolemic and cardiovascular shock
- ii) Muscle fasciculations
- iii) Generalized ecchymoses
- iv) Cardiac arrhythmias
- v) Hemoglobinuria
- vi) Neurologic signs and hypovolemic shock predominate following envenomation by the Mojave rattlesnake. This is also possible in eastern diamondback rattlesnake envenomation.

(3) Based on clinical signs, classification of envenomated patients given in Table 13-4 may help in deriving a treatment plan.

(4) If patients present for pit viper bite and no local swelling, pain or ecchymoses are present after 4 h, it can be assumed no envenomation has occurred.

(5) Diagnosis is based on history and clinical signs.

(6) Differential diagnosis:
- i) Angioneurotic edema
  - (*A*) Nonpainful swelling
  - (*B*) Lack of ecchymoses, fang marks
- ii) Bee/wasp sting

TABLE 13-4. CLASSIFICATION OF PIT VIPER ENVENOMATION ACCORDING TO SEVERITY OF SIGNS

Mild	Moderate	Severe
Fang marks and minimal pain	Fang marks and pain	Fang marks and pain
Local swelling and ecchymosis which are nonprogressive in 1 h	Progressive swelling and edema	Severe swelling and edema
Absence of systemic signs	Mild hypovolemic shock	Severe hypovolemic shock
	Signs of coagulation defects, including hemorrhage from venipuncture sites	Coagulation defects Generalized ecchymoses
	Very small patient, very large snake	Bleb/blister formation surrounding bite
		Muscle fasciculations
		Cardiac arrhythmias
		Very small patient, very large or dangerous snake

- (*A*) May be difficult to differentiate except by history
- (*B*) Lack of fang marks

iii) Cellulitis/abscess
- (*A*) Develops much less rapidly
- (*B*) Lack of fang marks

iv) Vasculitis
- (*A*) May be accompanied by swelling
- (*B*) Lack of fang marks

4. Treatment (See Tables 13-5 and 13-6.)
   a) First aid
      (1) Owners should be instructed to present the patient as quickly as possible without attempting first aid measures.
      (2) Immobilization of a bitten extremity may prevent venom spread.
   b) Hospital therapy
      (1) Perform physical examination and establish degree of envenomation (if any). Ex-

TABLE 13-5. PROTOCOL FOR PIT VIPER ENVENOMATION

1. Immobilize and transport animal to hospital.
2. If possible, identify snake.
3. Perform thorough physical examination.
   a. Find fang marks.
   b. Assess severity of envenomation (see Table 13-4)
   c. Evaluate systemic changes.
   d. Examine for arrhythmias, get baseline ECG if possible.
4. Draw laboratory samples.
5. Insert an IV catheter.
   a. Begin multiple electrolyte solution.
      i. Dog: 50–100 ml/kg over several hours
      ii. Cat: 100–200 ml/aliquot
   b. Treat shock if present (see Chapter 1)
      Corticosteroids ± sodium bicarbonate
6. Clip and clean bite wound. Immobilize limb.
7. If animal is seen within *30 min* of bite and envenomation is thought to be severe, consider anesthesia and aseptic incision and suction.
8. If more than *30 min* has passed since the bite, do not perform incision and suction.
9. For moderate to severe envenomation:
   a. Begin antivenom therapy as outlined in Table 13-6.
   b. Monitor closely for:
      i. Cardiac arrhythmias
      ii. Allergic reactions (anaphylaxis)
10. Consider analgesic for severe pain.
    a. Meperidine HCl
       i. Dog: 10 mg/kg IM PRN
       ii. Cat: 3 mg/kg IM PRN
    b. Morphine SO_4
       i. Dog: 1 mg/kg IM
       ii. Cat: 0.1 mg/kg IM
11. Provide supportive care
    a. Maintain patent upper airway.
       If upper airway obstruction is threatened, perform a tracheostomy.
    b. If hemodilution or hypoproteinemia occurs, consider:
       i. Whole blood transfusion
       ii. Plasma transfusion
    c. ± Antibiotics
12. Monitor
    a. PCV, TS q4–12h
    b. ECG continuously
    c. Urine output continuously
       If necessary, insert indwelling catheter.
    d. Progression of tissue necrosis at bite site
13. Consider surgical debridement of necrotic tissue during recovery period.

TABLE 13-6. ANTIVENOM THERAPY PROTOCOL FOR PIT VIPER ENVENOMATION

1. Mild envenomation (see Table 13-4)
   a. Establish IV catheter and begin infusion of a balanced electrolyte solution.
   b. Antivenom is not indicated unless signs progress or the patient deteriorates.
2. Moderate envenomation (see Table 13-4)
   a. Establish IV catheter and begin infusion of a balanced electrolyte solution.
   b. Administer three to five vials of antivenom IV slowly.
   c. Monitor for signs of anaphylaxis.
   d. Monitor for progression of signs.
   e. If the patient continues to deteriorate administer more antivenom.
3. Severe envenomation (see Table 13-4)
   a. Establish IV catheter and begin infusion of a balanced electrolyte solution.
   b. Administer five to eight vials of antivenom IV slowly.
   c. Monitor for signs of anaphylaxis.
   d. Monitor for progression of signs for 24 h.
   e. If the patient responds, then deteriorates or fails to respond, administer more antivenom to total dose of 15–20 vials.
4. See Table 13-13 for sources of antivenom.

amination should be performed at frequent intervals.

(2) Determine whether the patient has been previously treated with antivenom or tetanus antitoxin. (If so, adverse reactions to antivenom is more likely.)

(3) Draw blood for CBC, BUN, and clotting profile.

(4) Insert an IV catheter and begin administration of a balanced electrolyte solution (see Chapter 1).

(5) Clip hair and clean the bite site.

(6) Treat for shock if present (see Chapter 1).

  i) Prednisolone sodium succinate
  ii) Intravenous balanced electrolyte solution in shock dosage.

(7) If the bite has occurred *within* 30 min of presentation, aseptically prepare the bite site and make one continuous skin inci-

sion centered over fang wounds. The incision should penetrate the SQ tissue. Apply suction (mechanically) and liberally lavage the wound with normal saline.

i) If more than 30 min has elapsed since the bite DO NOT perform incision and suction.
ii) Apply a sterile dressing over the incision site.
iii) Remember this surgical procedure may result in *more* tissue morbidity locally. This should be reserved for situations judged to be life-threatening envenomations (large, dangerous snake; small patient).

(8) If the bite has occurred on an extremity, immobilize the leg in a splint and Robert Jones bandage.

(9) Antivenom therapy (See Table 13-6.) Antivenom given *early* is the basis for successful therapy of moderate to severe pit viper envenomation. A single polyvalent antivenom is available which is effective against the venoms of all North American pit vipers including the Mojave rattlesnake. (See Table 13-13). Published dosage schedules for companion animals are unavailable, however, the authors feel *underdosage* is a common mistake in therapy of envenomated patients.

i) Antivenom should be administered IV *only*.
ii) Antivenom is produced from horse serum, and anaphylaxis may occur following administration, especially at high doses or if the patient has been sensitized by previous drugs of equine origin.

(*A*) Treatment of anaphylaxis is with 1 : 1,000 epinephrine and corticosteroids (see section on Anaphylaxis, Chapter 6).

(*B*) Other allergic reactions including serum sickness, may occur 24–48 h to several days after administration. These respond to corticosteroids.

(10) If pain is severe, administer meperidine or morphine.

(11) Severe envenomation may require supportive therapy for several problems.

i) Upper airway obstruction caused by local swelling, although rare, may necessitate tracheostomy. Such treatment including artificial ventilation may also be required following envenomation by the Mojave rattlesnake.

ii) Cardiac arrhythmias, especially ventricular ectopic beats, may be encountered (see section on Cardiac Arrhythmias, Chapter 2).

iii) Blood transfusion, plasma, or colloidal fluids may be required to prevent hemodilution and hypoproteinemia associated with crystalloid fluid treatment of hypovolemic shock.

(12) Surgical debridement is indicated when tissue becomes necrotic during the recovery phase of envenomation.

(13) Antibiotics are not routinely administered; however, prolonged maintenance of IV catheters and/or the presence of devitalized tissue are indications for the use of a bactericidal antibiotic.

B. Coral snakes

Note: Coral snake envenomation of dogs or cats is rare to nonexistent. However, as people are generally aware of the extremely toxic potential of this colorful snake, the veterinary emergency clinician should be prepared to handle inquiries as well as potential envenomations.

1. Biology
   a) There are two species of coral snakes in the United States. *Micrurus fulvius* occurs in the southeastern United States from South Carolina southward and west into western Texas. *Micruroides euryxanthus*, the Arizona coral snake, occurs in Arizona, New Mexico, and western Texas. The latter is of little medical importance.
   b) Everyone is aware of the colorful red-, black-, and yellow-banded pattern of this snake. The black-on-yellow pattern is used to distinguish the coral snake from harmless imitators. There are also black and albino individuals, however. Although large coral snakes may be up to 18 cm long, most are much smaller.
   c) Coral snakes are secretive, nonaggressive burrowing animals. They are most likely to be encountered during gardening activities.
   d) The mouth and fangs of the coral snake are small enough that only the relatively hairless digits of pets are likely to be sites of effective bites. The snake must hold on to the victim for a short period in order to inject venom.
2. Pathophysiology of envenomation
   a) The coral snake is an elapid and possesses a very potent venom similar to cobra venom. The venom contains a neurotoxin and a cardiotoxin.
   b) The *neurotoxin* is a postsynaptic inhibitor which acts at the neuromuscular junction. As such, it possesses a curare-like action.

c) The *cardiotoxin* is a direct membrane-acting toxin which depolarizes membranes of cardiac, skeletal, and smooth muscles, and of neurons.

3. Clinical signs
   a) There is usually little pain or local tissue reaction associated with a bite. The bite wound consists of very small punctures.
   b) The systemic signs may be delayed for several hours. Once signs begin, they progress rapidly.
   c) Early systemic signs include:
      (1) Restlessness
      (2) Cranial nerve paresis causing ptosis
      (3) Inability to swallow (thus hypersalivation)
      (4) Ocular muscle derangements
   d) Laryngeal, pharyngeal, respiratory, and generalized paralysis develop rapidly.
   e) If respiratory function is artificially supported, victims then usually succumb to cardiovascular collapse.
4. Treatment (See Table 13-7.)
   a) The snake should be collected for positive identification.

TABLE 13-7. PROTOCOL FOR CORAL SNAKE ENVENOMATION

1. Wash wound thoroughly.
2. Identify the snake (black bands on yellow).
3. Determine likelihood of envenomation (fang marks, snake held on).
4. If envenomation likely, administer *Micrurus fulvius* antivenom (see Table 13-13).
   a. One to two vials IV or IM.
   b. If systemic signs are observed, five to seven vials IV, then PRN.
   c. Observe for adverse reaction (anaphylaxis).
5. Prepare for tracheostomy; intermittent positive pressure ventilation if needed. (See protocol for airway obstruction, Chapter 12.)
6. Monitor respiration, cardiovascular function for 48 h.
7. Treat cardiovascular collapse with protocol for congestive cardiomyopathy, Chapter 2.

b) The wound should be immediately and thoroughly washed.
c) No restrictive tourniquet or incision/suction procedure is indicated.
d) If a bite has definitely been observed to occur, especially if the snake was seen to hold on to the victim, *Micrurus fulvius* antivenom therapy should be instituted. (See Table 13-13)
   (1) At least two vials should be administered IV or IM.
   (2) If systemic signs are observed, up to five to seven vials may be indicated and should be administered IV.
   (3) Observations for adverse reactions to equine origin antivenom (anaphylaxis) should be made.
e) Preparations should be made for tracheostomy and IPPV support.
f) Cardiovascular support should be similar to that for congestive cardiomyopathy (see Chapter 2).
g) The patient should be monitored and supported as needed for 48 h.

C. Australian venomous snakes
1. Biology
a) The majority of venomous snakes of Australia are elapids.
b) Bites are most likely to occur between September and March with October and January being peak months.
c) Successful treatment of envenomation is based on the early administration of the correct antivenom.
d) The most important species and their geographic locations are:
   (1) Brown snakes
      (i) Common brown snake (*Pseudonaja textilis*) is found in eastern Queens-

land and the southeastern interior, in eastern New South Wales, the wheat belt and the Murrumbidgee area, the whole of Victoria, and in the southeast of South Australia.

(ii) Western brown snake (*P. nuchalis*) is found throughout Western Australia, Northern Territory, western Queensland, western New South Wales, northwestern Victoria, and South Australia.

(iii) Spotted brown snake or dugite (*P. affinis*) is found in southern parts of Western Australia only.

(2) Black snakes

(i) King brown snake (*Pseudechis australis*) is a member of the Black Snake genus. It is widely distributed throughout the mainland.

(ii) Red-bellied black snake (*Pseudechis porphyriacus*) is found in eastern Queensland, eastern New South Wales, Victoria, and southeastern South Australia.

(3) Copperhead (*Austrelaps spp.*) is found in cooler regions, Tasmania, Bass Strait islands, and alpine districts of southeastern Australia.

(4) Tiger snakes (*Notechis spp.*) are found in southern and southeastern areas, the southwest corner of Western Australia Bass Strait islands, and Tasmania.

(5) Death adder (*Acanthopis antarcticus*) is widely distributed over the mainland except the southeastern corner.

(6) Taipan (*Oxyuranus scutellatus*) is found

in the coastal areas of northern New South Wales, Queensland, and Northern Territory.

2. Pathophysiology of envenomation

Australian snake venoms have neurotoxic, hemolytic, coagulant, and cytotoxic properties. These properties differ from species to species.

a) *Neurotoxins* are responsible for the lethal action of Australian elapid venoms. They may work at either presynaptic or postsynaptic junctions causing muscular paralysis.
b) *Coagulants* cause activation of the clotting mechanism by converting prothrombin to thrombin. This paradoxically results in local bleeding from fang wounds or IV catheter placement, and hematuria.
c) *Hemolysins* cause red blood cell destruction resulting in jaundice or hemoglobinuria.
c) *Cytotoxins* may have myotoxic, nephrotoxic, or vasculotoxic effects.

3. Clinical signs

The predominant clinical signs of envenomation are *neurologic*, however, signs of hemorrhage are also seen. The most common signs are:

a) Local reactions at the bite site are rare. Fang marks are usually not seen.
b) Collapse
c) Ataxia or paralysis, of ascending type
d) Shaking
e) Mydriasis
f) Depressed or absent pupillary light reflex
g) Salivaton
h) Vomiting/diarrhea
i) Hematuria/hemoglobinuria/myoglobinuria
j) Bleeding from fang wounds or venipuncture sites
k) Death due to respiratory failure

4. Diagnosis
   a) Diagnosis is based on history of an observed bite or the clinical signs of paralysis and prolonged bleeding time.
   b) If expenses permit, venom detection kits may be used to aid diagnosis. Serum, urine, or tissue may be analyzed for the presence of specific venoms.
   c) Hemoglobinuria, myoglobinuria, abnormal clotting profile, and elevated plasma creatinine kinase levels may support the diagnosis of snakebite.
   d) Differential diagnosis
      (1) *Ixodes holocyclus* (bush tick) paralysis.
      (2) Botulism
      (3) Organophosphate intoxication
5. Treatment (See Table 13-8.)

   Treatment is based on administration of the correct antivenom.
   a) Every effort should be made to identify the species of offending snake.
      (1) Owners should present the snake if it has been killed.
      (2) Knowledge of the species in a given area may assist in identification. Color of the snake is of little value.
      (3) Professional advice for correct identification may be required.
   b) First aid
      (1) First aid measures are useless. Owners should be instructed to present their animal for treatment as quickly as possible.
      (2) Immobilize the bitten part if possible.
   c) Hospital therapy
      (1) Perform physical examination to determine if signs of envenomation are present. Clinical signs may be present acutely

TABLE 13-8. PROTOCOL FOR AUSTRALIAN ELAPID ENVENOMATION

1. Immobilize and transport animal to hospital.
2. If possible, identify snake.
3. Perform thorough physical and neurological examination.
   Assess for positive signs of envenomation. (Early signs—mydriasis, loss of pupillary light reflexes)
4. Draw laboratory samples.
5. Insert an IV catheter.
   a. Begin multiple electrolyte solution.
      Dog: 50–100 ml/kg over several hours
      Cat: 100–200 ml/aliguot
   b. Treat shock if present (see Chapter 1).
6. Apply Robert Jones dressing on affected extremity.
7. Administer appropriate antivenom IV (see Tables 13-9, 13-10, and 13-13)
8. Observe for adverse reaction (anaphylaxis).
9. Supportive care
   a. Maintain airway and respiration
      i. Tracheostomy if necessary
      ii. Intermitent positive pressure ventilation (IPPV) if necessary
   b. Monitor for development of shock and/or hypotension.
   c. Sedation or anesthesia if necessary:
      i. Acepromazine, 0.1–0.5 mg/kg SQ, IM, IV up to 6 mg
      ii. Na thiopental, 3–15 mg/kg IV, then to effect
      iii. Thiamylal Na, 8–20 mg/kg IV to effect
      iv. Na pentobarbital, Up to 30 mg/kg IV to effect
10. Monitor
    a. Respiration
    b. PCV, TS q 24 h
    c. Urine output
    d. Blood pressure (see Chapter 1)
    e. Progression of clinical signs
       Repeat antivenom, if necessary.
11. Surviving patients may take several weeks to return to normal neurologic function.

or commence several hours after the bite.

(2) Establish identity of the snake if possible.

(3) Determine whether the patient has been

previously treated with antivenom or tetanus antitoxin. If so, adverse reaction to antivenom is more likely.

(4) Draw blood for CBC, BUN, and clotting profile.

(5) Insert an IV catheter and begin administration of balanced electrolyte solution.

(6) If the bite has occurred on an extremity, absorption of venom may be delayed by a firmly applied Robert Jones dressing.

(7) Administer the appropriate monovalent antivenom IV. Polyvalent antivenom may be used if the species is unknown. (See Tables 13-9 and 13-10 for antivenom recommendations, Table 13-13 for antivenom sources.)

i) Observe for signs of anaphylaxis.

ii) Treat anaphylaxis with 1:1,000 ep-

TABLE 13-9. AUSTRALIAN ANTIVENOM PROTOCOL: CHOICE OF ANTIVENOM AND DOSAGE WHERE THE IDENTITY OF THE SNAKE IS UNCERTAIN

State	Recommended Antivenom for Veterinary Use	Initial Dose (U)	Recommended Antivenom for Human Use	Initial Dose (U)
Tasmania	Tiger snake	6,000	Tiger snake	6,000
Victoria	Tiger snake + brown snake	3,000 1,000	Tiger snake + brown snake	3,000 1,000
NSW SA WA NT	Tiger snake + brown snake + death adder	3,000 1,000	Polyvalent snake antivenom	Contents of one container
QLD-north of Rockhampton	Brown snake + death adder	1,000 6,000	Polyvalent snake antivenom	Contents of one container
QLD-south of Rockhampton	Tiger snake + brown snake + death adder	3,000 1,000 6,000	Polyvalent snake antivenom	Contents of one container

Abbreviations: NSW, New South Wales; NT, Northern Territory; QLD, Queensland; SA, South Australia; WA, West Australia.

(Lewis PF: Snake bite in animals in Australia. Twelfth Annu Rep Postgrad Found Vet Sci 36:287, 1977. Reprinted with permission)

TABLE 13-10. AUSTRALIAN ANTIVENOM PROTOCOL: CHOICE OF ANTIVENOM AND DOSAGE WHEN SNAKE HAS BEEN IDENTIFIED

Snake	Recommended Antivenom for Veterinary Use	Initial Dose (U)	Recommended Antivenom for Human Use	Initial Dose (U)
Tiger snake	Tiger snake antivenom	3,000	Tiger snake antivenom	3,000
Tasmanian tiger snake	Tiger snake antivenom	6,000	Tiger snake antivenom	6,000
Chappell Island black tiger snake	Tiger snake antivenom	12,000	Tiger snake antivenom	12,000
Death adder	Death adder antivenom	6,000	Death adder antivenom	6,000
Taipan	Taipan snake antivenom	12,000	Taipan snake antivenom	12,000
Copperhead	Tiger snake antivenom	3,000	Tiger snake antivenom	3,000
Brown snake dugite	Brown snake antivenom	1,000	Brown snake antivenom	1,000
Black snake	Tiger snake antivenom	3,000	Black snake antivenom	6,000
King brown or mulga snake	Tiger snake antivenom	9,000	Black snake antivenom	18,000

(Lewis PF: Snakebite in animals in Australia. Twelfth Annu Rep Postgrad Found Vet Sci 36:287, 1977 Reprinted with permission.)

inephrine and corticosteroids. (See section on Allergic Reactions, Chapter 6.)

(8) Supportive care

i) Respiration should be monitored closely. Supplemental O_2 or artificial ventilation in the form of tracheostomy and ventilator use may be required.

ii) Insert a urinary catheter to monitor urine output. Maintain high urine output.

iii) Keep the patient quiet. Sedate if necessary (narcotic analgesics may be contraindicated) with:

(*A*) Acepromazine
(*B*) Barbiturate anesthetic
(*1*) Pentobarbital Na
(*2*) Thiamylal Na
(*3*) Na Pentothal

(9) Monitor the patient closely. If initial improvement occurs following antivenom therapy followed by deterioration, additional antivenom is indicated.

TOAD POISONING

I. Definition

Many members of the genus Bufo contain toxins in their skin and parotid glands. Mouthing or ingestion of toads by dogs and cats may cause profuse salivation and irritation of oral mucosa. Only the large toad *Bufo marinus*, when mouthed or ingested by dogs may cause a potentially fatal intoxication.

II. *Bufo marinus* intoxication

1. Biology
   a) *Bufo marinus* is distributed worldwide in tropical coastal areas. Dogs are likely to encounter the toads at night under lights.
   b) *Bufo marinus* occurs in the tropical regions of Texas and Florida in the United States. It has been introduced and is well established in Hawaii.
   c) *Bufo marinus* occurs in tropical coastal areas of Australia.
2. Pathophysiology of intoxication
   a) The toxin is a complex of cardiovascular active components. The most important of the components exhibits a digitalis-like action on the myocardium. Another contains catecholamine-like activity.
   b) The *digitalis-like* factor is rapidly absorbed from oral and gastric mucosa.
   c) The *pressor amine* fraction is normally degraded rather than absorbed, so is important only in experimental settings.

d) The digitalis-like component is associated with progressive development of ventricular arrhythmias which may lead to ventricular fibrillation.

3. Clinical signs
   a) Slight to profuse salivation
   b) Mouthing, pawing at mouth and head-shaking
   c) Cyanosis
   d) Collapse
   e) Ventricular arrhythmias
   f) Seizure
   g) Cardiac arrest (ventricular fibrillation)
4. Treatment (See Table 13-11)
   a) If specific identification of the toad is lacking and if *B. marinus* intoxication is not common in the area, conservative management may be warranted:
      (1) Wash out buccal mucosa with water.
      (2) Obtain a baseline lead II ECG.
      (3) Acepromazine IM, SQ 0.2–1.0 mg/kg if needed.
   b) If *B. marinus* exposure is known or likely:
      (1) Propranolol HCl has been shown to be an effective antiarrhythmic agent in toad poisoning (see Palumbo et al., 1975, Bibliography).
      (2) Induce anesthesia with pentobarbital Na IV, and intubate. (See Table 13-12)

TABLE 13-11. PROTOCOL FOR *Bufo marinus* (TOAD) POISONING

1. Establish likelihood of exposure to *Bufo marinus*.
2. Administer propranolol HCl IV 1.5–5 mg/kg.*
3. Induce anesthesia with pentobarbital Na (up to 6 mg/kg IV, to effect), and intubate.
4. Place on an ECG monitor or obtain serial lead II ECG readings.
5. Wash oral cavity thoroughly with water.
6. Monitor ECG. If arrhythmias persist:
   a. Administer more propranolol HCl 0.2 mg/kg slowly IV.
   b. Consider the use of diphenylhydantoin or other antiarrhythmic agents as outlined in Chapter 2 under Ventricular Arrhythmias.

* Administer with caution in patients with antecedent heart disease.

TABLE 13-12. COMMERCIAL PRODUCTS USED IN ENVENOMATIONS OR TOAD POISONING (NORTH AMERICAN DRUGS AND SOURCES)

Acepromazine	Prom-Ace	Fort Dodge, Fort Dodge, IA 50501
Barbiturate anesthetics:		
Pentobarbital Na	Pentobarbital Na	Med-Tech, Elwood, KS 66024 Fort Dodge, IA 50501
Sodium thiopental	Pentothal	CEVA/Abbott Laboratories, Overland Park, KS 66212
Thiamylal Na	Surital	Parke-Davis, Morris Plains, NJ 07950
	Bio-Tal	Bio-Ceutic Laboratories, St. Joseph, MO 64502
10% Calcium gluconate	Calcium INJ-USP gluconate	Upjohn, Kalamazoo, MI 49001
Canine Hyperimmune serum for tick paralysis		See Table 13-13
Dexamethasone	Azium	Schering, Kenilworth, NJ 07033
	Dexate-SP	Burns-Biotec Laboratories, Omaha, NE 68103
	H-L Dex	Haver-Lockhart, Shawnee Mission, KS 66201
Diphenylhydantoin	Phenytoin Na INJ	Elkins-Sinn, Cherry Hill, NJ 08034
	Dilantin INJ	Parke-Davis, Morris Plains, NJ 07950
Hydrocortisone Na succinate	Solu-Cortef	Upjohn, Kalamazoo, MI 49001
Meperidine HCl	Demerol	Winthrop Laboratories, New York, NY 10016
	Meperidine HCl	Wyeth Laboratories, Philadelphia, PA 19101
Methocarbamol	Robaxin INJ	A.H. Robbins, Richmond, VA 23220
	SK Methocarbamol	Smith, Kline & French, Philadelphia, PA 19101
Morphine sulfate	Morphine sulfate Carpuject	Winthrop Laboratories, New York, NY 10016
Pentazocime lactate	Talwin-V	Winthrop Laboratories, New York, NY 10016
Phenoxybenzamine HCl	Dibenzyline	Smith, Kline & French, Philadelphia, PA 19101
Prednisolone sodium succinate	Solu-Delta-Cortef	Upjohn, Kalamazoo, MI 49001
Propranolol HCl	Inderal	Ayerst Laboratories, New York, NY 10017

TABLE 13-13. SOURCES FOR ANTIVENOMS

1. *Latrodectus spp*. (black widow, red-back spiders) antivenom
   Merck, Sharpe and Dohme, West Point, PA 19486; 215-699-5311
2. Atrax (Sydney funnel-web spider)
   Commonwealth Serum Laboratories, 212 Willoughby Rd., Naremburn, Australia 2065; Tel. 4397011
3. Loxosceles (brown recluse spider) antivenom
   None available
4. Centuroides (scorpion) antivenom
   Iatrics Laboratory, Arizona State University, Tempe, AZ 85282; 602-966-3116
5. Canine hyperimmune serum for Australian tick paralysis
   Commonwealth Serum Laboratories—see entry no. 8 for addresses.
6. North American pit viper (crotalid) polyvalent antivenom
   Wyeth Laboratories, Philadelphia, PA 19101; 215-688-4400
7. Micrurus (coral snake) antivenom
   Wyeth Laboratories, Philadelphia, PA 19101; 215-688-4400
8. Australian snake antivenoms
   a. Contact local human hospital or State Poison Information Centers for out-of-date antivenoms.
   b. Commonwealth Serum Laboratories, Australia
      Victoria—45 Poplar Rd., Parkville 3052; Tel. 3891385
      New South Wales—212 Willoughby Rd., Naremburn 2065; Tel. 4397011
      Queensland—86 Brookes St., Fortitude Valley 4006; Tel. 524392
      South Australia—282–284 Gilbert St., Adelaide 5000; Tel. 516556
      West Australia—416 Newcastle St., Perth 6000; Tel. 328281

(3) Place the patient on an ECG monitor or perform serial lead II ECG readings.
(4) Wash oral cavity thoroughly with water.
(5) If arrhythmias persist:
  i) Administer more propanolol HCl
  ii) Consider the use of diphenylhydantoin or other antiarrhythmic agents as outlined in Chapter 2 in the section on Ventricular Tachyarrhythmias.

BIBLIOGRAPHY

Anonymous [Editorial]. Spider bites. Lancet 2:133, 1980
Barsanti JA: Botulism, tick paralysis and acute polyradiculoneuritis.

p. 773. In Kirk RW (ed): Current Veterinary Therapy. Vol. 7. WB Saunders, Philadelphia, 1980

Foil LD, Norment BR: Envenomation by *Loxosceles reclusa*. J Med Entomol 16:18, 1979

Ilkiw JE: Tick paralysis in Australia. p. 691. In Kirk RW (ed): Current Veterinary Therapy. Vol. 8. WB Saunders, Philadelphia, 1983

Lewis PF: Snake bite in animals in Australia. p. 287. In Proceedings No. 36 of Course for Veterinarians—Fauna. Postgraduate Committee in Veterinary Science, Sydney, 1978

Murnaghan MF, and O'Rourke FJ: Tick paralysis. p. 419. In Bettini S (ed): Arthropod Venoms. Handbook of Experimental Pharmacology. Vol. 48. Springer-Verlag, New York, 1978

Palumbo NE, Perri S, Read G: Experimental induction and treatment of toad poisoning in the dog. J Am Vet Med Assoc 167(11):1000, 1975

Russell FE: Snake Venom Poisoning. JB Lippincott, Philadelphia, 1980

Stahnke HL: The genus Centuroides and its venom. p. 279. In Bettini S (ed): Arthropod Venoms. Handbook of Experimental Pharmacology. Vol. 48. Springer-Verlag, New York, 1978

Stone BF: Chemical characterization studies on salivary gland toxins of the paralysis tick. *Ixodes holocyclus*. p. 273. In Chubb IW, Geffen LB (eds): Neurotoxins—Fundamental and Clinical Advances. Adelaide University, Unron Press, Adelaide, 1979

Sutherland SK: Treatment of arachnid poisoning in Australia. Aust Fam physician 5:305, 1976

Sutherland SK: The management of bites by the Sydney funnel-web spider, *Atrax robustus*. Med J Aust 1:148, 1978

Sutherland SK: *Latrodectus mactans hasselti* bite in animals. p. 253. In Sutherland SK (ed): Australian Animal Toxins. Oxford University Press, Melbourne, 1983

Van Mierop LHS: Poisonous snake bite: a review. J Fla Med Assoc 63:191, 1976

Wright IG, Stone BF, Neish AL: Tick (*Ixodes holocyclus*) paralysis in the dog—induction of immunity by injection of toxin. Aust Vet J 60:69, 1983

14

Emergencies of Avian Species

Robert B. Altman
Eileen Rowan

I. NEUROLOGIC EMERGENCIES

A. Brain trauma
  1. Etiology
    a) Impact during flight
      (1) Mirrors
      (2) Windows
      (3) Walls
      (4) Closing doors
    b) Bites
      (1) Dog and cat
      (2) Large birds
    c) Human mishandling
    d) Dropped cage
  2. Clinical signs
    a) Varying degrees of consciousness
    b) On cage floor, reluctant to perch and grasp
    c) Torticollis, opisthotonos, abnormal head movements
    d) Blindness
    e) Drowsiness or stupor
    f) Seizures
  3. Diagnosis
    a) History of free flight and/or exposure to dogs, cats, birds, or children

- b) Necropsy findings
  - (1) Subdural hematoma
  - (2) Cerebral edema
  - (3) Skull fractures
  - (4) Must differentiate from hemorrhagic areas found within the calvarium, which is a common post mortem finding
4. Treatment
   - a) Cage rest confinement for minimum of 2 weeks
   - b) Dexamethasone
     - (1) Intramuscularly initial 48 h (see Table 14-1)
     - (2) Per os until clinical signs are no longer evident
   - c) Supportive care
     - (1) Increased ambient temperature (80–85°F; 27–30°C)
     - (2) Nutritional supplementation (tube feeding)
     - (3) Parenteral fluid administration (5% D/W)

B. Spinal cord lesions
1. Etiology
   - a) Trauma, impact
     - (1) Spinal cord contusion and/or hemorrhage
     - (2) Fracture of vertebrae
   - b) Mycotic infections (aspergillosis)
   - c) Tumor
     - (1) Primary spinal cord tumor (Metastatic secondary lesions very rare.)
     - (2) Bone tumor (osteogenic sarcoma)
2. Clinical signs

   Acute unilateral or more frequently bilateral paresis
3. Diagnosis
   - a) Acute loss of function and reflex of one or both legs
   - b) Radiology
4. Treatment
   - a) Trauma therapy

(1) Cage rest
(2) Function often returns within 8–24 h in raptors.
(3) Parenteral dexamethasone (see Table 14-1)

TABLE 14-1. MISCELLANEOUS DRUGS

Acetyl cysteine 10% (Mucomyst-Mead Johnson Pharmaceutical)
  Dose: 1 drop SID-BID

Atropine sulfate
  Dose: 0.1–0.2 mg/kg SQ or IM

Calcium glycerophosphate 50 mg and calcium lactate 50 mg—10 mg/ml (Calphosan-Carlton)
  Dose: 0.5–1 ml BID IM, SQ

Calcium gluconate 10%
  0.05 ml/30 g diluted 1:9 with electrolyte solution
  SQ several sites

Glubionate calcium (Neocalglucon-Dorsey Laboratories)
  1–2 tsp/4 oz drinking water
  2–20 drops PO BID

Calcium EDTA (Haver-Lockhart Laboratories) OR
Calcium disodium versenate (Riker Laboratories)
  35 mg/kg BID IM
  Dilute with saline since irritating

Dexamethasone (Shering)
  Injectable:
    0.01 mg/30 g IM
    1 mg/kg in raptors
  Oral: 0.01 mg/30 g or one drop of 1% solution/oz water

Diazepam (Valium-Roche) 5 mg/ml
  Dose: 0.001 mg/g body weight as often as needed

Doxapram (Dopram-Robins)
  1–2 mg IV raptors

Furosemide (Lasix-Hoechst) 50 mg/ml
  Injectable dose:
    0.005 ml/30 g IM
    4–6 mg/kg raptors SID-BID
  Oral dose: 0.025 mg/30 g/day

Hydrocortisone (Upjohn)
  10 mg/kg raptors IM

Ipronidazole (Hoffman LaRoche)
  0.58 g/gal water

TABLE 14-1. *(Continued)*

Kaopectate (Upjohn)
    Two drops/30 g PO SID
    2 ml/kg PO BID-TID

Lactobacillus acidophilus (Lactinex-Hynson, Westcott and Dunning)
    One tablet crushed on seeds daily × 3 days

Lugol's iodine
    One drop/8 oz drinking water
    Dilute by: 2 parts Lugol's to 28 parts water
    Use 1 drop/oz SID for therapy and weekly for prevention.

Oxytocin (Pitocin-Parke-Davis) 20 U/ml
    0.015 ml/30 g IM
    Repeat in 2 h for egg binding.

Tincture of paregoric (Rexall)
    1–6 drops direct PO BID

Elix Phenobarbital 20 mg/5 ml
    1-6 drops PO BID-TID

Pralidoxine chloride (Protopam, 2 PAM-Ayerst)
    100 mg/kg IM

Prednisolone sodium succinate (Solu Delta Cortef-Upjohn)
    5–10 mg/kg SID raptors

Proparacaine HCl (Ophthaine-Squibb) 0.5% solution
    Can be toxic to cornea if used long-term
    Local anesthesia in less than 30 sec
    Lasts 15 min

Vitamin A and D_3 Injecom (Roche)
    Vitamin A 100,000 IU/ml, Vitamin D_3 10,000 IU/ml
        Dose: 0.01 ml/100 g q7d

Vitamin B complex
    B_1, B_2, B_{12}, Niacin, Panthotenic acid
        Dose: 0.025 ml–0.25 ml depending on size of bird q7d

Vitamin K
    Aquamephyton (Merck Sharp & Dohme)
        2 mg/kg IM
    Synkayvite (Roche) 5 mg/ml
        0.05 mg/30 g

Vidarabine (Vira-A-Parke Davis)
    Ophthalmic TID

b) Mycotic and tumor therapy
   (1) By the time clinical signs appear, treatment is futile.
   (2) Recommend euthanasia

5. Prognosis
   If no return to function after 48 h, prognosis is poor.

C. Seizures

1. Etiology
   a) Toxicity
      (1) Chlorinated hydrocarbons
      (2) Organophosphates
      (3) Lead toxicosis
      (4) Strychnine
      (5) Hair spray
   b) Hypoglycemia
   c) Hypocalcemia
   d) Head trauma
   e) Idiopathic epilepsy
2. Clinical signs
   a) Mild
      (1) Tremors
      (2) Maintains ability to perch
   b) Moderate
      (1) In the budgerigar spastic twitch of one leg with concurrent head jerk to the same side as the affected leg. Bird will emit a characteristic "chirp" with each spastic movement.
      (2) Appears to have full consciousness
   c) Severe
      (1) Inability to perch
      (2) Violent flapping of wings accompanied by leg movements
      (3) Loss of consciousness
3. Diagnosis
   a) Toxicity
      (1) History of exposure

(2) Lead poisoning diagnosis
  i) Radiographic evidence of metallic density, primarily in gizzard, but even lead shot found in the muscle has caused toxicity.
  ii) Serum blood lead levels

   Accuracy and normal levels vary with individual laboratories.

b) Hypoglycemia
  (1) Serum glucose determination (normal 250–550 mg/dl)
  (2) Seizures can occur with blood glucose levels below 100 mg/dl.

c) Hypocalcemia
  (1) Blood calcium determination (normal 7–13 mg/dl)
  (2) Radiographic evidence of secondary nutritional hyperparathyroidism seen as decalcification of the cortices of the long bones. The cortices become thin and decrease in density.

d) Head trauma

   History of trauma

e) Idiopathic epilepsy

   Absence of definitive diagnosis with transient recurrent episodes responsive to anticonvulsant therapy

4. Treatment
  a) General treatment
    (1) Parenteral diazepam (see Table 14-1)
    (2) Supportive therapy
      i) Administration of SQ or IV 2.5% dextrose in half-strength saline
      ii) Increase environmental temperature.
      iii) Maintain a quiet and dark environment.
      iv) Supplemental alimentation after return of all reflexes if anorexic

b) Specific treatment for toxicity
   (1) Chlorinated hydrocarbons
      i) Wash bird.
      ii) Calcium gluconate 5% IV (see Table 14-1)
   (2) Organophosphate
      Atropine sulfate (See Table 14-1)
   (3) Lead toxicosis
      i) Calcium EDTA until cessation of neurologic signs
      ii) May require second course of treatment if signs reappear (see Table 14-1)

   Repeat radiographs to determine passage of lead.
   (4) Metaldehyde
      Gastrointestinal (GI) lavage
c) Specific treatment for hypoglycemia
   5% D/W IV or IM (see Table 14-2)
d) Specific treatment for hypocalcemia
   (1) Calcium gluconate (see Table 14-1)
   (2) Vitamin D_3 supplementation (IM) to en-

TABLE 14-2. AVERAGE VOLUME IN MILLILITERS FOR FLUID ADMINISTRATION

SPECIES	PO (SID-TID)	SQ (SID-TID)
Finch	0.25–0.5	0.05
Canary	0.5	0.5–1
Budgerigar	0.5–1.5	1–2
Cockatiel	2–3	3
Amazon Parrot	6–10	6–10
Cockatoo	8–15	8–15
Macaw (large)	12–15	15–20
Mynah	5	4–6
Dabbling ducks (Teal, Black, Mallard, Pintail, Gadwall)	25	10–15
Diving ducks (Ruddy, Oldsquaw)	8–10	5–8

hance absorption of calcium (see Table 14-1)

e) Specific treatment for epilepsy
(1) Control with IM diazepam (see Table 14-1).
(2) Maintenance with oral elixer phenobarbital (see Table 14-1)

D. Renal adenocarcinoma in budgerigars

Included in this section because the bird presents with neurologic signs.

1. Clinical signs
a) Unilateral or bilateral leg weakness with diminished grasping reflex progressing to paresis
b) Inability to bear weight or extend or flex toes
c) Polyuria/polydipsia
d) Progressive weight loss
e) Posterior abdominal distension
2. Diagnosis
a) Atrophy of leg musculature
b) Weak or no grasping reflex
c) ± Palpable posterior abdominal mass
d) Radiographic evidence of enlarged anterior kidney lobe
3. Treatment—none

Suggest euthanasia.

II. OCULAR EMERGENCIES

A. Proptosis—rarely occurs because of the anatomy of the eye and orbit.

1. Etiology
a) Traumatic postorbital hemorrhage usually follows attack by other birds or animals, or flight into mirror or window.
b) Postorbital tumor
c) Postorbital abscess
2. Diagnosis based on history of acute trauma or gradual bulging of eye with no history of trauma.

3. Treatment
    a) If there is laceration of globe, suture and do tarsorrhaphy.
    b) Always stain cornea with fluorescein to look for abrasion or ulcer.
    c) If no trauma to globe or cornea
        (1) Reduce proptosed eye if possible.
        (2) Apply topical corticosteroid and antibiotic ointment.
        (3) Perform tarsorrhaphy
            i) Suture lids together using 3-0–5-0 nylon sutures.
            ii) Remove sutures in 10–14 days.
        (4) If corneal surface abraded, do not use corticosteroids.
    d) If postorbital abscess or tumor, enucleation of the eye is necessary.

B. Burns—rarely occur.

Occasionally birds will develop severe conjunctivitis and keratitis from smoke when exposed to a smoky fire.

C. Acute blepharitis

1. Clinical signs
    a) Swelling and inflammation of the lids causing a great deal of discomfort
    b) Squinting and rubbing lids
2. Etiology
    a) Avian pox—primarily in psittacines
        (1) Clinical signs
            i) Blepharitis is usually the first lesion seen.
            ii) Can be unilateral or bilateral
            iii) Serous ocular discharge
            iv) Lids swell and can paste together.
            v) Can get secondary corneal ulceration
            vi) Ocular lesions can last up to 6 weeks.
        (2) Treatment

i) Systemic and topical antibiotics
ii) Vitamin A
iii) Mercurochrome eyewash 2%—mix 1 oz to 4 oz of eyewash solution

b) Lovebird eye disease

Seen only in lovebirds, primarily Peach Face mutations (*Agaporius roseicollis sp.*). This disease is a fatal systemic disease which has ocular manifestations of blepharitis.

(1) Clinical signs
i) Depression
ii) Blepharitis
iii) Serous ocular discharge
iv) Lids become hyperemic and swollen
v) Death in a few days

(2) Etiology

Appears to be stress related (shipping)

(3) Treatment
i) None successful
ii) Try to minimize stress.

D. Conjunctivitis in cockatiels—seen most commonly in albino mutations
1. Etiology unknown
2. Clinical signs
   a) Early in course of disease (acute)
      (1) Serous ocular discharge
      (2) Blepharitis
   b) Later in course of disease (chronic)
      (1) Progressive conjunctivitis
      (2) Upper and lower respiratory infection
      (3) Sneezing, nasal discharge, coughing
3. Treatment
   a) Tylosin eye spray BID (Table 14-3)
   b) Corticosteroid/antibiotic ophthalmic ointment BID-TID
   c) Electrosurgical removal of hypertrophied conjunctival tissue
4. Conjunctivitis secondary to bacterial, mycoplasmal, chlamydial, or viral disease

TABLE 14-3. ANTIBIOTICS

Amikacin sulfate (Bristol Laboratories) 250 mg/ml
 Dose: 0.01 mg/g IM SID-BID

Amoxicillin suspension (Beecham) 50 mg/ml
 Dose: 5 mg/30 g BID (most species)

Ampicillin (Bristol Laboratories)
 Dose:
  Oral suspension—150–200 mg/kg BID-TID (parrots)
  Injectable IM—100 mg/kg every 4 h (parrots)

Cefotaxime sodium (Dista Products) 1-g vials
 Dose: 100 mg/kg QID IM

Chloramphenicol (Parke Davis)
 Dose:
  Succinate 100 mg/ml: 80 mg/kg IM BID-TID
  Palmitate oral suspension: 0.1 mg/30 g BID-TID

Gentamycin (Schering) 50 mg/ml
 Dose: 10 mg/kg IM SID-BID
  Note: SQ fluids given at same time helps to decrease nephrotoxicity.
  PO: 40 mg/kg SID for 2–3 days

Kanamycin (Bristol Laboratories) 50 mg/ml
 Dose:
  10 mg/kg IM BID
  1–5 ml/gal water × 3 days

Neomycin solution with methscopolamine bromide (50 mg/ml)
 Dose:
  1–10 drops/oz water × 1–3 days
  ½–4 drops direct PO BID

Tetracycline HCl (Upjohn)
 Dose:
  Oral suspension:
   75 mg/300 g SID or
   25–50 mg/300–500 g TID

Tylosin (Corvel Laboratories)
 Dose:
  Injectable (50 mg/ml): 0.01–0.025 mg/g IM BID-TID
  Oral soluble powder (250 g/8.81 oz): 1 tsp/5 oz water
  Ophthalmic: mix powder with water in 1:10 dilution; spray in eyes.

a) Clinical signs similar to above (see Section 2b, above)
b) Treatment
 (1) As above (3b)
 (2) Treat specific infectious disease.

E. Corneal emergencies
  1. Lacerations
    a) Etiology
      (1) Trauma
      (2) Conjunctival or corneal foreign bodies
    b) Diagnosis
      (1) Lacrimation and unilateral squinting
      (2) Collapse and indentation of cornea
    c) Treatment
      (1) Suture cornea.
      (2) Topical antibiotics
  2. Corneal ulcers
    a) Etiology
      (1) Trauma
      (2) Foreign body
      (3) Secondary to infectious disease
    b) Clinical signs
      (1) Squinting and lacrimation
      (2) Rubs eye
    c) Diagnosis—positive fluorescein staining
    d) Treatment (see Table 14-1)
      (1) Acute—topical antibiotics BID-TID
      (2) Chronic
        i) Mechanical debridement of loose epithelial tags at margin of ulcer with a dry cotton tipped applicator.
        ii) SID-BID antibiotic eye drops
        iii) SID-BID collagenase inhibitor
        iv) Suture the eyelids together if ulcers are recurring.
        v) In nonhealing chronic ulcers, topical application of an antiviral agent before suturing the lids is sometimes of value.
  3. Keratitis
    a) Etiology
      (1) Chronic corneal ulcers
      (2) In mynah birds the cause is unknown—possibly related to shipping

(3) Amazon parrots can develop a punctate keratitis of unknown etiology.

b) Treatment

(1) Treat as chronic corneal ulcer

(2) Treat any infectious disease

F. Uveitis

1. Etiology usually associated with systemic disease
2. Clinical signs

a) Photophobic ophthalmia

b) Hyperemic iris

c) Aqueous flare

d) "Steamy" cornea

e) May have hypopyon

f) Can develop synechiae (iris to lens)

3. Treatment

a) Topical steroids TID

b) Treat primary disease

G. Emergencies of the adnexa

1. Lacerations of the eyelids

a) Etiology

(1) Are traumatic in origin and uncommon

(2) Primarily caused by cats and other birds

b) Treatment

(1) Suture with 3-0–5-0 nonabsorbable suture material, using a cutting needle.

(2) Remove sutures in 10–14 days.

2. Lacerations of the membrana nictitans

a) Etiology—the same as above

b) Treatment

(1) If not extensive, suture with 5-0 absorbable suture material.

(2) If tear leaves a large devascularzied flap, it is advisable to surgically excise the flap.

H. Acute blindness

1. Etiology

a) Trauma—concussion

b) Lead poisoning

c) Chlorinated hydrocarbon intoxication

d) Hexachlorophene toxicity

2. Diagnosis
   Based on lack of menace response
3. Treatment
   a) If caused by trauma:
      (1) Furosemide (see Table 14-1)
      (2) Systemic corticosteroids
      (3) Maintain food and water consumption
   b) If caused by toxic agents—see section on Toxic Emergencies, below.

III. ORTHOPEDIC EMERGENCIES

A. Trauma causing luxations and fractures in both pet and wild bird populations are the most common traumatic injuries seen by the veterinarian. It is essential that the entire bird be evaluated before focus is directed to the fractured area. Initial stabilization of the patient, with respect to shock, internal injuries, and soft tissue damage, is more important than immediate stabilization of the fracture segments.

B. Once the patient's status has been evaluated, it is essential to consider the primary function of the patient. If the bird is a pet or companion, prime consideration in approaching the injury is toward the safety and survival of the patient. If, however, the prime consideration is the return to function enabling the bird to return to the wild, emphasis must be placed on the repair, sometimes compromising the bird's well-being.

C. Initial approach to patient
   1. Complete physical examination of the entire body.
   2. Diagnostic evaluation
      a) Packed cell volume
      b) Blood glucose
      c) Radiographic evaluation—radiographs should be taken even if the fracture is readily palpable, since long bone cortices are often thin and decalcified as the result of secondary nutritional hyperparathyroidism.

3. If a compound fracture is present, evaluate the extent of soft tissue damage:
    a) Nerves
    b) Blood vessels
    c) Tendons
    d) Ligaments

D. Treatment
1. For shock
    a) Corticosteroids (see Table 14-1)
    b) Antibiotics (see Table 14-3)
    c) 2.5% dextrose in half-strength saline SQ
    d) Keep ambient temperature between 80 and 88°F.
2. For soft tissue damage
    a) Must preserve the integrity of major nerves, blood vessels, tendons, and joints.
        (1) If flight and return to wild is required, repair with microsurgery may be essential.
        (2) If flight and return to wild is not essential, a standard surgical closure of the wound should be performed after debridement and surgical cleansing.
3. For fractures of the extremities
    a) Simple fracture
        (1) Attempt manual reduction.
        (2) Immobilization by
            i) Taping to body
            ii) Adhesive tape splint
            iii) Polymer orthopedic tape (Hexalite) (see Table 14-4)
    b) Compound or comminuted fractures
        (1) Do not attempt to reduce manually.
        (2) Immobilize as above until permanent surgical fracture repair can be undertaken.
4. General considerations
    a) Remove grating from bottom of cage.
    b) Lower perches to a few inches above floor of cage. Do not remove perches.

TABLE 14-4. EQUIPMENT

Polyglycolic sutures—(Vicryl-Roche)
Desseret, short IV catheter Angio-Set short 22 × $\frac{3}{4}$ in. Cat. no. 6022
Hexalite (Hexcel Medical Products)
Monsells (Ferric Subsulfate-Amend)
Clotisol—Pet Care Industries

c) Be sure food and water are accessible.
d) Remove all swinging perches and movable toys.
e) Remove gravel or gravel paper from floor and perches.

5. Luxations
   a) Uncommon in birds
   b) Should be reduced as quickly as possible.

IV. INTEGUMENT EMERGENCIES

A. Laceration and punctures

1. Etiology
   a) Cat bites and scratches
   b) Impact
   c) Miscellaneous
2. Clinical signs
   Laceration of skin with or without blood loss
3. Diagnosis
   a) History
   b) Physical examination
4. Treatment
   a) Cat bites and scratches
      (1) *Immediate* injections of broad spectrum antibiotics are indicated since Pasteurella from a cat's mouth is often fatal within 24 h.
      (2) Suture when stable with 5-0 polyglycolic

suture material (Vicryl) in a continuous pattern. Larger-gauge vicryl for birds over 500 g. (See Table 14-4.)

b) Impact
   (1) The skin over the sternum will split on impact and will not heal without suturing. Debridement is necessary if wound is over 24 h duration.
   (2) The ventral tail base can split between the cloaca and tail, requiring suturing.

B. Self-mutilation
1. Etiology
   a) "Feather picker"
   b) Infection
   c) Allergy
   d) Parasites
   e) Foreign substances on feathers
   f) Unknown chronic intermittent necrotising dermatitis of possible immune deficiency syndrome
2. Clinical signs
   a) "Feather pickers" and allergic birds: feathers chewed to varying degrees on any of the following areas: legs, wings, tail, general body. The head and neck will have normal feathering.
   b) Infected and immune-deficient birds: specific area of skin infected with yellow crusting and feather picking localized to involved area only. Can develop superficial or deep necrosis resulting in sloughing.
   c) Allergic and parasitized birds: constant or nervous picking at feathers
3. Diagnosis
   a) History
   b) Physical examination
   c) Response to steroids
   d) Lack of response to any treatment for immune-deficient birds

e) Biopsy of chronic lesions
f) White towel over cage technique for red mites (*Dermanyssus sp.*)

4. Treatment
   a) General
      (1) Elizabethan collar
      (2) Insure proper diet and vitamin supplementation.
   b) Specific
      (1) "Feather picker"
         i) Eliminate any psychological stress bothering bird.
         ii) Insure proper caging, freedom, and toys.
         iii) Increase attention spent on bird.
         iv) Squirt with water bottle when picking attempts are made.
         v) Psychological stress can occur from the absence or presence of another bird.
      (2) Infection
         i) Systemic antibiotics (see Table 14-3)
         ii) Topical antibiotic/steroid creams
         iii) Ointments and creams when applied topically must be used judiciously and applied only to the lesion. Excessive application can cause pasting and subsequent feather loss leading to increased picking.
      (3) Allergy
         Systemic steroids (see Table 14-1)
      (4) Parasites
         i) Mite/lice spray (rotenone and pyrethrum) at weekly intervals for 3 weeks
         ii) For *Dermanyssus* use Vapona strip outside cage.

- (5) Foreign substances on feathers
  - i) Commercial bird "bath sprays" often cause picking at feathers because they leave a film. Attempt to rinse off spray with warm water and/or mild detergent (Dawn dishwashing liquid).
  - ii) Oiled feathers—see section on oiled birds in Toxic Emergencies section below.
- (6) Chronic intermittent necrotising dermatitis
  - i) Long-term treatment with systemic antibiotics and topical antibiotic/steroid ointments.
  - ii) Systemic steroid (see Table 14-1)
  - iii) Once infection under control, local debridement and suturing often speeds recovery.
  - iv) Recurrence is possible.

C. Burns

1. Etiology
   - a) Hot substances in kitchen contacted during flight
   - b) Chemical
   - c) Electrical
2. Clinical signs
   - a) Peeling of skin of feet and distal legs most often seen
   - b) Discoloration of toes, feet, legs from burn with eventual necrosis
3. Diagnosis
   - a) History
   - b) Examination
4. Treatment
   - a) Supportive care if appetite affected
   - b) Systemic and topical antibiotics
   - c) Elizabethan collar if self-mutilation has begun

D. Ulcerations
   1. Etiology
      a) In budgerigars, ulcerated fatty granulomas are common.
      b) Tumors
   2. Clinical signs
      a) Blood loss
      b) Picking at affected area
      c) Excoriations
   3. Diagnosis
      Physical examination
   4. Treatment
      a) Surgical excision of ulcerated granuloma
      b) Surgical excision of tumor

E. Ingrown feathers—Not a true emergency, but owners often assume they are more serious.
   1. Etiology—unknown
   2. Clinical signs
      a) Enlarging mass often on wings, but can be anywhere on body
      b) Picking at affected site
   3. Diagnosis
      Physical examination
   4. Treatment
      a) Lance and curettage
      b) Electro- or chemical cautery to try to prevent recurrence (silver nitrate)
      c) Surgical excision if recurs

F. Subcutaneous emphysema—see section on Respiratory Emergencies, below.

V. GASTROINTESTINAL EMERGENCIES

A. Bloody stool
   1. Etiology
      a) Gram-negative bacterial overgrowth
      b) Lead poisoning

c) Allergic reactions
d) Parasitism
(1) Coccidia
(2) Capillaria
(3) Ascarids
(4) Tapeworms
e) Tumors of intestinal tract
Cloacal polyps
f) Viral diseases
(1) *Chlamydia psittaci*
(2) Viscerotropic Velogenic Newcastle's Disease (VVND)
(3) Herpes
g) Chronic inflammatory hyperplasia of the cloacal mucosa
h) Warfarin—see section on Toxic Emergencies, below.

2. Clinical signs
a) Trace to excessive blood in stool
b) Straining to defecate is occasionally present.
c) Concomitant signs of systemic disease
d) Diarrhea
e) Eversion of cloacal mucosa

3. Diagnosis
a) Fecal culture and sensitivity (C & S)
b) Gram stain stool for immediate confirmation of bacterial overgrowth
c) Cloacal examination with an otoscope
d) Fecal smears and flotation for detection of parasites
e) Radiology
(1) Diagnostic for presence of lead (metallic density)
(2) Can reveal gas or fluid-filled bowels from gram-negative bacterial overgrowth or tumor
f) Diagnosis of allergy based on response to steroids

g) Culture and complement fixation serology for Chlamydiosis
h) Viral isolation from cloacal swabs for VVND
i) Histopathologic evidence for VVND and herpes

4. Treatment
   a) General
      (1) Replace fluid loss (see Table 14-2)
         i) Subcutaneous fluids
         ii) Tube feeding
         iii) Monitor PCV and TS
   b) Specific
      (1) Gram-negative bacterial overgrowth
         i) Appropriate antibiotics as indicated on C & S
            Used IM or PO (see Table 14-3)
         ii) Repeat C & S until negative for growth
         iii) Increase gram-positive bacterial intestinal flora
            (*A*) Lactobacillus (see Table 14-1)
            (*B*) Plain yogurt
      (2) Lead poisoning
         Calcium EDTA (see Table 14-1)
      (3) Allergic reactions
         Corticosteroids IM or PO (See Table 14-1)
      (4) Parasitism (see Table 14-5)
         i) Coccidia
            (*A*) Amprolium
            (*B*) Sulfadimethoxine
            (*C*) Sulfamethazine
         ii) Capillaria
            (*A*) Ivermectin
            (*B*) Levamisole HC1
         iii) Ascarids
            (*A*) Piperazine
            (*B*) Levamisole
            (*C*) Ivermectin

TABLE 14-5. ANTHELMINTICS

Amprolium (Corid-MSD AGVET) 9.6% solution
  Coccidia: 2 ml/gal water × 5 days or longer

Dimetridazole (Emtryl—Salsbury Laboratories), 182 g/6.42 oz
  Trichomonas: 1 tsp/gal water × 5 days
  Giardia: 1 tsp/gal water or 1.5 mg/30-g bird—repeat 3× every 12 h by direct lavage.

Ivermectin (Eqvalan-MSD AGVET)
  Coccidia and Capillaria: 200 μg/kg IM once or 0.10 ml/kg of a 2 mg/ml concentration
    Note:
      Light-sensitive, so a fresh solution should be made every dosage
      Approved only for horses
      May be toxic

Levamisole HCl 13.65% injectable (Professional Veterinary Pharmaceuticals)
  Capillaria:
    20 mg/kg SQ; Repeat in 10 days
    5–10 ml/gal water for 1–3 days
  Ascarids:
    15 mg/kg gavage to crop; repeat in 3 weeks
    5–10 ml/gal water for 24 h; repeat in 3 weeks

Niclosamide (Yomesan-Haver Lockhart)
  Tapeworms: 200 mg/kg in food or crop by gavage; repeat in 2 weeks

Piperazine (Burns-Biotech Laboratories)
  Raptors 100 mg/kg PO
  4 g piperazine citrate/qt water × 3–4 days; repeat in 2 weeks
  200–1000 mg/kg single dose PO
  0.3–0.5 mcg/g single dose PO

Sulfadimethoxine (Roche)
  Coccidia:
    0.05% powder dose:
      1 pkg/50 gal water
      ¼ tsp/oz water
    Solution 12.5%:
      Use 1 oz to 2 gal water
    Oral suspension (100 mg/ml):
      Dose: 0.01 ml/30 g BID PO
      Dose: 0.1 ml/lb PO

Sulfamethazine solution (30 mg/oz)
  Coccidia: full strength in place of drinking water

Vapona strip
  Hang outside of cage where bird cannot come into direct contact—3–5 days

iv) Tapeworms
Niclosamide
v) Giardia
(*A*) Ipronidazole (see Table 14-1)
(*B*) Dimetridazole
(5) Tumor
Attempt surgery.
(6) Chronic inflammatory hyperplasia of the cloacal mucosa
See section on Prolapsed Cloaca versus Hyperplastic Tissue, below.

B. Advanced chronic diarrhea
1. Etiology
a) Gram-negative bacterial overgrowth
b) Parasitism
(1) Coccidia
(2) Capillaria
(3) Ascarids
(4) Tapeworms
(5) Giardia
(6) Trichomoniasis
c) Chlamydial infection
d) Tuberculosis
2. Clinical signs
a) Emaciation
b) Pasty vent can lead to pseudocoprostasis.
c) Often a ravenous appetite
3. Diagnosis
a) Culture and sensitivity of cloaca and feces; acid fast stains
b) Fecal smear and fecal flotation (fresh mount for Trichomonas)
c) Psittacosis titer if other signs or history compatible
d) For tuberculosis, postmortem findings may be suggestive but only microscopic identification of the organism can confirm the disease.
4. Treatment

- a) General
  - (1) Fluid administration
    - i) Subcutaneous
    - ii) Tube feeding
  - (2) Paregoric (see Table 14-1)
  - (3) Kaopectate (see Table 14-1)
  - (4) Neomycin solution with methscopolamine bromide (see Table 14-3)
- b) Specific
  - (1) Gram-negative bacterial overgrowth
    For treatment, see section on Bloody Stool, above.
  - (2) Parasitism
    - i) See treatment under section on Bloody Stool, above.
    - ii) For Trichomonas—dimetridazole (Table 14-5)
  - (3) Chlamydial infections
    Tetracycline HCl PO (see Table 14-3)
  - (4) Tuberculosis—no treatment

C. Crop laceration

1. Etiology
   - a) Bite wounds
   - b) Foreign body
   - c) Iatrogenic
     - (1) Subcutaneous injections
     - (2) Tube feeding
   - d) Flying into sharp object
2. Clinical signs
   - a) If full-thickness skin and crop laceration, food will be discharged through the opening.
   - b) Few signs may occur if only the crop is lacerated until food accumulates and causes a caseous abscess.
   - c) Crop and esophageal iatrogenic lacerations may cause acute hemorrhage.
3. Diagnosis
   - a) Presence of food in fistula

b) Postmortem finding of acute severe hemorrhage
c) Palpation of mass not in crop
4. Treatment
a) Suture with polyglycolic material (see Table 14-4) in separate crop and skin layers.

D. Foreign body (partial or complete obstruction)
1. Etiology
a) Lead ingesta
b) Crop calculi
c) Ventricular grit impaction
d) Other foreign bodies
2. Clinical signs
a) Occasionally bloody droppings
b) Regurgitation
c) Anorexia
d) Depression
3. Diagnosis
a) Survey radiographs
b) Barium series for partial or complete obstruction

Obstruction by foreign body often found in proventriculus.
4. Treatment
a) Lead

Calcium EDTA until signs abate (see Table 14-1)
b) Foreign material, if unlikely to pass, will require surgical intervention.
c) Ventricular grit impaction
(1) Mineral oil PO for one to 3 days
(2) Supportive hyperalimentation
(3) Within 7–10 days, if there is no sign of clinical improvement or radiographic evidence of passage of grit, then a ventriculotomy should be considered.

E. Pseudocoprostasis

1. Etiology
    a) Chronic diarrhea
    b) Egg binding
2. Clinical signs
    a) Pasted vent
    b) Depression
    c) Occasionally anorexia
    d) Tenesmus
3. Diagnosis
    Based on physical examination
4. Treatment
    a) Gentle cleansing with warm water and mild soap
    b) If cloaca is very irritated, use topical antibiotic/steroid cream.

F. Persistent regurgitation
1. Etiology
    a) Crop infection
        (1) Candida
        (2) Trichomonas
        (3) Gram-negative bacterial overgrowth
    b) Foreign body in crop, proventriculus, or gizzard
    c) Crop calculi
    d) Tumors
    e) Hepatonecrosis
    f) Sexual display
    g) Crop dilation and atony
2. Clinical signs
    a) Regurgitation
    b) Weight loss is common.
    c) Crop distended with fluid and seed
3. Diagnosis
    a) Crop C & S
    b) Crop wash
        (1) Microscopic examination
        (2) Gram stain

c) Radiographs for grit impaction, crop calculi, tumors

4. Treatment
   a) General
      (1) Supportive therapy with SQ 2.5% dextrose in half-strength saline and tube feeding until signs abate.
   b) Specific
      (1) Infection
         i) Candida
            (*A*) Nystatin (see Table 14-6)
            (*B*) Ketoconazole (see Table 14.6)
         ii) Trichomonas
            Dimetridazole (see Table 14-5)
         iii) Gram-negative bacterial overgrowth
            Antibiotics as determined by C & S
      (2) Foreign body
         i) Supportive therapy until it passes
         ii) Surgery if won't pass
      (3) Crop calculi
         Surgery

TABLE 14-6. ANTIFUNGALS

For Candida:

Nystatin (Mycostatin oral suspension, Squibb) 100,000 U/ml
  Dose: 1 ml/300–350 g PO SID-BID × 7 days

Ketoconazole (Nizaral-Janssen) 200-mg tablet
  Dose: dissolve one tablet in 1 qt drinking water—treat 7–14 days; stir frequently

For Aspergillus:

Amphotericin B (Fungizone-Squibb) 50-mg vials; refrigerate after reconstitution
  Intratracheal SID 0.001 mg/g until bird is asymptomatic
  Nebulize 15 min BID: 1 mg/ml sterile saline
  IV for raptors: 1.5 mg/kg TID × 3 days
  3% Lotion—SID oral application
    Note: Potentially nephrotoxic

5-Fluorocytosine (Ancobon-Roche) 250 mg/capsule
  Dose
    0.25 mg/g BID by tube (psittacine)
    0.12 mg/g raptors PO TID
      Note: Safe for extended periods

(4) Tumors
Usually too advanced to treat by surgery
(5) Hepatonecrosis
Antibiotics

G. Prolapsed cloaca versus hyperplastic tissue
1. Etiology
a) Prolapsed cloaca
(1) Chronic diarrhea
(2) Straining from egg laying
(3) Diminished cloacal muscle tone
b) Hyperplastic tissue
Cause unknown
2. Clinical signs
a) Prolapsed tissue (hyperemic to necrotic) protruding from cloaca
b) Blood in stool
c) Straining
d) Droplets of blood on perch and cage bottom
3. Diagnosis
a) Prolapse
Tubular prolapse obvious on examination, usually edematous
b) Hyperplastic tissue
(1) Hyperemic ring of hyperplastic mucosa, usually at mucocutaneous junction
(2) Tissue intermittently prolapses from cloaca.
4. Treatment
a) Prolapse
(1) If viable, reduce and insert pursestring suture for 3 days.
i) Topical antibiotics and steroids applied through pursestring
ii) Topical anesthetic to prevent tenesmus
iii) May need to be repeated if reprolapses when pursestring removed

iv) Pursestring must be loose enough for stool to pass.

v) Surgical tacking of cloaca to body wall

(2) If prolapsed mucosa is nonviable, resection is indicated.

b) Hyperplastic tissue

(1) Surgical removal

i) Electrosurgery

ii) Cryosurgery

(2) Tissue is vascular, therefore hemostasis is essential.

5. Prognosis

a) Prolapse

(1) Good chance for recurrence

(2) If viable and short duration, prognosis is good

(3) If viability is questionable or prolapse is old, prognosis is less favorable.

(4) If surgery indicated, prognosis is poor.

b) Hyperplastic tissue

(1) Prognosis good, low mortality

(2) May require additional surgery to remove all hyperplastic tissue

(3) Can recur

VI. ENDOCRINE EMERGENCIES

A. Hypoglycemia—normal serum glucose levels for most avian species is 200–550 mg/dl. Birds with serum glucose levels below 150 mg/dl require immediate glucose supplementation. Birds with levels below 70 mg/dl usually die.

1. Etiology

a) Starvation—glycogen storage in the liver can be depleted in 12–48 h in most avian species.

b) Chronic disease

c) Stress

d) Prolonged anesthesia and recovery
e) Excessive insulin administration
f) Insulinoma

2. Clinical signs
    a) Weakness
    b) Ataxia
    c) Collapse
    d) Seizure
3. Diagnosis is based on history and blood glucose levels below 150 mg/dl.
4. Treatment
    a) If blood glucose is between 150 and 200 mg/dl give:
        (1) Saturated sugar solution 0.5–5 ml PO (stomach tube).
        (2) Karo syrup or honey—use stomach tube
    b) If blood glucose is less than 150 mg/dl, administer 5% D/W IM or IV to effect.
    c) Treat cause appropriately.
5. Prevention: birds that are anorexic or stressed undergoing surgery or have chronic disease but have blood glucose levels above 200 ml/dl should get oral or SQ glucose supplementation.

B. Hyperglycemia
1. Etiology
    a) Idiopathic transient hyperglycemia
    b) Diabetes mellitus
2. Clinical signs
    a) Polyuria (appearing as watery droppings)
    b) Polydipsia
    c) Lethargy
    d) Ataxia
3. Diagnosis
    a) Elevated urine glucose
    b) Elevated blood glucose (usually above 800 mg/dl)—can reach levels of 2,000 mg/dl
    c) Blood glucose levels must be elevated for 24–48 h to consider a diagnosis of diabetes. Therefore, daily repeated sampling is necessary.

4. Treatment

NPH insulin given once daily IM. Dilute U40 NPH insulin to 0.04 U/ml for a 30- to 40-g parakeet. Start with 0.002 U (0.05 ml). Increase by 0.002 U until serum glucose has been reduced to normal levels. Blood glucose determinations should be evaluated daily. When glucose levels have dropped below 600 mg/dl, urine glucose can be monitored.

C. Hypocalcemia
1. Etiology—this condition has been reported in the literature and has been seen in parrots, particularly African Grey parrots. The true etiology is not known but suggested theories are:
   a) Secondary nutritional hyperparathyroidism
   b) Parathyroiditis
2. Clinical signs
   a) Anorexia
   b) Depression
   c) Seizures
   d) Death
   e) Low blood calcium (<6 mg/dl)
3. Treatment
   a) Intravenous or IM calcium (see Table 14-1)
   b) Oral glubionate calcium (see Table 14-1) in the drinking water
   c) Supportive therapy as needed

VII. UROGENITAL EMERGENCIES

A. Cloacal prolapse

Note: True prolapse needs to be differentiated from hyperplastic tissue of cloacal mucosa. For etiology, clinical signs, diagnosis, and treatment, see section on Gastrointestinal Emergencies, above.

B. Egg binding
1. Etiology
   a) Excessively large egg; rough or irregular surface of egg

   - b) Ruptured oviduct
   - c) Lack of tone of oviduct
   - d) Calcium depletion
   - e) Spasticity of oviduct around egg
2. Clinical signs
   - a) Straining to pass egg
   - b) Depressed and puffed
   - c) Anorexia
   - d) Scant droppings
   - e) Posterior abdominal distention
   - f) Prolapsed tissue seen protruding from cloaca
3. Diagnosis
   - a) History of behavior and prior problems with passing eggs
   - b) Gentle physical palpation
   - c) Radiology
     - (1) To determine if egg is broken
     - (2) To count number of eggs
     - (3) To ascertain the calcification of egg shell
4. Treatment
   - a) Increase heat to high 80s, low 90s (°F).
   - b) Place several drops of mineral oil into cloaca.
   - c) If egg is broken, laparotomy is necessary. See section on Egg Yolk Peritonitis, below.
   - d) Calcium injection (see Table 14-1)
   - e) Oxytocin injection (See Table 14-1)
   - f) If not successful in passing egg with above methods, try manual cloacal dilatation.

     If unable to reach egg, transcloacal approach or laparotomy is needed.

C. Egg yolk peritonitis
1. Etiology
   - a) Poor shell calcification leads to broken egg
   - b) Rough palpation of egg
   - c) Ruptured oviduct allows egg to pass to abdominal cavity without shell formation
2. Clinical signs
   - a) Depression

b) Anorexia
c) Possibly diarrhea

3. Diagnosis
   Radiology
   (1) Ground glass appearance to abdomen
   (2) May or may not see broken egg
   (3) Paracentesis of abdomen
4. Treatment
   a) Systemic antibiotics
   b) Supportive care
   c) Laparotomy
      (1) Flush abdomen to remove all debris.
      (2) Remove as much of oviduct as possible if badly torn; otherwise, repair.
      (3) Usually cannot remove ovary

VIII. BLEEDING EMERGENCIES

A. Beak
1. Types of injuries
   a) Cracks
   b) Broken tip
   c) Partial or total avulsion of beak
2. Clinical signs
   Obvious bleeding and damage to beak
3. Diagnosis
   a) History of injury
   b) Obvious trauma on physical examination
4. Treatment
   a) Control bleeding
      (1) Topical hemostatic agents
         i) Ferric subsulfate solution (see Table 14-4)
         ii) Clotisol
         iii) Silver nitrate

(2) Electrocautery

b) Determine severity of blood loss.

(1) Measure PCV

(2) If PCV is below 10%, consider transfusion.

c) Prevent hypovolemic shock by administration of IV fluids (see Table 14-7).

d) Institute tube feeding if bird not eating.

e) Repair damaged beak where applicable with dental acrylics.

B. Nail

1. Types of injuries

a) Broken nail

b) Torn nail

c) Avulsed nail

2. Treatment

a) Cut or remove nail.

b) Cauterize to stop bleeding.

c) Monitor blood loss.

d) Bandage if necessary.

C. Feather

1. *Note:* Only broken immature feathers will bleed.

2. Treatment

a) Remove broken feather shaft.

b) Apply pressure on follicle to prevent oozing after shaft removal.

D. Legs and toes

1. Lacerations are the primary type of injury.

2. Treatment

a) Begin compression to stop bleeding instantly.

TABLE 14-7. IV EMERGENCY FLUID THERAPY FORMULA

50% glucose	two parts
Ringers solution	three parts
Amino acid electrolyte solution	one part
Dose: Give 10 ml/450 g over 2–5 min with IV catheter if possible	

b) Suture and ligate where indicated.
c) Apply pressure bandages as needed.
d) With deep lacerations it is sometimes necessary to amputate a toe.

E. Mouth
1. Etiology
a) Bleeding from mouth only
(1) GI tract
(2) Bitten or lacerated tongue
b) Bleeding from mouth and nose
Usually from respiratory tract
2. Treatment
a) If tongue badly lacerated, suture.
b) Since blood loss can only be estimated, must monitor PCV
c) Supportive therapy

F. Tumors
1. Causes of bleeding
a) All superficial tumors can ulcerate and bleed.
b) Some tumors (xanthomas) become necrotic, break down, and bleed.
c) Birds may pick and traumatize themselves resulting in hemorrhage.
2. Treatment
a) Stop bleeding
(1) Cautery
(2) Ligation
(3) Local hemostasis
b) Surgical removal of tumor

G. Acute hemorrhagic syndrome
1. Etiology unknown
2. Clinical signs
a) Occurs in Amazon parrots
b) Acute onset
c) Reddish-orange fluid urine (hemoglobinuria)
d) Tomato soup droppings as a result of the hemoglobin mixing with urates

e) Depression—mild to severe
f) Regurgitation
g) Anorexia
h) Death within 24–72 h

3. Diagnosis based on:
   a) Clinical signs
   b) Laboratory findings
      (1) Low PCV
      (2) Hemolysis
      (3) Negative radiographic evidence of foreign bodies or lead in the GI tract
   c) No RBCs are found in the droppings, since the color results from hemoglobinuria rather than hemorrhage.
4. Differential diagnosis
   a) Gastrointestinal hemorrhage from:
      (1) Trauma
      (2) Foreign body
      (3) Parasites
   b) Cloacal bleeding
   c) Warfarin poisoning
   d) Lead poisoning
   e) Viral and bacterial septicemias
5. Treatment
   a) Antibiotics (see Table 14-3)
   b) Corticosteroids (see Table 14-1)
   c) Injacom 100 (see Table 14-1)
   d) Vitamin B complex supplementation (see Table 14-1)
   e) Subcutaneous fluid therapy (see Table 14-2)
   f) Maintain ambient temperature at 85–90°F (29–32°C).
   g) If PCV drops below 10%, a blood transfusion is indicated.
      (1) Use a pigeon as donor
         i) Collect blood in heparin-washed syringe with a 22-gauge needle.

ii) Collect via cardiac puncture.
iii) Can safely draw 3 ml
(2) Cross-match recipient sera-donor red cells on a slide and look for agglutination.
(3) Inject slowly via superficial ulnar or medial tibiotarsal vein with a butterfly catheter (Desseret) (see Table 14.4).

6. *Note:* If treatment is instituted early, response to therapy is generally good. An intensive therapeutic regimen is essential.

H. Acute hemorrhagic disease in canaries (*Sernius canarius*)

1. Etiology

Is caused by an unknown hemoparasitic protozoa. This parasite is morphologically similar to the megaloschyzonts of Leucocytozoan infections seen in other species.

2. Clinical signs
   a) Acute death
   b) Abdominal distention with blood
3. Postmortem Findings
   a) Thoraco-abdominal hemorrhage
   b) Acute hepatocellular necrosis and petechiation
   c) Cysts resembling megaloschyzonts of a hemoparasite in the liver
4. Diagnosis
   a) Based on acute death with extravasation of blood in the thoraco-abdominal cavity
   b) The histopathologic identification of cysts (megaloschyzonts) in the liver
5. Treatment of exposed birds
   a) Dimetridazole (0.04% in drinking water for 5 days)
   b) Blood transfusions

I. Toxicities causing hemorrhagic enteritis

1. Lead poisoning (see section on Toxic Emergencies, below)

2. Warfarin (See section on Toxic Emergencies, below)

IX. RESPIRATORY EMERGENCIES

A. Airway obstruction
  1. Etiology
    a) Secretions
      Most common is vomitus obstructing the glottis.
    b) Foreign body
      Most common is seed hull
    c) Parasitic
      (1) *Syngamus trachea*
      (2) Trichomoniasis
    d) Fungal
      Aspergillus colonies in trachea and syrinx
    e) Viral
      Exudative plugs from avian pox
    f) Thyroid hyperplasia
  2. Clinical signs
    a) Open-mouth breathing and gaping
    b) Inspiratory and expiratory wheeze
    c) Rhythmic tail bob
    d) Cyanosis
    e) Coughing
  3. Diagnosis
    a) Obstruction of glottis
      History and evidence of vomitus in pharyngeal area and glottis
    b) Foreign body
      (1) Evidence of foreign body in trachea on bronchoscopic examination
      (2) Often found only at necropsy
    c) Parasitic obstruction
      (1) *Syngamus trachea*
        i) Can sometimes see adult worms at-

tached to tracheal wall through glottis
- ii) Fecal flotation
- (2) Trichomoniasis
  - i) Fresh wet mount smear of tracheal exudative plaque
  - ii) Often found at necropsy

d) Fungal obstruction
- (1) Most often found at necropsy
- (2) Positive agar gel diffusion

e) Viral obstruction
- (1) Exudative plugs of trachea usually accompanied by other evidence of pox, including oral and ocular lesions
- (2) Postmortem confirmation with viral isolation

f) Thyroid hyperplasia
- (1) Occasional radiographic confirmation of thyroid enlargement

  Nodular densities lateral to the trachea and anterior to the syrinx
- (2) Lack of immediate response to corticosteroids

  Clinically is similar to asthma but asthma responds to corticosteroid therapy.
- (3) Long-term response to iodine therapy

4. Treatment

a) General
- (1) Attempt to remove obstructing agent
- (2) Oxygen

b) Specific
- (1) Obstruction of glottis

  Irrigation of pharyngeal area to clear obstructive material
- (2) Parasitic
  - i) *Syngamus trachea*

(*A*) Mechanical removal where applicable
(*B*) Levamisole IM (see Table 14-5)
ii) Trichomoniasis
Dimetridazole (see Table 14-5)
(3) Fungal—Aspergillosis
i) By the time lesions are evident, response to treatment is unlikely.
ii) Amphotericin B (see Table 14-6)
(*A*) Injectable
(*B*) Intratracheal
(*C*) Nebulization
(4) Viral—pox
i) Attempt to aspirate exudate
ii) Supportive therapy
(5) Thyroid hyperplasia
Iodine supplementation in drinking water (see Table 14-1)

B. Lung lesions and air sacculitis
1. Etiology
a) Bacterial lung abscess
b) Aspergillosis
c) Parasitic
(1) *Sternastoma tracheacolum* (trachea or air sac mite)
(2) *Cytodites nudus*
d) Inhalation pneumonia
(1) Aspiration of vomitus
(2) Aspiration of drugs
e) Idiopathic hemorrhage
2. Clinical signs
a) Dyspnea, cyanosis
b) Open-mouth breathing
c) Tail bob
d) Exaggerated thoracic movement
e) Bleeding from mouth and nares

3. Diagnosis

   NOTE: In any bird showing a significant degree of respiratory embarrassment, unless immediate drug therapy is deemed necessary as a life saving procedure, it is propitious to place the bird in O_2 prior to examination. This will increase the patient's ability to withstand the stress of examination and can decrease the chance of respiratory arrest.

   a) Auscultation
      (1) Abnormal air sac sounds can be of a moist type or a friction-like sound.
      (2) Sounds are dull or absent in consolidated areas.
   b) Thoracic radiography
   c) Laparoscopy
      (1) Visual confirmation
      (2) Culture and sensitivity
   d) Bacterial C & S
   e) Positive Aspergillus titer and culture
   f) Fecal flotation for mite identification
   g) Postmortem examination
   h) Idiopathic hemorrhage diagnosed on basis of hemorrhage with no other diagnostic criteria—confirmed at necropsy.

4. Treatment
   a) General

      Oxygen therapy when dyspnea is evident
   b) Specific
      (1) Bacterial and inflammatory lesions:

          Antibiotics
          i) Systemic
          ii) Inhalation
      (2) Aspergillus:

          Amphotericin B (see Table 14-6)
          i) Intratracheal
          ii) Inhalation
          iii) Systemic

(3) Parasitic:
Vapona strip inhalation (see Table 14-5)
(4) Inhalation pneumonia
i) Antibiotics
ii) Supportive therapy
(5) Idiopathic hemorrhage
i) Maintain in dark quiet environment.
ii) Blood transfusions if needed
5. Prognosis
a) Lung abscess—grave
b) Aspergillosis—grave
c) Parasites—fair
d) Inhalation pneumonia—guarded depending on volume of material inhaled
e) Idiopathic hemorrhage
(1) If bleeding can be stopped and bird is maintained for 24 h with no bleeding, prognosis is fair.
(2) Recurrence is possible.

C. Acute asthma
1. Etiology
Thought to be allergic.
2. Clinical signs
a) Acute onset of respiratory distress of varying degree
b) Characteristic respiratory "click" (sounds like crying)
Occurs in budgerigars, large psittacines, and canaries
c) Open-mouth breathing
d) Wings held away from body
3. Diagnosis
a) Primarily based on immediate response to steroids
b) Differentiate from thyroid hyperplasia
4. Treatment

- a) Intramuscular corticosteroids (see Table 14-1)
  - (1) Response to corticosteroids usually dramatic
  - (2) Occurs within 1–3 h
- b) Oxygen if severe

5. Prognosis

   Good to excellent

D. Subcutaneous emphysema

1. Etiology
   - a) Thought to be leakage of air from air sac system
   - b) Possibility of superinflation of SQ air sac system
   - c) Trauma with penetrating wound through air sac
2. Clinical signs
   - a) Emphysematous air bubble usually in the head and cervical region
   - b) In acute severe cases the SQ emphysema can be generalized.
3. Diagnosis

   Puncture with 21-gauge needle and aspirate air.
4. Treatment
   - a) Incise skin over air bubble avoiding cutaneous vascular pattern and decompress. Leave a sizeable opening. Do not suture. It is essential if incising over the dorsal thoracic inlet to be sure that the incision avoids the crop which is in close approximation to the skin in this area.
   - b) With chronic recurrence, insert gauze seton to release air.
5. Prognosis
   - a) Excellent
   - b) Recurrence is frequent.

E. Ascites

Though not specifically a respiratory problem, the air sac system is compromised since a bird has no diaphragm and ascitic fluid will encroach upon all air sacs up to the lung margin.

1. Etiology
   a) Liver disease
   b) Cysts
      (1) Renal
      (2) Ovarian
   c) Heart disease
   d) Tumors
2. Clinical signs
   a) Abdominal distension
   b) Dyspnea
   c) Open-mouth breathing
3. Diagnosis
   a) Abdominal palpation
   b) Paracentesis of abdomen and analysis of ascitic fluid
      (1) Culture and sensitivity
      (2) Cytology
   c) Radiology
      Typical ground glass appearance of abdomen
   d) Diminished air sac sounds on auscultation
   e) Liver biopsy
4. Treatment
   a) General
      Abdominal paracentesis and removal of as much fluid as possible. Bird usually shows immediate relief.
   b) Specific
      (1) Liver disease
         Systemic antibiotics (see Table 14-3)
      (2) Cardiac origin
         i) Furosemide (See Table 14-1)
         ii) Digitalis
            Oral digitalis of questionable value

F. Respiratory arrest
 1. Etiology
  a) Anesthetic apnea
   (1) Direct result of anesthetic agent
   (2) In small psittacines such as budgerigars, when placed in ventrodorsal recumbency, the tongue falls over the glottis occluding it.
   (3) Occlusion of endotracheal tube from viscid respiratory secretions associated with the preanesthetic administration of atropine
  b) Handling and shock
   When handling severely stressed or debilitated birds, respiratory arrest can occur. It is therefore imperative to evaluate the patient prior to examination.
 2. Clinical signs
  Cessation of respiration
 3. Prevention
  a) Anesthetic apnea
   (1) Careful monitoring during anesthetic administration
   (2) Intubation of any bird where feasible
   (3) Maintaining as light a plane of anesthesia as possible and minimizing anesthetic time
   (4) Careful examination of endotracheal tube prior to intubation for patency
  b) Handling and shock
   (1) Administer oxygen prior to handling birds with moderate to severe respiratory distress.
   (2) Minimize handling time with gentle restraint.
   (3) During examination careful observation of bird's postural attitude and reflexes

will give early recognition of stress induced apnea.

4. Treatment
   a) Anesthetic apnea
      (1) Intubated birds
         i) Turn off anesthesia
         ii) Assist in ventilation by gentle compression of rebreathing bag to cause minimal sternal elevation. (Excessive pressure will rupture air sacs.)
         iii) Fifteen to 20 respirations/min
         iv) Doxapram (see Table 14-1)
      (2) Nonintubated birds
         i) Turn off anesthesia
         ii) Maintain O_2 flow
         iii) Artificial respiration by gentle compression over the pectoral muscles with the bird in ventrodorsal recumbency at rate of 15 respirations/min.
         iv) Doxapram (See Table 14-1)
   b) Handling and stress arrest
      (1) At first evidence of reflex change, the bird should be IMMEDIATELY released and placed in O_2.
         i) Loss of grasping reflex
         ii) Cessation of blink reflex
         iii) Loss of body rigidity
      (2) If not responsive or apnea is evident, follow procedure for nonintubated birds (as above).

X. TOXIC EMERGENCIES

A. Lead toxicosis—there are many sources of lead which pet owners are unaware of: stained glass windows and window ornaments, Tiffany lamps, lead-based paint, old sheet rock, lead-weighted plastic pop-up toys, backing of mirrors, curtain and drapery weights, solder, oil paint and paintings, foil from wine and champagne bottles, spent pellets from pellet guns, and fishing sinkers.

1. Clinical signs
   a) Depression
   b) Occasionally regurgitation and diarrhea
   c) Anorexia
   d) Neurologic signs
      (1) Ataxia
      (2) Tremors or seizures
      (3) Head tilt
      (4) Blindness
   e) Acute intravascular hemolysis
2. Diagnosis
   a) Based on history of ingestion or access to lead
   b) Evidence of neurologic signs
   c) Radiographic evidence of radiodense metallic objects in the GI tract
   d) If there is no radiographic confirmation, blood lead levels should be assayed (>20 μg/dl should be considered positive).
   e) Response to chelating agents
3. Treatment
   a) Ca EDTA (see Table 14-1)
   b) 2.5% dextrose in half-strength saline SQ (See Table 14-2)
   c) Hyperalimentation
   d) For seizures, administer Diazepam IM (Table 14-1)

B. Polytetrafluoroethylene (PTFE) becomes a highly toxic gas when subjected to temperatures greater than 280°C. Polytetrafluoroethylene is a synthetic polymer used to coat "nonstick" cooking utensils (Teflon).

1. Clinical signs
   a) Acute respiratory distress

b) Ataxia
c) Death shortly after onset of above symptoms
2. Diagnosis is based on history of burning a PTFE-coated pot or pan.
3. Treatment
a) There is rarely enough time or any effective treatment regimen
b) Discontinue burning the pot.
c) Immediate ventilation and aeration of room

C. Smoke inhalation is rapidly fatal, particularly in small species.
1. Clinical signs
a) Dyspnea
b) Ataxia
c) Coughing
d) Ocular discharge and squinting
2. Treatment
a) Place in O_2 until dyspnea improves
b) Systemic corticosteroids (see Table 14-1)
c) Systemic antibiotics (see Table 14-3)
d) Topical antibiotic ophthalmic ointment

D. Chlorinated hydrocarbons are found in pesticides and can be sprayed on a pet bird by an uninformed pet owner.
1. Clinical signs
a) Ataxia and incoordination
b) Regurgitation
c) Seizures
2. Diagnosis is based on history and clinical signs.
3. Treatment
a) Wash bird.
b) 5% D/W SQ or IV (see Tables 14-2, 14-7).
c) 5% calcium gluconate SQ or IV (see Table 14-1)
d) Diazepam IM if seizuring (see Table 14-1)

E. Organophosphates are found in many common household insecticides, flea collars, and pest strips.

1. Clinical signs
    a) Bradycardia
    b) Paralysis
    c) Rarely seizures
2. Diagnosis based on history
3. Treatment
    a) Pralidoxine iodine used in raptors (see Table 14-1)
    b) Atropine sulfate—efficacy questionable
    c) Supportive therapy

F. Ethyl alcohol intoxication is caused by beer, wine, and mixed alcoholic beverages, particularly when mixed with fruit punch.
1. Clinical signs
    a) Anorexia
    b) Lethargy
    c) Ataxia
    d) Occasionally regurgitation
    e) Coma and death
2. Treatment consists of support with fluids and gavage feeding.

G. Warfarin
1. Etiology
    Impregnated seeds used for rodent control
2. Clinical signs
    a) Bloody droppings
    b) Weakness
    c) Regurgitation
    d) Low PCV
3. Diagnosis
    Based on history
4. Treatment
    a) Vitamin K IM (see Table 14-1)
    b) Supportive therapy
        (1) Fluids
        (2) Hyperalimentation
        (3) Blood transfusions when indicated

H. Oiled bird emergencies

1. Etiology
   a) Wildlife land in waters contaminated by industrial oil spill (toxic oils)
   b) Pet birds become oiled during free flight around cooking oils (nontoxic oils) or motor oil (toxic oils).
2. Clinical signs
   a) Varying degrees of oiling of feathers
   b) Loss of flotation leading to drowning
   c) Loss of insulation leading to hypothermia in cold months
   d) Conjunctivitis
   e) Enteritis
   f) Toxicity from skin and GI absorption
      (1) Central nervous system disturbances
      (2) Depression
3. Diagnosis
   a) Physical examination

      Visual examination is not always reliable. If there is any question about oiling, test for waterproofing by spraying with water to be sure water beads up.
   b) Full extent of toxicity of oil is shown on postmortem and histopathology.
4. Treatment
   a) Rehydrate (SQ and oral fluids) (see Table 14-2).
      (1) Oral fluid supplementation of 2.5% dextrose in half-strength saline
      (2) Add Pepto Bismol to tubing solution at first to coat GI track.
   b) Flush eyes with Dacriose.
   c) Clean nares and mouth of oil.
   d) Warm to normal temperature for species with heat lamps (101–106°F). There is wide species variation!
   e) Bathe in warm (103°F) soapy (3–10%) water
      (1) Stroke feathers in proper direction *only*

(2) Use *only* recommended soap solutions—Dawn dishwashing soap is considered safe.

f) Rinse *thoroughly* until water beads on back and abdominal feathers.

g) Dry under heat lamps or ambient warm air.

h) Provide housing in unstressful conditions

(1) Provide clean water for swimming to encourage preening essential to restore waterproofing (Usually in 1–5 days).

(2) Provide food *appropriate* for species and in a manner *appropriate* for species (i.e., feed in deep water for diving ducks).

i) Check to be sure is free of disease before releasing

j) When self-feeding and waterproofing has returned, and outdoor conditions are favorable, release to a suitable habitat.

BIBLIOGRAPHY

Altman RB: Avian medicine. Syllabi CVMA 13:417, 1982

Altman RB: Heterologous blood transfusions in avian species. Proc American Association of Zoo Veterinarians, New Orleans, 1982

Altman RB: Heterologous blood transfusions in avian species. Proc AAV: 28, 1983

Arnall L, Keymer IF: Bird Diseases. TFH Publishing, Neptune City, NJ, 1975

Clubb S: The use of antibiotics in birds. Proc AAV San Diego, Calif. 110, 1982

Clubb S: The Bristol Veterinary Handbook of Antimicrobial Therapy. Veterinary Learning Systems, Syracuse, NY, 1982

Doyle JR: Introduction to microsurgery. Proc Association of Avian Veterinarians 50:13, 1983

Fowler M: Diseases of the integument. Syll CVMA: 440, 1982

Frink L: Tri State Bird Rescue and Research, Wilmington, DE, personal communication, 1984

Galvin C: Avian Drugs and Dosages. Wildlife Rehabilitation Council, Walnut Creek, CA, 1976

Galvin C: Acute Hemorrhagic Syndrome of Birds. p. 617. In Kirk RW (ed): Current Veterinary Therapy. Vol. 8. WB Saunders, Philadelphia, 1983

Karpinski L, Clubb S: Clinical aspects of ophthalmology in caged birds. Proc AAV: 216, 1983

Langenberg J: Parasitology. Mid Atlantic States Avian Medicine Seminar, Atlantic City, NJ, April, 1983

McCluggage D: Emergency fluid therapy. AAV Newsletter IME no. 325, 4(1):23, 1983

McDonald SE: Lead toxicosis in psittacine birds. Proc AAV: 77, 1983

Panigraphy B, Harmon BG, Grumbles LC: Hemorrhagic disease in canaries (*Serinus canarius*) (in press)

Pasco JW: Avian therapeutic agents. Proc AAV: 272, 1983

Pasco JW, Hickman G, Levine B: Emergency care and protocol for pet birds: the first 24 hours. Proc AAV: 231, 1983

Rosskopf WJ, Woerpel RW, Monohan-Brenna M: Seizures induced by hypocalcemia in an African Grey parrot associated with an adrenalopathy and parathyroid hyperplasia. Proc AAV: 267, 1983

Small E, Burke T: Diseases of the organs of special sense p. 491. In Petrak M. (ed): Diseases of Cage and Aviary Birds. 2nd Ed. Lea & Febiger, Philadelphia, 1982

Soifer F: AAV Newsletter, IME no. 164, 3(1):12, 1982

Wells RE: Fatal toxicosis in pet birds caused by an overheated cooking pan lined with polytetrafluoroethylene. J Am Vet Med Assoc 182(11):248, 1983

15

Emergency Treatment of Poisonings

Gregory F. Grauer

The symptoms of intoxications in small animals are often severe and rapid in onset. These circumstances are usually extremely distressing to the owner as well. A preplanned course of action and ready availability of equipment and drugs is essential. This chapter discusses the source, action, clinical signs, diagnosis, and treatment of the more frequently encountered intoxications in small animal medicine. An attempt is made to list clinical signs and treatment objectives in chronological order. A general protocol for emergency treatment of poisonings as well as a list of equipment and drugs for an "antitoxin crash cart" are outlined in Tables 15-1 and 15-2. For further information regarding toxins not specifically addressed, the reader is encouraged to contact the National Animal Poison Control Center [(217) 333-3611].

RODENTICIDES

I. Strychnine
  A. Source
    1. Alkaloid used for rat, mole, gopher, and coyote poison
    2. Sweet-tasting pellets or coating on rodent food, usually dyed purple, red, or green
    3. Toxic dose
      a) Dogs 0.75 mg/kg
      b) Cats 2.0 mg/kg
  B. Action

TABLE 15-1. EMERGENCY TREATMENT OF POISONINGS PROTOCOL

1. Preliminary instructions to owner to prevent further exposure to toxicant
    a. Bathe with large volumes of water when skin or eyes exposed.
    b. Induction of emesis—best if within 2 h of ingestion
        i. Contraindications—CNS depression and ingestion of petroleum distillates, acids, alkali, tranquilizers, or other emetics
        ii. Household remedies—syrup of ipecac (1 tbsp), hydrogen peroxide (1 tsp), table salt (1 tsp), mustard (1 tsp), sticking a finger in back of mouth—these are only about 50% effective and may be dangerous.
    c. Owner can allow animal to drink water.
    d. Owner should be instructed to bring vomitus and/or suspected material with the animal for possible analysis.

2. Prevent further absorption of toxicant.
    a. Induction of emesis
        i. Make sure stomach contains food material or liquids before inducing emesis.
        ii. Apomorphine is most effective emetic, however, it may aggrevate CNS depression.
            Dose—0.04 mg/kg IV or 0.08 mg/kg IM, a tablet placed in the conjunctival sac will induce vomiting but can result in moderate to severe conjunctivitis.
        iii. Antagonists to apomorphine
            (*A*) Naloxone 0.04 mg/kg IV
            (*B*) Levallorphan 0.02 mg/kg IV
            (*C*) Nalorphine 0.1 mg/kg IV
    b. Gastric lavage—best if within 2 h of ingestion
        i. Anesthesia with cuffed endotracheal tube in place—tube should extend 2 in. beyond teeth to prevent aspiration.
        ii. Use large-bore stomach tube.
        iii. Premeasure tube from nose xiphoid.
        iv. Lower head slightly below body.
        v. Do not force stomach tube.
        vi. Use 5–10 ml lavage solution/kg body weight for each washing—use low pressure.
        vii. Aspirate with large bulb or 60-ml syringe.
        viii. Repeat 10 times.
    c. Gastrointestinal absorbants
        i. Activated charcoal is best—tablets are easiest to handle
        ii. Slurry—1 g activated charcoal/5 ml water
        iii. Dose: 10 ml slurry/kg body weight
        iv. Allow last lavage to sit 30 min then give a cathartic.
    d. Cathartics
        i. Sodium sulfate is best
        ii. Dose 1 gm/kg orally
    e. Enemas, use warm soapy water—avoid hexachlorophene soaps.

3. Specific antidotes—covered under individual poisonings.

TABLE 15-1. EMERGENCY TREATMENT OF POISONINGS PROTOCOL (*Continued*)

4. Hasten elimination of absorbed toxicant.
   a. Maintain renal function and urine output.
      i. Fluid therapy
      ii. Diuretics—be sure animal is well hydrated first
         (*A*) Mannitol 2 mg/kg/h IV
         (*B*) Furosemide 4 mg/kg IV
   b. Ion trapping—ionized compounds traverse cell membranes less readily than do nonionized compounds hence ionized compounds are poorly reabsorbed by renal tubules.
      i. Alkaline urine facilitates ionization of acid compounds, e.g., aspirin, barbiturates
         Sodium bicarbonate 5 mEq/kg/h IV
      ii. Acidic urine tends to ionize basic compounds, e.g., amphetamines, strychnine
         Ammonium chloride 200 mg/kg/day in divided doses
   c. Peritoneal dialysis
5. Supportive therapy
   a. Respiratory support
      i. Airway
      ii. Oxygen and artificial respiration if necessary
   b. Cardiovascular support
      i. Treat shock.
      ii. Correct cardiac arrhythmias.
      iii. Correct electrolyte abnormalities.
      iv. Correct acid-base imbalances.
      v. Maintain normal hydration.
   c. Body temperature control
      i. Hypothermia—blankets, heat lamps, circulating water pads
      ii. Hyperthermia—fans, cold water baths
   d. Central nervous system
      i. Depression—O_2 and respiratory support is best
      ii. Hyperactivity and/or seizures
         (*A*) Diazepam 2.5–20 mg IV as needed
         (*B*) Phenobarbital 2–4 mg/kg IV
         (*C*) Pentobarbital to effect IV
         (*D*) Seizures may cause cerebral edema and therapy with mannitol and/or dexamethasone may be appropriate.
   e. Control of pain—meperidine HCl
      i. Dogs 5–10 mg/kg IM
      ii. Cats 1–2 mg/kg IM

1. Interferes with postsynaptic neuronal inhibition in spinal cord and medulla
2. Antagonizes glycine in spinal cord and medulla where glycine is an inhibitory transmitter
3. Allows spinal reflex activity to proceed unchecked

TABLE 15-2. ANTITOXIN CRASH CHART

Equipment list

1. Endotracheal tubes—several sizes
2. Laryngoscope, with light
3. Oxygen source
4. Mechanical respirator or respirator (AMBU) bag
5. Gauze and tape
6. Intravenous catheters
7. Needles
8. Syringes
9. Fluid administration sets and IV extension tubing
10. Thermometer
11. Large funnel or pump for stomach tube
12. Stomach tubes—several sizes
13. Aspirator bulb
14. Enema bag and hose
15. Urinary catheters—several sizes
16. Small sterile surgery kit for venostomy or tracheostomy
17. Mild soap or detergent
18. Pen light
19. Blanket, heat lamps, circulating water heating pad
20. Clean specimen vials

Drug List

1. Acetylcystine (Mucomyst)
2. Acetylpromazine maleate (Acepromazine)
3. Activated charcoal
4. Ammonium chloride
5. Amphetamine sulfate (Benzedrine)
6. Apomorphine
7. Ascorbic acid (Vitamin C)
8. Atropine sulfate
9. Barbiturates, phenobarbitol, pentobarbitol (Nembutal)
10. Calcium EDTA (Versenate)
11. Calcium gluconate 10%
12. 5% Dextrose/Water
13. Dimercaprol (BAL)

TABLE 15-2. ANTITOXIN CRASH CHART (*Continued*)

14. Diphenylthiocarbazone (Dithizone)
15. Diazepam (Valium)
16. 20% ethanol
17. Ferric cyanoferrate (Prussian blue)
18. Furosemide (Lasix)
19. Glyceryl guiaicolate (Geocolate)
20. Glyceryl monoacetate
21. Kaolin (Kaopectate)
22. Lactated ringers solution
23. Levallorphan (Lorfan)
24. Lidocaine (Xylocaine)
25. Lime water
26. 20% mannitol
27. 10% methocarbamol (Robaxin)
28. Meperidine HCl (Demerol)
29. Nalorphine HCl (Nalline)
30. Naloxone HCl (Narcan)
31. Nicotinamide (Nictinic acid, Niacin)
32. Normal saline
33. *d*-Penicillamine (Cuprimine)
34. Phenylephrine (Neosynephrine)
35. Phenytoin (Dilantin)
36. Potassium chloride, oral (Kay Ciel) and IV
37. Potassium permangante (1:10,000)
38. Pralidoxime chloride (2PAM, Protopam)
39. Propranolol (Inderal)
40. Pyridoxine HCl (Vitamin B_6)
41. Sodium bicarbonate, oral and IV
42. Sodium sulfate (Glauber's salt)
43. 10% sodium thiosulfate
44. Thiamine (Vitamin B_1)
45. Vitamin K_1 (Aqua-mephyton)
46. Whole, fresh blood (less than 2 weeks old)
47. Xylaxine (Rompum)

C. Clinical signs
   1. Appear within 10 minutes to 2 h postingestion
   2. Early—apprehension, nervousness, stiffness
   3. Rigid abdominal and cervical musculature
   4. Violent tetanic seizures appear spontaneously or secondary to stimuli—bright light, sound, touch
   5. All striated muscle affected but more powerful extensors predominate giving rigid, symmetric "saw horse" stance
   6. Tetanic spasms become more frequent and powerful.
      a) Legs and body are stiff
      b) Ears are erect
      c) Lips are pulled back over teeth (risus sardonicus)
      d) Pupils dilate
      e) Breathing stops
   7. Death is due to exhaustion and/or hypoxia.
   8. Postmortem
      a) No gross or microscopic lesions
      b) Stomach is usually full of undigested food or bait.

D. Diagnosis
   1. Based on history of ingestion or exposure, characteristic clinical signs, absence of lesions—often large-breed, male dogs
   2. Hyperesthetic response to sharp handclap can be diagnostic aid.
   3. Chemical analysis of stomach contents
   4. Caution—analysis of liver from dogs treated with pentobarbital may give false-positive results.
   5. Differential diagnosis—hypocalcemia, chlorinated hydrocarbons, lead, zinc phosphide, metaldehyde, Compound 1080, tetanus

E. Treatment
   1. Prevent absorption
      a) Induce vomiting if animal is not hyperesthetic or convulsive.

b) Gastric lavage with 1–2% tannic acid or 1:2,000 potassium permanganate, followed by activated charcoal and sodium sulfate

2. Maintain relaxation and prevent hypoxia.
   a) Pentobarbital IV to effect
   b) Endotracheal tube, O_2, and artificial respiration for respiratory failure
   c) Inhalation anesthesia, or
   d) Diazepam 2.5–20 mg IV as needed, or
   e) Glyceryl guaiacolate 110 mg/kg IV as needed (c–e used to prevent exposure to barbiturates for long periods and possible respiratory depression)
   f) Caution—morphine is contraindicated because of its spinal cord stimulant and respiratory depressant properties.
3. Hasten elimination of absorbed toxicant.
   a) Diuresis
   b) Urinary acidification with 200 mg/kg/day NH_4Cl PO in divided doses. Do not administer NH_4Cl until diuresis is established.
   c) Elimination usually complete by 24–48 h

II. Sodium fluoroacetate—Compound 1080

A. Source
1. Available only to licensed exterminators
2. Usually used in commercial or industrial settings—grain elevators, mills, railroad yards, shipyards, sewers
3. Usually mixed with a black dye and added to bread, bran, carrots, or cereal—the compound itself is colorless, odorless, and tasteless.
4. Secondary intoxications are possible if pets eat rodents or birds killed by Compound 1080.
5. Toxic dose for dogs 0.05–0.10 mg/kg

B. Action
1. Fluoroacetate replaces acetyl CoA which combines with oxaloacetic acid in the citric acid cycle to form fluorocitric acid.

2. Fluorocitric acid blocks the citric acid cycle by inhibiting the enzyme aconitase.
3. Citric acid builds up and cellular energy production and respiration is blocked affecting the heart and CNS predominantly.

C. Clinical signs
1. Latent period of $\frac{1}{2}$–2 h
2. Very acute syndrome with violent signs which progress rapidly
3. Dogs
   a) Initial apprehension, hyperirritability, and vomiting
   b) Repeated urination, defecation, and vomiting—tenesmus continues after bowel and bladder are empty.
   c) Dyspnea, frothing at nostrils and mouth
   d) Running fits with abnormal barking and howling
   e) Cyanosis
   f) Intermittent tonic-clonic seizures with paddling
   g) Collapse from exhaustion between running fits or seizures with no response to stimuli
   h) Cycle repeats itself with duration becoming shorter.
   i) Death in 2–12 h due to respiratory failure
   j) Rigor mortis develops rapidly with limbs rigidly extended.
4. Cats—similar to signs in dogs without the marked activity
   a) Cardiac arrhythmias
   b) Hyperesthesia
   c) Abnormal vocalization

D. Diagnosis
1. Usually based on history and characteristic clinical signs—frenzied running and yelping fits, tenesmus, and lack of response to stimuli

2. Hyperglycemia is often present due to poor utilization of glucose.
3. Analysis of suspected bait or vomitus
4. Differential diagnosis—strychnine, chlorinated hydrocarbon, organophosphates, lead, hypocalcemia, garbage intoxication

E. Treatment
1. Prevent absorption—induce emesis and/or gastric lavage with milk or lime water.
2. Specific antidotes—glyceryl monoacetate (monacetin) 0.55 g/kg IM or 8 ml/kg 50% ethanol and 8 ml/kg 5% acetic acid orally may help block the acetate to citrate synthesis.
3. Supportive care
    a) Control seizures—short-acting barbiturates—try to avoid complete anesthesia and respiratory depression.
    b) Oxygen and artificial respiration for respiratory failure
    c) Monitor ECG for arrhythmias.

III. Coumarins and related compounds

A. Source
1. Warfarin—D-Con; brodifacoum—Talon
2. Indandione products
    a) Pindone—Pival
    b) Diphacinone—Diphacin
3. Most frequently used class of rodenticide—usually corn or other grain baits
4. Some products also incorporate sulfonamides
5. Single toxic dose
    a) 5–50 mg/kg warfarin for dogs and cats
    b) 3 and 15 mg/kg indandione for dogs and cats, respectively
6. Cumulative toxic dose
    a) 1–5 mg/kg warfarin for 5–15 days for dogs
    b) 1 mg/kg warfarin for 7 days for cats

B. Action

1. Coumarins inhibit activation of vitamin K which is necessary for hepatic synthesis of coagulation factors II, VII, IX, and X.
2. Sulfonamides can inhibit synthesis of vitamin K by intestinal bacteria.

C. Clinical signs
   1. Hemorrhage—clinical signs depend on amount and source of hemorrhage
   2. Latent period of 2–5 days before coagulation defects occur
   3. Acute onset—animals may be found dead especially with brain, pericardial, or intrathoracic hemorrhage.
   4. Subacute onset
      a) Anemia, weakness
      b) External hemorrhage—epistaxis, hematemesis, hematuria, melena, hematachezia
      c) Internal hemorrhage
         (1) Dyspnea with thoracic and or abdominal hemorrhage
         (2) Neurologic signs with brain and/or spinal cord hemorrhage
         (3) Lameness with hemarthrosis
         (4) Subcutaneous hematomas and ecchymoses secondary to minor trauma or handling

D. Diagnosis
   1. Hemostasis profile
      a) Prolonged one-stage prothrombin time (OSPT) occurs first inasmuch as factor VII has shortest $T_{\frac{1}{2}}$ (6.2 h) of affected factors.
      b) Prolonged APTT (early in intoxication may be normal)
      c) Prolonged activated clotting (early in intoxication may be normal)
      d) Platelet count, fibrinogen, and FSP are usually normal.
      e) Caution—-use peripheral vein not jugular for

venapuncture since it is easier to control cephalic and saphenous bleeding than jugular bleeding.

2. Plasma or liver warfarin levels
3. Response to vitamin K
4. Differential diagnosis for vitamin K responsive coagulopathies—chronic cholestasis, cirrhosis, malabsorption syndromes, gut sterilization with antibiotics

E. Treatment
1. Prevent absorption—induce vomiting if early after ingestion.
2. Acute cases
   a) Handle animal gently to prevent bruising, avoid IM injections.
   b) Fresh whole blood transfusion 10–20 ml/kg IV, give first half rapidly and second half at 20 drops/min.
   c) Oxygen if hypoxic
   d) If dyspneic consider radiographs and thoracentesis for intrathoracic hemorrhage.
   e) Vitamin K (see below)
3. Subacute cases
   a) Vitamin K_1 IV *slowly* in 10 ml 5% D/W
      (1) Dogs 10 mg q12h
      (2) Cats 2–5 mg q12h

      Repeat until coagulation times are normal.
   b) Caution—anaphylactoid reactions have been reported secondary to IV vitamin K.
   c) Follow with daily oral vitamin K_1 2.5–5.0 mg/kg divided TID for 4–6 days—some long-acting coumarins may require treatment for up to 30 days (Talon and Diphacin).
   d) Caution—vitamin K_3 is much less effective than vitamin K_1.
4. Hasten elimination of absorbed toxicant
   a) Sedation or light anesthesia with barbiturates may aid gentle handling of animals and also

increase hepatic biotransformation of warfarin.

b) Warfarin is highly protein bound (inactive) in plasma; drugs that displace warfarin from albumin (phenylbutazone, aspirin, sulfonamides, corticosteroids) may aggravate hypoprothrombinemia as well as hasten elimination.

c) Elimination of warfarin is usually complete within 48–96 h, however, diphacinone may have a half-life of 15–20 days.

IV. Thallium

A. Source

1. U.S. Department of Agriculture (USDA) halted manufacture of thallium pesticides in 1972; still used in Europe and other countries.
2. Thallium acetate and sulfate used to be sold in combination with corn, oats, and peanuts as rodenticides.
3. Preparations were also used for roaches, waterbugs, ants, and silverfish.
4. LD_{50} for most species is 10–15 mg/kg; 20–25 mg/kg is fatal in almost all cases.

B. Action

1. Thallium interacts with structural and enzymatic proteins at the cellular level combining with mitochondrial sulphydryl enzymes and hence interferes with oxidative phosphorylation.
2. Thallium also exchanges for potassium in excitable tissues such as muscle and nerve.

C. Clinical signs

1. Acute form
   a) Signs appear 1–4 days postingestion
   b) Severe gastroenteritis—hematemesis, hemorrhagic diarrhea, abdominal pain, anorexia—if animal survives there is an apparent spontaneous recovery for 1–2 days then relapse.
   c) Dyspnea, cough, nasal discharge—thallium

destroys respiratory epithelial cilia—secondary pneumonia may develop.

d) Nervous system—trembling, ataxia, paralysis, convulsions, and coma are possible.

e) Brick-red mucous membranes 2–4 days postingestion

2. Subacute form
   a) Three to 7 days postingestion
   b) Gastrointestinal and nervous signs are similar to acute phase but milder.
   c) Brick-red mucous membranes
   d) Renal damage—proteinuria, glycosuria with casts, RBC, WBC, and epithelial cells in urine sediment
   e) Skin—erythema and pustule formation first on ears and nose then inguinal and axillary regions, then interdigital areas which progresses to serum oozing and crust formation—spontaneous hair loss begins about seventh day.
   f) Mucopurulent conjunctivitis
3. Chronic form
   a) Seven to 10 days postingestion
   b) Mild gastrointestinal and nervous involvement
   c) Skin—pronounced hair loss with drying and scaling of skin

D. Diagnosis
   1. History and clinical signs—gastrointestinal disturbance prior to dyspnea and brick-red mucous membranes followed by skin changes
   2. Thallium detection in urine
   3. Differential diagnosis—distemper, heavy metal intoxication, gastrointestinal and bullous skin diseases

E. Treatment
   1. Prevent absorption early after ingestion
   2. Specific antidotes
      a) Diphenylthiocarbazone (Dithizone) chelates and detoxifies thallium—dose for dogs 50–70

mg/kg TID orally for a period up to 5 days—best if initiated within 36 h of ingestion
            (1) Cataracts and blindness have been reported in dogs treated with Dithizone.
            (2) Not currently recommended for cats
        b) Potassium chloride supplementation may be necessary to maintain plasma potassium levels as chelated thallium is displaced from cells and replaced by potassium—2–6 g KCl orally/day or 20–30 mEq/L IV fluids; be sure adequate renal function exists.
    3. Hasten elimination—ferric-cyanoferrate (Prussian blue) interferes with enterohepatic circulation of thallium, increasing fecal excretion—100 mg/kg TID orally—may be more effective than Dithizone after initial 24 h of treatment.
    4. Supportive care

V. Vacor (N-3-pyridylmethyl N′-p-nitrophenyl urea)
  A. Source
    1. 2% bait and 10% tracking powder; over the counter, single-dose, quick-kill rodenticide
    2. Taken off the market in 1979
    3. Toxic dose
        a) Dog 0.5–1.0 g/kg
        b) Cat 62–200 mg/kg
  B. Action
    1. Interferes with nicotinamide metabolism
    2. Has caused diabetes mellitus in humans by destroying pancreatic β islet cells
  C. Clinical signs
    1. Initial—vomiting and abdominal pain
    2. Muscular trembling and weakness
    3. Collapse 12–24 h postingestion
    4. Coma, respiratory and cardiovascular failure, and death
  D. Diagnosis
    1. Known exposure

2. Laboratory analysis probably not available
3. Differential diagnosis—hypocalcemia, garbage intoxication

E. Treatment
1. Cleansing of gastrointestinal tract if early after ingestion
2. Specific antidotes have not been very effective in dogs and cats—niacinamide (nicotinamide) 500–1,000 mg IM, then 200–300 mg IM q4h for 48 h, then 200 mg SID orally for 2 weeks in animals that recover.
3. Supportive care
4. Caution owners of surviving animals about possibility of diabetes mellitus—frequent urinalyses should be checked for glycosuria.

VI. ANTU (alpha-naphthyl thiourea)

A. Source
1. White or blue-grey bitter-tasting powder which is not water soluble
2. Usually prepared in bread or sausage baits
3. Limited usage as rodenticide due to development of more effective compounds
4. Toxic dose
   a) Dogs 10–40 mg/kg—younger dogs are more resistant
   b) Cats 75–100 mg/kg

B. Action
1. Increases permeability of pulmonary capillaries, causing edema
2. Strong emetic, however, vomiting is less likely to occur if there is food in stomach.

C. Clinical signs
1. Initial gastric irritation—vomiting, salivation
2. Restlessness with increased heart and respiratory rate
3. Depression, weakness, coughing, and cyanosis
4. Dogs often sit with forelegs extended and elbows

rotated outward, head and neck are extended in effort to reduce dyspnea.

5. Coma and death usually by 12 h due to hypoxia
6. Survival beyond 12 h warrants more favorable prognosis.

D. Diagnosis
   1. History and characteristic clinical signs
   2. Post mortem—pulmonary edema, pericardial and pleural effusion, hyperemia of trachea, gastrointestinal tract, and kidneys
   3. Laboratory analysis for ANTU usually not helpful
   4. Differential diagnosis—other causes of pulmonary edema; organophosphates may cause similar pulmonary lesions.

E. Treatment
   1. Cleansing of gastrointestinal tract—caution: apomorphine may cause respiratory depression.
   2. Supportive care
      a) No specific antidotes available.
      b) Oxygen—surfactant aerosols (silicone), nebulization with 30–50% ethanol to reduce foaming
      c) Corticosteroids
      d) Postural drainage
      e) Thoracentesis
      f) Diuretics
      g) Antibiotics

VII. Zinc phosphide

A. Source
   1. Grey-black powder, water-insoluble, incorporated into bread, sugar, and grain baits at 2–5%
   2. The compound has a faint acetylene or rotten fish odor.
   3. Toxic dose for most animals is 20–40 mg/kg.

B. Action
   1. Phosphine gas is released from zinc phosphide in the presence of acid pH, leading to asphyxia.

2. Intact phosphide may also cause liver and kidney damage.

C. Clinical signs
   1. Onset of signs is usually within 15 min to 4 h.
   2. Anorexia and lethargy followed by dyspnea
   3. Vomiting—often dark blood with abdominal pain
   4. Ataxia and running and yelping fits have been observed.
   5. Terminal gasping and struggling—hyperesthesia and convulsions may also occur.
   6. Death is due to hypoxia

D. Diagnosis
   1. Phosphine or acetylene odor to breath or vomitus
   2. Analysis of stomach contents
   3. Differential diagnosis—strychnine, Compound 1080

E. Treatment
   1. Prevention of absorption
      a) Gastrointestinal cleansing
      b) Oral 5% sodium bicarbonate to increase gastric pH
   2. No specific antidotes
   3. Supportive care

PESTICIDES

I. Metaldehyde
   A. Source
      1. Snail, slug, and rat poison especially common in the Southern lowlands, Pacific coastal areas, and Hawaiian Islands
      2. Palatable liquid, powder, or pelleted bait used around vegetable and ornamental gardens
      3. Older preparations also contained arsenic compounds
      4. Toxic dose for dogs is 100–1,000 mg/kg

B. Action
   1. Thought to be due to acetaldehyde which is released by hydrolysis of metaldehyde in the acidic stomach.
   2. Some effects may be due to metaldehyde itself.
   3. Severe metabolic acidosis also plays a role.

C. Clinical signs
   1. Appear within 1–4 hours
   2. Anxiety, hyperesthesia, and ataxia
   3. Muscle fasciculations and tremors—not responsive to external stimuli
   4. Nystagmus in cats
   5. Severe hyperthermia, as high as 108°F (42°C)
   6. Severe metabolic acidosis
   7. Loss of consciousness, decreased respiration, cyanosis
   8. Death due to respiratory failure

D. Diagnosis
   1. Geographic region and compatible clinical signs
   2. Bait may be found in vomitus or lavage material
   3. Acetaldehyde odor on breath or from stomach contents
   4. Laboratory analysis of stomach contents
   5. Differential diagnosis—strychnine, Compound 1080, chlorinated hydrocarbons, organophosphates

E. Treatment
   1. Prevent absorption
      a) Induce vomiting if animal is conscious
      b) Gastric lavage—milk or lime water decreases absorption.
   2. Maintain relaxation and prevent hypoxia
      a) Diazepam 2.5–20 mg IV as needed
      b) Muscle relaxants
         (1) Methocarbamol 150 mg/kg IV
         (2) Xylazine 1.1 mg/kg IV
      c) Pentobarbitol IV to effect may be necessary.
      d) Endotracheal intubation, O_2, and artificial respiration for respiratory failure
   3. Supportive care

II. Organophosphates and carbamates
   A. Source
      1. Veterinary products—dips, sprays, powders, flea collars, and oral products
         a) Organophosphates (OP)
            (1) Dichlorvos
            (2) Trichlorfon
            (3) Dimethoate
            (4) Ruelene
            (5) Malathion
            (6) Parathion
            (7) Ronnel
            (8) Diazinon
            (9) Chlorpyrifos
            (10) Dyfonate
            (11) Phosmet
            (12) Di-syston
         b) Carbamates
            (1) Carbaryl (Sevin)
            (2) Methomyl (Lannate)
            (3) Propoxur (Baygon)
            (4) Bendiocarb (Ficam)
            (5) Aldicarb (Temik)
            (6) Carbofuran (Furdan)
      2. Numerous agricultural insecticides and home and garden insecticides
      3. Toxic dose is variable depending on the product.
   B. Action
      1. Organophosphates and carbamates inhibit acetylcholinesterase enzymes at the myoneural junction allowing acetylcholine to accumulate at the synapse.
      2. Inhibition of cholinesterase enzymes by OP tend to be irreversible with time whereas inhibition by the carbamates is reversible.
   C. Clinical signs
      1. Signs may appear within minutes to several hours after exposure.

2. Overstimulation of the parasympathetic nervous system and skeletal muscles:
   a) Muscarinic effects
      (1) Salivation
      (2) Lacrimation
      (3) Defecation—watery diarrhea, urination
      (4) Gastrointestinal hypermotility—abdominal pain
      (5) Miosis
      (6) Pallor
      (7) Cyanosis
      (8) Dyspnea
   b) Nicotinic effects

      Twitching of facial and tongue muscles progressing to all musculature followed by paralysis
   c) Central nervous system effects
      (1) Extreme depression
      (2) Tonoclonic seizures
3. Death is due to hypoxia—respiratory muscle paralysis, bronchoconstriction, excessive pulmonary secretions, pulmonary edema, and bradycardia.

D. Diagnosis
1. History of exposure and characteristic clinical signs
2. Analysis of stomach contents
3. Evaluation of cholinesterase activity in whole blood—25% of normal activity suggests excessive exposure.
4. Response to atropine
5. Differential diagnosis—strychnine, Compound 1080, ANTU, chlorinated hydrocarbons, metaldehyde

E. Treatment
1. Prevent further exposure and absorption.
   a) Remove flea collar.
   b) Bathe skin with soapy water if exposure is topical.

c) Induce emesis if ingestion is witnessed.
d) Activated charcoal slurry—lavage of stomach

2. Specific antidotes
   a) Atropine sulfate does not counteract the cholinesterase inhibitor but blocks the effect of accumulated acetylcholine at the synapse.
      (1) Dose 0.2–0.5 mg/kg to effect (mydriasis and reduced salivation) usually $\frac{1}{4}$ dose is given IV and $\frac{3}{4}$ SQ—may need to repeat at 3–6 h for 1–2 days depending upon response
   b) Oximes—pralidoxime chloride (2PAM) acts on the OP-enzyme complex binding the phosphate and thereby releasing the cholinesterase—early treatment before the OP-enzyme has stabilized or "aged." Usually requires only 24–36 h of therapy whereas the stabilized complex may require therapy for several days—dose 20 mg/kg IV BID.

      Caution—some authors indicate 2PAM should not be used in cases of carbamate toxicity since 2PAM may increase the toxicity by developing a more stable carbamate—enzyme complex.
3. Supportive care
   a) Ventilation and oxygen for respiratory failure
   b) Contraindicated drugs
      (1) Morphine
      (2) Succinylcholine
      (3) Phenothiazine tranquilizers

III. Chlorinated hydrocarbons
   A. Source
      1. Veterinary products—powders, sprays, dips
         a) Methoxychlor
         b) Toxaphene
         c) Lindane
         d) Chlordane

2. Agricultural products—insecticides
   a) Diphenyl aliphatics (DDT)
   b) Dieldrin
   c) Aldrin
   d) Endrin
3. Toxic dose is variable depending on product—cats are particularly susceptible.

B. Action
1. Lipid-soluble products absorbed through skin or ingested
2. Diffuse stimulants or depressants of CNS—exact mechanism is unknown (except DDT)
3. DDT decreases nerve membrane action potential threshold.

C. Clinical signs
1. Onset can be within minutes to days of exposure, however, usually within several hours
2. Apprehension, hypersensitivity, exaggerated response to stimuli, vomiting if toxin was ingested
3. Muscle twitching of face and neck that progresses posteriorly to severe fasciculations and tremors
4. Intermittent clonic—tonic seizures with paddling and foaming from the mouth
5. Elevated body temperature
6. These compounds are stored in fat and the clinical course may be protracted.

D. Diagnosis
1. History of exposure and characteristic clinical signs
2. Analysis of stomach contents, brain, or SQ fat
3. Differential diagnosis—strychnine, Compound 1080, metaldehyde, garbage intoxication, lead, organophosphates

E. Treatment
1. Prevent further exposure and absorption.
   a) Bathe with soapy water.
   b) Induction of emesis may initiate seizures.
   c) Gastric lavage with saline and activated charcoal

2. Control seizures.
    a) Specific antidotes do not exist.
    b) Diazepam 2.5–20 mg IV as needed
    c) Barbiturates IV to effect
3. Sedatives for excitability if seizures not present
    a) Diazepam 2.5–20 mg IV as needed
    b) Do not use phenothiazines as they lower seizure threshold.
4. Supportive care—maintain hydration and urine output as the chlorinated hydocarbons are primarily eliminated in the urine.

IV. Arsenic
  A. Source
    1. Inorganic arsenicals—arsenic trioxide, sodium arsenite, sodium arsenate
        a) Insecticides—ant and roach poisons
        b) Herbicides—crabgrass killers
        c) Preservatives on wooden building materials
    2. Organic arsenicals
        a) Sodium caparsolate
        b) Filcide
    3. Toxic dose—1–25 mg/kg of sodium arsenite, arsenic trioxide is one tenth to one third as toxic, 7–14 mg/kg sodium arsenate
  B. Action—arsenicals inhibit the sulfhydryl enzyme systems which are essential for normal cellular respiration and for fat and carbohydrate metabolism.
  C. Clinical signs
    1. Onset is usually within 30 min to several hours of ingestion.
    2. Restlessness, salivation, nausea, and repeated vomiting
    3. Severe abdominal pain with watery, often bloody diarrhea, that may contain mucosal tags
    4. Muscle weakness, trembling, staggering, ataxia
    5. Polyuria and proteinuria often precede anuric renal failure.

6. Severe dehydration, hypovolemic shock
7. Paralysis, coma, and death

D. Diagnosis
1. History of exposure
2. Rapid onset of severe hemorrhagic gastroenteritis
3. Analysis of gastrointestinal contents or urine
4. Analysis of liver and kidney tissue at postmortem
5. Differential diagnosis—thallium, lead, garbage intoxication, hemorrhagic gastroenteritis, viral gastroenteritis

E. Treatment
1. Prevent further absorption if soon after ingestion.
   a) Induction of emesis
   b) Gastric lavage, activated charcoal, and cathartic
2. Specific antidotes
   a) Dimercaprol (BAL) chelates arsenic, hastening elimination —dose: 4mg/kg IM q4–6h. Due to the toxicity of BAL it should not be given continuously for more than 4 days.
   b) Ten percent sodium thiosulfate—wide margin of safety compared to BAL-1 g/day divided into four doses given IV.
3. Supportive care
   a) Fluid, electrolyte, sodium bicarbonate therapy for shock and/or renal failure
   b) Blood transfusions
   c) Digestive tract protectants

BACTERIAL TOXINS

I. Enterotoxemias—garbage- and food-borne intoxication

A. Source
1. Ingestion of food or garbage which contains preformed toxins (*C. perfringens, C. botulinum*, Staphylococcus)
2. Ingestion of food which is grossly contaminated with bacteria (*E. coli*, Salmonella)

B. Action
   1. Most enterotoxins activate intestinal epithelial secretory mechanisms causing loss of fluid and electrolytes—absorptive mechanisms are usually intact.
   2. Some enterotoxins cause morphologic changes in the mucosa.
   3. *C. botulinum* produces a neurotoxin causing generalized neuromuscular blockade due to inhibition of the presynaptic release of acetylcholine—this syndrome is rare in dogs and cats, however, due to relatively high resistance to the toxin.

C. Clinical signs
   1. Signs usually appear within 2–6 h postingestion.
   2. Vomiting, cranial abdominal pain
   3. Diarrhea—may be hemorrhagic
   4. Restlessness, weakness, ataxia
   5. Shock can result from hypovolemia or toxemia.

D. Diagnosis
   1. History of ingestion of garbage or dead animals
   2. Abdominal radiographs may reveal bones or garbage material in the gastrointestinal tract.
   3. Bacterial culture or serologic identification of Staph or Clostridial toxins
   4. Differential diagnosis—viral gastroenteritis, thallium, lead, arsenic, hemorrhagic gastroenteritis (*C. botulinum* differential diagnosis—tick paralysis, polyradiculoneuritis)

E. Treatment
   1. Cleansing of the gastrointestinal tract
      a) Emetics
      b) Gastric lavage
      c) Enemas
   2. Supportive therapy
      a) Treat shock
         (1) Fluid, electrolyte, acid-base therapy
         (2) Corticosteroids
         (3) Parenteral antibiotics
      b) Gastrointestinal protectants

II. Tetanus—*Clostridium tetani*
   A. Source
      1. Gram-positive spore forming anaerobic bacteria
      2. Found in soil and feces of various animals
      3. Germination occurs in necrotic or infected wounds.
      4. Dogs and cats are relatively resistant to the disease.
   B. Action
      1. The bacteria produces a neurotoxin which reaches the CNS via peripheral nerves and the circulation.
      2. The toxin inhibits the activity of inhibitory interneurons (Renshaw cells) in the CNS which function to limit duration, intensity, and distribution of motor neuron discharges.
      3. Persistent increased motor reflex excitability results.
   C. Clinical signs
      1. Incubation period is usually 5–8 days
      2. Localized spasms of facial and cervical musculature
         a) Elevation of upper eyelids
         b) Wrinkling of forehead skin
         c) Retraction of lipfolds (risus sardonicus)
         d) Erect ear carriage
         e) Prolapse of third eyelid
         f) Masticatory and pharyngeal muscle spasms resulting in trismus (lockjaw)
      3. Exaggerated response to external stimuli
      4. Generalized muscle spasticity
         a) Exaggerated clonus in response to tendon motor reflexes
         b) Rigid extension of limbs and tail (sawhorse stance)
      5. Death due to respiratory paralysis
   D. Diagnosis
      1. History of laceration, puncture wound, or recent surgery
      2. Characteristic clinical signs—continuous spasticity versus the alternating periods of spasticity seen with strychnine
      3. Anaerobic and aerobic bacterial cultures
      4. Differential diagnosis—strychnine, canine distem-

per, rabies, meningitis, chlorinated hydrocarbons, metaldehyde, hypocalcemia

E. Treatment
   1. Relaxation and maintenance of respiration—similar to strychnine therapy
   2. Specific therapy
      a) Systemic penicillin G
         Dose 1,000,000 U IV initially, followed by daily IM procaine penicillin G
      b) Tetanus antitoxin will neutralize free or unbound toxin before it reaches the CNS but it is ineffective against toxin already in nerve cells.
         Dose 30,000–100,000 U IV after a test dose of 0.1–0.2 ml SQ and 30 min observation for anaphylactic reaction
   3. Surgical debridement of wound and local installation of 10,000 U of tetanus antitoxin and 1,000,000 U of aqueous penicillin G
   4. Supportive care
      a) Quiet, darkened kennel
      b) Fluid therapy
      c) Alimentation
      d) Corticosteroids may have some antitoxin effects.
      e) Endotracheal intubation, O_2 and artificial respiration for respiratory failure

HOUSEHOLD TOXINS

I. Lead
   A. Source
      1. Lead is ubiquitous in the environment.
         a) Household items
            (1) Linoleum
            (2) Rug padding
            (3) Lead toys
            (4) Drapery weights
            (5) Lead base paints
            (6) Decorative glazes
         b) Construction items

(1) Putty and caulking material
(2) Plumbing materials
(3) Solder
(4) Roofing materials
(5) Lead base paint

c) Automotive items
(1) Batteries
(2) Wheel weights
(3) Antiknock gasoline additives
(4) Crankcase oil
(5) Grease

d) Sporting goods
(1) Fishing sinkers
(2) Pellets and lead shot
(3) Golf balls

2. Toxic dose—10–25 mg/kg is lethal to dogs.

B. Action
1. Lead interferes with thiol-containing enzymes
2. Anemia—usually mild
a) Increased RBC fragility and premature destruction
b) Inhibition of hemoglobin synthesis in bone marrow
3. Central nervous system is affected by decreased blood supply due to damaged capillaries.
4. Peripheral nerves undergo segmental demyelination causing slowed nerve conduction.

C. Clinical signs
1. Usually appear within 3–15 days after ingestion
2. Gastrointestinal
a) Anorexia
b) Abdominal pain, "lead colic"
c) Vomiting and diarrhea
d) Megaesophagus
3. Neurologic
a) Hysteria, aggression, nervousness, barking
b) Ataxia, tremors
c) Clonic-tonic seizures
d) Blindness, deafness, dementia

D. Diagnosis
   1. History
      a) Usually a younger animal, less than 1 year old—except in high-lead environments
      b) Often from inner city environment where buildings and furnishings are old
      c) Recent home remodeling
   2. Clinical signs—gastrointestinal and nervous involvement
   3. Laboratory tests
      a) Basophilic stipling and inappropriate numbers of nucleated RBCs for degree of anemia—look at fresh blood smears as anticoagulants can interfere with visualization of basophilic stipling.
      b) Heparinized blood lead levels—0.35 ppm (35 μg/dl) has been suggested as the upper limit of normal with greater than 0.60 ppm diagnostic of lead toxicity, however, clinical signs have been observed in dogs with blood lead levels of 0.20–0.30 ppm.
      c) Increased levels of amino levulinic acid in urine
      d) Increased free RBC protoporphyrin
   4. Radiography
      a) Diffuse radiopaque material (lead) in the gastrointestinal tract
      b) Lead lines may develop in the metaphyses of long bones in chronically exposed immature dogs.
   5. Differential diagnosis—canine distemper, epilepsy, thallium, strychnine, Compound 1080, chlorinated hydrocarbons, arsenic

E. Treatment
   1. Prevent further absorption from gastrointestinal tract.
      a) Emetics
      b) Gastric lavage and activated charcoal
      c) Enemas
      d) Surgery may be necessary if large lead objects are present in the stomach.

2. Specific antidotes
   a) Ca EDTA (Versenate) chelates lead and hastens excretion. Be sure there is no lead in the gastrointestinal tract before using chelating agents.
      (1) Dose 100 mg/kg divided into four daily doses given SQ in 5% D/W for 5 days. Some dogs may require an additional 5-day treatment after ending the first treatment—especially if blood lead is greater than 1.0 ppm.
      (2) Daily dose should not exceed 2 g and should not be continued for more than 5 consecutive days inasmuch as Ca EDTA may cause renal or gastrointestinal damage.
   b) Penicillamine is an oral chelating agent which may be used as an alternate or adjunct to Ca EDTA.

      Dose 33 mg/kg/day divided QID for 7 days, this can be repeated after 7 days off therapy. If vomiting occurs Dramamine (2–4 mg/kg) PO $\frac{1}{2}$ h prior to the penicillamine is often helpful.
3. Supportive care
   a) Fluid, electrolyte, and acid-base therapy
   b) Control seizures
4. Prevent reexposure and ensure client education.
   a) The source of the lead should be identified if at all possible.
   b) Owners of lead-poisoned animals with young children should be advised to consult with their pediatrician.

II. Ethylene glycol
   A. Source
      1. Automobile antifreeze—antiboil radiator solutions which are 95% ethylene glycol
      2. Color film processing solutions in home darkrooms
      3. Toxicity—minimum lethal dose

a) Dogs 6.6 ml/kg
b) Cats 1.5 ml/kg

B. Action
1. Ethylene glycol is oxidized by liver into toxic metabolites.
2. Glycoaldehyde is CNS toxin.
3. Glycolate and glyoxylate contribute to metabolic acidosis.
4. Pulmonary edema is common—mechanism is unknown.
5. Glycolate and oxalate are severe renal tubular epithelial toxins.

C. Clinical signs
1. Signs vary with stage of intoxication.
2. Stage one occurs 30 min to 12 h postingestion—similar to alcohol intoxication—CNS signs predominate.
   a) Polydipsia, polyuria
   b) Nausea and vomiting
   c) Ataxia
   d) Metabolic acidosis
   e) Coma and death with ingestion of large doses
3. Stage two occurs 12–24 h postingestion—signs in animals are indistinct and animals often appear to be recovering.
4. Stage three occurs 24–48 h postingestion—renal signs predominate.
   a) Severe depression
   b) Oliguria, anuria
   c) Anorexia and vomiting
   d) Death due to acute anuric renal failure and acidosis

D. Diagnosis
1. History of ingestion or exposure
2. Usually a young animal
3. Severe metabolic acidosis
4. High serum osmolality and large anion and osmolal gap

5. Calcium oxalate and/or hippuric acid crystalluria may occur 6 h postingestion.
6. Serum or urine ethylene glycol levels
7. Acute, anuric renal failure. Early after ingestion there is a marked polyuria—azotemia does not occur until 24–48 h postingestion in dogs.
8. Examination of renal biopsy under polarized light for presence of calcium oxalate crystals
9. Differential diagnosis—other causes of acute renal failure, ketoacidotic diabetes mellitus, pancreatitis, gastroenteritis, garbage intoxication

E. Treatment
1. Prevent gastrointestinal absorption if early after ingestion.
   a) Emesis
   b) Gastric lavage and activated charcoal
2. Specific antidotes block metabolism of ethylene glycol by inhibiting liver alcohol dehydrogenase, allowing the intact ethylene glycol to be excreted by the kidneys. Prognosis varies inversely with time between ingestion and initiation of therapy. Therapy to block metabolism beyond 24 h postingestion is of questionable value.
   a) Twenty percent ethanol
      (1) Dose for dogs 5.5 ml/kg IV q4h for five treatments, then q6h for four more treatments.
      (2) Dose for cats 5.0 ml/kg IV q6h for five treatments, then q8h for four more treatments.
   b) Thirty percent 4-methylpyrazole is a potent alcohol dehydrogenase inhibitor which has been used experimentally in dogs with good success. It does not depress the CNS like ethanol.

      Dose used experimentally in dogs—20 mg/kg IV, then 15 mg/kg IV at 24 h, then 5 mg/kg IV at 36 h
   c) Thiamine and pyridoxine do not inhibit alcohol

dehydrogenase but facilitate conversion of glyoxylate to nontoxic metabolites.

Dose 25–50 mg IV per average-sized dog daily during therapy

3. Supportive care
    a) Fluid and electrolyte therapy to maintain urine output
    b) Sodium bicarbonate to combat the metabolic acidosis
        (1) Dosage is best based on plasma bicarbonate levels.
        (2) If blood gases are unavailable—6.0 mEq/kg IV slowly q4–6h
    c) Diuretics may be used to maintain urine output if patient is well hydrated.
    d) Peritoneal dialysis is best therapy if animal presents in renal failure. The nephrosis may be reversible with time.

III. Phenolic compounds

A. Source
1. Wood preservatives—creosote, creosol, pine tar
2. Solvents—toluene, xylene
3. Disinfectants, sanitizers—phenol, cresol, hexachlorophene
4. Herbicides, fungicides, insecticides—dinitroorthocresol
5. Moth balls—naphthalene
6. Toxicity—cats and young dogs are especially susceptible due to a deficiency of metabolizing enzymes.

B. Action
1. Phenolic compounds are rapidly absorbed from the gastrointestinal tract or through intact skin.
2. Phenolic compounds cause necrosis of mucous membranes, cerebral edema, hepatopathies, and nephropathies.
3. Phenolic metabolites inhibit mitochondrial respiration and result in methemoglobin formation.

4. Also hypothesized that phenol causes accumulation of acetylcholine at the myoneural junction

C. Clinical signs
 1. With ingestion of concentrated solutions there is corrosion of oral mucous membranes.
 2. Depression, vomiting
 3. Incoordination, ataxia
 4. Muscle fasciculations, seizures
 5. Coma, respiratory failure
 6. With slower absorption from chronic skin exposure there is increased RBC fragility, hemolysis, and icterus.

D. Diagnosis
 1. History and clinical signs
 2. Urine test for phenols—add 1 ml of 20% ferric chloride to 10 ml of urine; a blue-purple color is positive.
 3. Differential diagnosis—chlorinated hydrocarbons, hypocalcemia, garbage intoxication, metaldehyde, vacor

E. Treatment
 1. Prevent further absorption.
  a) Bathe with soap and water if skin exposed
  b) If there is evidence of corrosion of mouth induction of vomiting is contraindicated—milk or egg whites should be given immediately to decrease corrosive action.
  c) Gastric lavage with activated charcoal
 2. Supportive therapy
  a) Fluids, electrolytes, acid-base therapy
  b) Gastrointestinal protectants
  c) Control seizures

HOUSEHOLD DRUGS

I. Acetaminophen and other oxidant drugs
 A. Source
  1. Acetaminophen analgesic—antipyretic drugs
   a) Tylenol

   b) Excedrin
   c) Anacin-Three
   d) Datril
2. Phenazopyridine—urinary analgesic
3. Methylene blue—urinary antiseptic
4. Allyl propyl disulfide (onions raw and cooked)
5. Naphthalene (moth balls)
6. Cats are particularly susceptible to these drugs due to the high sulfhydryl content in feline hemoglobin.
7. Toxic dose—for cats 163–650 mg acetaminophen one-time dose and 65 mg/kg/day phenazopyridine for 3 days.

B. Action
1. Ferrous iron Fe^{2+} is oxidized to ferric iron Fe^{3+} converting hemoglobin to methemoglobin which does not carry O_2.
2. Oxidation of hemoglobin also forms disulfide bonds resulting in hemoglobin precipitation and Heinz body (erythrocyte refractile body) formation.
3. Heinz bodies are removed by macrophages in the spleen and liver causing the RBC to lose surface area and decreasing its life span.
4. Some of these drugs also cause liver damage.

C. Clinical signs
1. Facial edema (acetaminophen)
2. Depression, weakness, anorexia
3. Tachypnea, tachycardia
4. Cyanosis, brown mucous membranes
5. Naphthalene may also cause seizures or CNS depression.
6. Acute hemolytic anemia (acetaminophen)

D. Diagnosis
1. History of administration of the drugs or feeding table scraps containing onions.
2. Heinz bodies on RBCs
3. Elevated methemoglobin levels (normal is 0–1%)
4. Icterus and elevated serum glutamic-pyruvic transaminase (alanine aminotransferase) may occur.

- E. Treatment
  1. Induce emesis if early after ingestion, followed by activated charcoal and cathartic.
  2. Specific antidotes
     - a) Acetylcystine (Mucomyst)—probably works by increasing conjugation and excretion of acetaminophen metabolites.

       Dose 140 mg/kg orally initially and then 70 mg/kg orally q6h for up to 36 h.
     - b) Ascorbic acid reduces methemoglobin to oxyhemoglobin—dose 100 mg/kg BID.
  3. Hasten elimination—alkaline urine will increase excretion of naphthalene.

     Sodium bicarbonate 5 mEq/kg/h IV
  4. Supportive care
     - a) Transfusions
     - b) Fluid, electrolyte, acid-base therapy

II. Aspirin—salicylates

- A. Source
  1. Accidental ingestion or administration of improper dose
  2. Cats and young dogs are more susceptible due to a deficiency in metabolizing enzymes—particularly those responsible for glucuronide formation.
  3. Potentially toxic dose in dogs and cats is 60 mg/kg.
- B. Action
  1. Initial stimulation and then depression of respiration
  2. Metabolic acidosis
  3. Gastric ulceration
  4. Decreased platelet aggregation
  5. Bone marrow hypoplasia
- C. Clinical signs
  1. Tachypnea early, then respiratory depression
  2. Hyperthermia
  3. Anorexia, vomiting, hemorrhagic gastritis
  4. Metabolic acidosis which can lead to coma
  5. Renal damage
  6. Hemorrhage

7. Nonregenerative anemia occurs with long-term administration.

D. Diagnosis
1. History is usually helpful
2. Metabolic acidosis, aciduria, increased anion gap
3. Serum or urine salicylate levels
4. Add three drops of 10% ferric chloride to 1 ml acidified urine—dark red color indicates salicylates are present.
5. Differential diagnosis—other causes of gastritis and severe metabolic acidosis, ethylene glycol

E. Treatment
1. Prevent absorption if early after ingestion with induction of emesis, gastric lavage, and cathartics.
2. Hasten elimination with alkalinization of urine for 36–48 h.
   Sodium bicarbonate 5 mEq/kg/h IV
3. Supportive care
   a) Fluid, electrolyte, acid-base therapy
   b) Gastrointestinal protectants

III. Xanthines

A. Source
1. Caffeine
   a) Over-the-counter and prescription preparations
      (1) Diet pills
      (2) Mood elevators
      (3) Fatigue reduction
   b) Tea leaves, coffee beans
2. Theobromine—chocolate and cocoa
3. Toxic dose of caffeine for dogs is 100–150 mg/kg.

B. Action
1. Caffeine is a powerful CNS stimulant which can cause hyperesthesia and spinal cord reflex excitability.
2. Xanthines inhibit phosphodiesterase and therefore increase c-AMP concentrations.
   a) Xanthines stimulate the myocardium directly, causing increased rate and force of contraction.

b) Xanthines strengthen skeletal muscle contraction, probably through increased release of acetylcholine at the neuromuscular junction.
c) Xanthines increase gastric secretion and may cause mucosal ulceration.
3. Diuresis occurs due to increased cardiac output and increased urinary sodium and chloride excretion.

C. Clinical signs
1. Restlessness, hyperesthesia, hyperirritability
2. Tachycardia with pounding heartbeat, extrasystoles
3. Vomiting
4. Polyuria
5. Tense skeletal musculature
6. Convulsions—may be epiletiform or tetanic
7. Death due to cardiac and respiratory arrest

D. Diagnosis
1. History of ingestion or exposure and characteristic clinical signs
2. Differential diagnosis—strychnine, zinc phosphide, nicotine, amphetamines, metaldehyde

E. Treatment
1. Prevent absorption if early after ingestion
   Emesis, gastric lavage, cathartics
2. Supportive therapy
   a) Oxygen and artificial respiration for respiratory arrest
   b) Control seizures
      (1) Diazepam 2.5–20 mg IV as needed
      (2) Barbiturates to effect IV
   c) Fluid, electrolyte, acid-base therapy
   d) Gastrointestinal protectants

IV. Nicotine

A. Source
1. Nicotine containing darts used by dog wardens
2. Ingestion of cigarettes and/or cigars (0.5–2 mg/cigarette)
3. Certain insecticides (Black Leaf 40)
4. Toxicity—minimum lethal dose for dogs and cats is 20–100 mg.

B. Action
  1. Small doses stimulate autonomic ganglia.
  2. Large doses block the autonomic ganglia and myoneural junction.

C. Clinical signs
  1. Salivation, excitement, tachypnea, tachycardia
  2. Vomiting, diarrhea
  3. Muscle tremors, ataxia, seizures
  4. Slow and shallow respiration, flaccid paralysis
  5. Death due to respiratory arrest

D. Diagnosis
  1. History, characteristic clinical signs
  2. Parts of cigarettes and/or cigars in vomitus or stomach contents
  3. Differential diagnosis—strychnine, xanthines, organophosphates—carbamates

E. Treatment
  1. Prevent absorption.
    a) Emesis
    b) Gastric lavage with 1:10,000 potassium permanganate solution
    c) Dermal exposure—wash with soap and water
  2. Supportive care
    a) Oxygen and artifical respiration for respiratory arrest
    b) Sedation early
       Diazepam 2.5–20 mg IV as needed
    c) Stimulants later
      (1) Phenylephrine—0.15 mg/kg IV
      (2) Amphetamine sulfate 0.5–1.0 mg/kg SQ
    d) Fluid, electrolyte, acid-base therapy

V. Marijuana—hashish
  A. Source—*Cannabis sativa* (hemp plant)
  B. Action—active ingredient tetrahydrocannabinol causes CNS depression, visual hallucinations, changes in sensory perception, and psychic exhilaration in humans.
  C. Clinical signs
    1. Drowsiness, depression, hypothermia
    2. Ataxia, poor vision

3. Salivation, vomiting
4. Mydriasis is common.
5. Bradycardia
6. Signs can rapidly change in nature.

D. Diagnosis
1. History from owner
2. Differential diagnosis—ethanol or early ethylene glycol, ingestion of tranquilizers, depressants, muscle relaxants

E. Treatment
1. Prevent absorption—gastrointestinal cleansing
2. Supportive care
    a) Time in quiet, darkened environment
    b) Maintain temperature
    c) Bradycardia may respond to atropine.

VI. Amphetamines

A. Source
1. Amphetamine sulfate, dextroamphetamine, methamphetamine
2. Diet pills, mood elevators, fatigue reduction
3. Toxicity—minimum lethal dose 10–23 mg/kg

B. Action
1. Potent stimulants of central nervous and cardiovascular systems
2. Amphetamines increase the amount of catecholamine at nerve endings by increasing release and inhibiting reuptake and metabolism.

C. Clinical signs
1. Hyperexcitability, hyperesthesia
2. Tachycardia, hypertension
3. Hyperthermia, panting
4. Mydriasis
5. Vomiting, diarrhea
6. Trembling, seizures

D. Diagnosis
1. History and clinical signs
2. Laboratory analysis of urine or stomach contents
3. Differential diagnosis—strychnine, zinc phosphide, metaldehyde, nicotine, xanthines

E. Treatment
   1. Prevent absorption—emesis, gastric lavage, activated charcoal, cathartics
   2. Sedation
      a) Acetylpromazine maleate has been recommended, although this may lower seizure threshold.
      b) Diazepam 2.5–20 mg IV as needed
      c) Barbiturates to effect IV—*caution*: this may deepen poststimulant CNS depression.
   3. Hasten elimination of amphetamine.
      Acidify urine—200 mg NH_4Cl/kg/day orally divided QID
   4. Supportive care—cold water baths may be necessary for severe hyperthermia—however, they should be used with caution as hypothermia may follow these baths.

TOXIC PLANTS

Ingestion of plants by cats and dogs occurs fairly frequently. The incidence appears to increase during winter months when both plants and pets are likely to be indoors. Boredom has been implicated as a cause of plant ingestion. Diagnosis is often difficult unless ingestion is witnessed or plant material is found in vomitus or gastric contents. Therapy is usually symptomatic and supportive after cleansing the gastrointestinal tract to prevent further absorption

I. Oxalate-containing plants—cause severe oral and pharyngeal irritation due to needle-like crystals of calcium oxalate. Oxalate nephrosis is also possible.
   A. Source
      1. Philodendron
      2. Dieffenbachia—dumb cane
      3. Schefflera
      4. Large-leaf ivies
   B. Clinical signs
      1. Hypersalivation, swelling of tongue and throat, possible dyspnea

2. Anorexia, vomiting
3. Tongue paralysis is possible
4. Renal failure occurs rarely

C. Treatment
1. Induce emesis, gastric lavage
2. Rinse mouth, cold pack lips.
3. Tracheostomy may be necessary in cases of severe pharyngeal swelling.
4. Gastrointestinal demulcents such as kaolin and activated charcoal
5. Fluid therapy for renal failure

II. Gastrointestinal irritants

A. Source
1. Poinsettia
2. Mistletoe—may also cause cardiovascular collapse

B. Clinical signs
1. Irritation, vesiculation of mucous membranes
2. Gastroenteritis
3. Slowed pulse occurs with mistletoe similar to digitalis intoxication; cardiac arrhythmias.

C. Treatment
1. Gastric lavage or emesis to prevent further absorption
2. Monitor ECG
   a) Evaluate serum potassium—hypokalemia and hyperkalemia can contribute to arrhythmias.
   b) Phenytoin, propranolol, or lidocaine may be useful in controlling ventricular arrhythmias. See section on Arrhythmias, Chapter 2.
3. Gastrointestinal demulcents—kaolin, activated charcoal

III. Taxine alkaloid—depresses cardiac conduction

A. Source
1. European yew
2. Japanese yew

B. Clinical signs
1. Trembling, weakness, collapse
2. Dyspnea

        3. Bradycardia, asystole
        4. Coma, convulsions, sudden death
    C. Treatment
        1. Gastric lavage or emesis
        2. Symptomatic and supportive with IV fluids and cardiac stimulants

IV. Cardiac glycosides—similar to digitalis intoxication
    A. Source
        1. Oleander
        2. Lily of the valley
    B. Clinical signs
        1. Depression, dizziness, mydriasis
        2. Gastroenteritis
        3. Cardiac arrhythmias, tachycardia, bradycardia
        4. Coma, convulsions
        5. Respiratory and cardiac arrest
    C. Treatment
        1. Gastric lavage or emesis to prevent further absorption
        2. Monitor ECG.
            a) Evaluate serum potassium—hypokalemia and hyperkalemia can contribute to arrhythmias.
            b) Phenytoin, propranolol, or lidocaine may be useful in controlling ventricular arrhythmias.
        3. Symptomatic and supportive

V. Mushrooms
    A. Source—usually genus *Amanita*—gastrointestinal and nervous system signs
    B. Clinical signs
        1. Muscarinic
            a) Hypersalivation
            b) Vomiting and diarrhea—often with mucus and blood
        2. Ataxia, paralysis, coma
        3. Liver and kidney damage may occur.
            a) Icterus
            b) Azotemia
    C. Treatment

1. Emesis and gastric lavage with 1:10,000 potassium permanganate followed by cathartics
2. Atropine may alleviate symptoms in some cases.
3. Symptomatic and supportive

VI. Blue-green algae endotoxin
- A. Source
  1. Most commonly *Microcytis aeruginosa* or *Anabena flos-aquae*
  2. Algae blooms on lakes or ponds in upper Midwest during hot, dry, summer weather.
  3. Pets ingest the endotoxin while drinking pond water.
- B. Clinical signs
  1. Vomiting
  2. Muscle trembling and ataxia, followed by paralysis and seizures
  3. Death frequently occurs within 1–2 h of ingestion.
- C. Treatment—symptomatic and supportive only

VII. Aflatoxins
- A. Source
  1. Toxins are produced by growth of *Aspergillus flavis* and *Penicillium spp.* on feeds.
  2. Usually requires repeated exposure for 20–30 days at a minimum of 1 ppm in diet
- B. Clinical signs
  1. Anorexia, weakness, depression
  2. Diarrhea—frequently bloody
  3. Icterus due to fatty liver degeneration and bile duct proliferation
  4. May see blood clotting abnormalities
  5. Prostration and death may occur within 7-10 days of onset.
- C. Treatment—symptomatic and supportive only

BIBLIOGRAPHY

Arena JM: Poisoning: Toxicology, Symptoms, Treatments. 4th Ed. Charles C Thomas, Springfield, IL, 1979

Aronson CE: Thallium intoxication p. 124. In Kirk RW (ed): Current Veterinary Therapy. Vol. 6 WB Saunders, Philadelphia, 1977

Atkins CE, Johnson RR: Clinical toxicities of cats. Vet Clin N Am 5:623, 1975

Baily EM: Emergency and general treatment of poisonings. p. 105. In Kirk RW (ed): Current Veterinary Therapy. Vol. 7. WB Saunders, Philadelphia, 1980

Barsanti JA, Walser M, Hatheway CL, et al: Type C botulism in American foxhounds, J Am Vet Med Assoc 172:809, 1978

Bellah JR, Weigel JP: Hemarthrosis secondary to suspected warfarin toxicosis in a dog. J Am Vet Med Assoc 182:1126, 1983

Blakely BR: Epidemiologic and diagnostic considerations of strychnine poisoning in the dog. J Am Vet Med Assoc 184:46, 1984

Buck WB, Osweiler GD, Van Gelder GA: Clinical and Diagnostic Veterinary Toxicology. 2nd Ed. Kendall-Hunt Publishing Co., Dubuque, IA, 1976

Buck WB: Household poisons and the veterinarian. 75th Annual Conference for Veterinarians. Ithaca, NY January 1983

Carson TL: Organophosphate and carbamate insecticide poisoning p. 147. In Kirk RW (ed): Current Veterinary Therapy. Vol. 7. WB Saunders, Philadelphia, 1980

Center SA: Suspected calcium EDTA intoxication in a dog. J Am Vet Med Assoc 183:884, 1983

Clarke EGC, Clarke ML: Veterinary Toxicology. Williams and Wilkins, Baltimore, 1975

Clay BR: Poisoning and injury by plants. p. 179. In Kirk RW (ed): Current Veterinary Therapy. Vol. 6. WB Saunders, Philadelphia, 1977

Davis LE: Clinical pharmacology of salicylates. J Am Vet Med Assoc 176:65, 1980

Eberhart GW: Garbage- and food-borne intoxications (enterotoxemias). p. 176. In Kirk RW (ed): Current Veterinary Therapy. Vol. 6. WB Saunders, Philadelphia, 1977

Edwards WC: Sodium fluoroacetate (Compound 1080) poisoning p. 119. In Kirk RW (ed): Current Veterinary Therapy. Vol. 6. WB Saunders, Philadelphia, 1977

Fenner WR: Intoxications. p. 565. In Fenner WR (ed): Quick Reference to Veterinary Medicine. JB Lippincott, Philadelphia, 1982

Foor J, Stowe CM: Acute fatal caffeine toxicosis in a dog. J Am Vet Med Assoc 167:379, 1975

Furr A: Arsenic poisoning. p. 134. In Kirk RW (ed): Current Veterinary Therapy. Vol. 6. WB Saunders, Philadelphia, 1977

Gaunt SD, Baker DC, Green RA: Clinicopathologic evaluation of N-acetylcysteine therapy in acetaminophen toxicosis in the cat. Am J Vet Res 42:1982, 1981

Glauberg A, Blumenthal HP: Chocolate poisoning in the dog. J Am Anim Hosp Assoc 19:246, 1983

Godbold JC, Hawkins BJ, Woodward MG: Acute oral marijuana poisoning in the dog. J Am Vet Med Assoc 175:1101, 1979

Goodman LS, Gilman A: The Pharmacologic Basis of Therapeutics. 5th Ed. Macmillan, New York, 1975

Grauer GF, Thrall MA: Ethylene glycol (antifreeze) poisoning in the dog and cat. J Am Anim Hosp Assoc 18:492, 1982

Green RA, Buck WB: Warfarin and other anticoagulant poisonings. p. 131. In Kirk RW (ed): Current Veterinary Therapy. Vol. 7. WB Saunders, Philadelphia, 1980

Hardin JW, Arena JM: Human poisoning from native and cultivated plants. 2nd Ed. Duke University Press, Durham, NC, 1974

Harris WF: Clinical toxicities of dogs. Vet Clin N Am 5:605, 1975

Harris WF: ANTU poisoning. p. 117. In Kirk RW (ed): Current Veterinary Therapy. Vol. 6. WB Saunders, Philadelphia, 1977

Harvey JW, Kornick HP: Phenazopyridine toxicosis in the cat. J Am Vet Med Assoc 169:327, 1976

Koch-Wesen J, Sellers EM: Drug interactions with coumarin anticoagulants (parts 1 and 2). N Engl J Med 285:487, 547, 1971

Knecht CD, Crabtee J, Katherman A: Clinical, clinicopathologic and electroencephalographic features of lead poisoning in dogs. J Am Vet Med Assoc 175:196, 1979

Kowalczyk DF: Lead poisoning. p. 136. In Kirk RW (ed): Current Veterinary Therapy. Vol. 7. WB Saunders, Philadelphia, 1980

Kowalczyk DF: Lead poisoning in dogs at the University of Pennsylvania Veterinary Hospital. J Am Vet Med Assoc 168:428, 1976

Lees GE, Polzin DJ, Perman V, et al: Idiopathic Heinz body hemolytic anemia in three dogs. JAAHA 15:143, 1979

LeWitt PA: The neurotoxicity of the rat poison vacor. N Engl J Med 302:73, 1980

Mount ME, Feldman BF: Mechanism of diphacinone rodenticide toxicosis in the dog and its therapeutic implications. Am J Vet Res 44:2009, 1983

Mull RL: Metaldehyde poisoning. p. 135. In Kirk RW (ed): Current Veterinary Therapy. Vol. 7. WB Saunders, Philadelphia, 1980

Oehme FW: Emergency kit for treatment of small animal poisoning (antidotes, drugs, equipment). p. 201. In Kirk RW (ed): Current Veterinary Therapy. Vol. 7. WB Saunders, Philadelphia, 1980

Oehme FW: Poisonings from phenolic chemicals. p. 145. In Kirk RW (ed): Current Veterinary Therapy. Vol. 6. WB Saunders, Philadelphia, 1977

Oehme FW: Toxicologic problems. p.173. In Ettinger SJ (ed): Textbook of Veterinary Internal Medicine, Diseases of the Dog and Cat. 2nd Ed. WB Saunders, Philadelphia, 1983

Osweiler GD: Sources and incidence of small animal poisoning. Vet Clin N Am 5:589, 1975

Osweiler GD: Strychnine poisoning. p. 122. In Kirk RW (ed): Current Veterinary Therapy. Vol. 7. WB Saunders, Philadelphia, 1980

Stephans HA: Poisonous Plants of the Central United States. Regents Press of Kansas, Lawrence, 1980

Stowe CM, Fangmann G: Schefflera toxicosis in a dog. J Am Vet Med Assoc 167:74, 1975

Stowe CM, Metz AL, Arendt TD, et al: Apparent brodifacoum poisoning in a dog. J Am Vet Med Assoc 182:817, 1983

Stowe CM, Nelson R, Werdin R, et al: Zinc phosphide poisoning in dogs. J Am Vet Med Assoc 173:270, 1978

Stowe CM, Werdin RE, Barnes DM, et al: Amphetamine poisoning in dogs. J Am Vet Med Assoc 168:504, 1976

Thrall MA, Grauer GF, Mero KN: Clinicopathologic findings in dogs and cats with ethylene glycol intoxication. J Am Vet Med Assoc 184:37, 1984

Tsukamoto H, Parker HR, Gribble DH, et al: Nephrotoxicity of sodium arsenate in dogs. Am J Vet Res 44:2324, 1983

Van Gelder GA: Chlorinated hydrocarbon insecticide toxicosis. p. 141. In Kirk RW (ed): Current Veterinary Therapy. Vol. 6. WB Saunders, Philadelphia, 1977

Appendix I. Commonly Used Abbreviations

ACD	Acid citrate dextrose solution
ACT	Activated clotting time
ACTH	Adrenocorticotropic hormone
ADP	Adenosine diphosphate
AGD	Acute gastric dilatation-torsion (volvulus)
AIHA	Autoimmune hemolytic anemia
ANA	Antinuclear antibody
APTT	Activated partial thromboplastin time
ARF	Acute renal failure
AV	Atrioventricular
BAL	Dimercaprol
BP	Blood pressure
BSP	Sulfobromophthalein
BUN	Blood urea nitrogen
Ca^{+2}	Calcium
cAMP	Cyclic adenosine monophosphate
CBC	Complete blood count
CHF	Congestive heart failure
Cl^-	Chloride
CNS	Central nervous system
CP	Conscious proprioception
CPR	Cardiopulmonary resuscitation
CRF	Corticotropin releasing factor
CRT	Capillary refill time
CVP	Central venous pressure
DIC	Disseminated intravascular coagulopathy
DKA	Diabetic ketoacidosis
DPP	Deep pain perception
D/W	Dextrose and water

ECG	Electrocardiogram
EDTA	Ethylenediamine tetracetate
EEG	Electroencephalogram
ELIZA	Enzyme-linked immunoadzorbant assay
ERG	Electroretinogram
FeLV	Feline leukemia virus
FIP	Feline infectious peritonitis
FSP	Fibrin split products
HE	Hepatic encephalopathy
Hgb	Hemoglobin
IgG	Immunoglobulin G
IgM	Immunoglobulin M
IVP	Intravenous pyelogram
K^+	Potassium
KCl	Potassium chloride
LHF	Left heart failure
MCHC	Mean corpuscular hemoglobin concentration
MCV	Mean corpuscular volume
MS	Musculoskeletal system
Na^+	Sodium
NH_4Cl	Ammonium chloride
NS	Normal saline
nRBC	Nucleated red blood cell
O_2	Oxygen
OP	Organophosphates
OSPT	One-stage prothrombin time
PCV	Packed cell volume
PD	Polydipsia
PF_3	Platelet factor 3
PRN	Administer as needed
PT	Prothrombin time
PTH	Parathormone

PTT	Partial thromboplastin time
PU	Polyuria
RBC	Red blood cell
RF	Rheumatoid factor
RVVT	Russell's viper venom time
SALT	Serum alananine aminotransferase (SGPT)
SAP	Serum alkaline phosphatase
SAST	Serum aspartate aminotransferase (SGOT)
SGGT	Serum glutamyl transpeptidase
SGOT	Serum glutamic oxaloacetic transaminase (SAST)
SGPT	Serum glutamic pyruvic transaminase (SALT)
SPP	Superficial pain perception
TS	Total solids
TT	Thrombin time
TTA	Transtracheal aspirate
UA	Urinalysis
VM	Voluntary motor or movement
WBC	White blood cell

Appendix II. Units Used in Text

Weights	kg	kilograms (10^3 g)
	gm	gram (1 g)
	mg	milligram (10^{-3} g)
	μg	microgram (10^{-6} g)
	ng	nanogram (10^{-9} g)
	pg	picogram (10^{-12} g)
	1 grain = 65 mg	
Fluids	L	liter (10^3 ml)
	dl	deciliter (10^2 ml)
	ml	milliliter (1 ml)
Pressure	mm Hg	millimeters of mercury
	cm H_2O	centimeters of water
Distance	mm	millimeters
	cm	centimeters
	in	inches
Time	sec	second
	min	minute
	h	hour
	q	every
Concentration of Solutions	m Eq/L	milliequivalent per liter
	mg/dl	milligrams per deciliter
	mOsm/kg	milliosmoles per kilogram
	μU/ml	microunits per milliliter
	μg/dl	micrograms per deciliter
	μM/L	microMoles per liter

Appendix III. Treatment Abbreviations

Routes of administration	PO	Per os, oral
	IC	Intracardiac
	IM	Intramuscular
	IV	Intravenous
	SQ	Subcutaneous
Dosage schedules	QID	four times daily; every 6 hours
	TID	three times daily; every 8 hours
	BID	twice daily; every 12 hours
	SID	once daily; every 24 hours
	QOD	once every other day; every 48 hours

Appendix IV. Centigrade and Fahrenheit Temperatures

°C	°F
23	73.4
24	75.2
25	77.0
26	78.8
27	80.6
28	82.4
29	84.2
30	86.0
31	87.8
32	89.6
33	91.4
34	93.2
35	95.0
36	96.8
37	98.6
38	100.4
39	102.2
40	104.0
41	105.8
42	107.6
43	109.4
44	111.2
45	113.0
46	114.8

INDEX

Page numbers followed by f represent figures; those followed by t represent tables.